Donald School

Fetal Brain Functioning

Donald School
Fetal Brain Functioning

Editor

Asim Kurjak MD PhD
Professor
Department of Obstetrics and Gynecology
Medical School University of Zagreb
Zagreb, Croatia
Professor Emeritus
University Sarajevo School of Science and Technology
Sarajevo, Bosnia and Herzegovina

Foreword
Frank A Chervenak

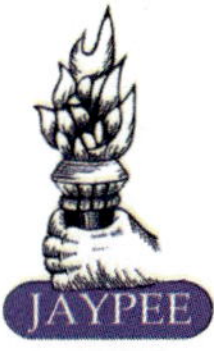

JAYPEE BROTHERS MEDICAL PUBLISHERS
The Health Sciences Publisher
New Delhi | London

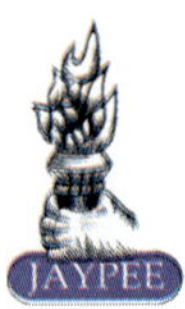 **Jaypee Brothers Medical Publishers (P) Ltd**

Headquarters

Jaypee Brothers Medical Publishers (P) Ltd
EMCA House, 23/23-B
Ansari Road, Daryaganj
New Delhi 110 002, India
Landline: +91-11-23272143, +91-11-23272703
+91-11-23282021, +91-11-23245672
Email: jaypee@jaypeebrothers.com

Corporate Office

Jaypee Brothers Medical Publishers (P) Ltd
4838/24, Ansari Road, Daryaganj
New Delhi 110 002, India
Phone: +91-11-43574357
Fax: +91-11-43574314
Email: jaypee@jaypeebrothers.com

Overseas Office

JP Medical Ltd
83 Victoria Street, London
SW1H 0HW (UK)
Phone: +44 20 3170 8910
Fax: +44 (0)20 3008 6180
Email: info@jpmedpub.com

Website: www.jaypeebrothers.com
Website: www.jaypeedigital.com

Donald School Fetal Brain Functioning

First Edition: **2022**

ISBN: 978-93-5465-646-0

Printed at: Sterling Graphics Pvt. Ltd. India.

Dedicated to

Biserka, Igor and Alan, and
Dea, Lina, Dal and Din

Contributors

Aida Salihagić Kadić MD PhD
Professor of Physiology and Neuroscience
Department of Physiology
Medical School University of Zagreb
Zagreb, Croatia

Anja Šurina MD
Resident
Department of Pediatric Infectious Diseases
University Hospital for Infectious Diseases
"Dr Fran Mihaljević"
Zagreb, Croatia

Asim Kurjak MD PhD
Professor
Department of Obstetrics and Gynecology
Medical School University of Zagreb
Zagreb, Croatia
Professor Emeritus
University Sarajevo School of Science and
Technology
Sarajevo, Bosnia and Herzegovina

Aya Koyanagi RMS
Sonographer
Department of Obstetrics and Gynecology
Miyake Clinic
Okayama-shi, Okayama, Japan

George Daskalakis MD PhD
Professor
Department of Obstetrics and Gynecology
Alexandra Maternity Hospital
University of Athens
Athens, Greece

Lara Spalldi Barišić MD PhD candidate
Specialist Obstetrician and Gynecologist
Department of Obstetrics and Gynecology
Private Clinic "Veritas"
Zagreb, Croatia

Maciej Bieliński MD PhD
Chair, Department of Clinical Neuropsychology
Collegium Medicum in Bydgoszcz
Nicolaus Copernicus University in Toruń
Department of Cardiac Rehabilitation and
Experimental Cardiology
Dr W Biegański Regional Specialist Hospital
in Grudziądz
Bydgoszcz, Poland

Maria Papamichail MD
Research Fellow
Department of Obstetrics and Gynecology
Alexandra Maternity Hospital
University of Athens
Athens, Greece

Marianna Theodora MD PhD
Professor
Department of Obstetrics and Gynecology
Alexandra Maternity Hospital
University of Athens
Athens, Greece

Milan Stanojević MD PhD
Professor
Neonatal Unit
Department of Obstetrics and Gynecology
Medical School University of Zagreb
Sveti Duh Hospital
Zagreb, Croatia

Miro Jakovljević MD PhD
Professor
Department of Psychiatry and
Psychological Medicine
University Hospital Centre Zagreb
Zagreb, Croatia

Natalia Lesiewska MD
Chair, Department of Clinical Neuropsychology
Department of Obstetrics and Gynecology
Collegium Medicum in Bydgoszcz
Nicolaus Copernicus University in Toruń
Jan Biziel University Hospital No 2
Bydgoszcz, Poland

Oliver Vasilj MD PhD
Specialist
Department of Obstetrics and Gynecology
Polyclinic "Medifem"
Zagreb, Croatia

Panagiotis Antsaklis MD PhD
Assistant Professor
Department of Obstetrics and Gynecology
Department of Fetal Maternal Medicine
Alexandra Maternity Hospital
University of Athens
Athens, Greece

Riko Takayoshi MD
Consultant
Department of Obstetrics and Gynecology
Miyake Clinic
Okayama-shi, Okayama, Japan
Research Student
Department of Perinatology and Gynecology
Kagawa University Graduate School of Medicine
Miki, Kagawa, Japan

Ritsuko K Pooh MD PhD MSc LLB
Professor and Director
Fetal Diagnostic Center, Fetal Brain Center
CRIFM Prenatal Medical Clinic
Osaka, Japan

Takahito Miyake MD PhD
President
Department of Obstetrics and Gynecology
Miyake Clinic
Okayama-shi, Okayama, Japan
Clinical Associate Professor
Department of Perinatology and Gynecology
Kagawa University Graduate School of Medicine
Miki, Kagawa, Japan

Toshiyuki Hata MD PhD
Special Adviser
Department of Obstetrics and Gynecology
Miyake Clinic
Okayama-shi, Okayama, Japan
Professor Emeritus
Department of Perinatology and Gynecology
Kagawa University Graduate School of Medicine
Miki, Kagawa, Japan

Yasunari Miyagi MD PhD
Director
Department of Gynecology
Miyake Ofuku Clinic
Okayama-shi, Okayama, Japan

Foreword

Since Ian Donald began his pioneering studies of ultrasound examination of the fetal patient, the brain has always been the main focus of attention. After decades of studying many and varied aspects of brain morphology, thanks to advances in four-dimensional ultrasound, science has advanced to now permit an in-depth study of brain function during the perinatal period.

Professor Asim Kurjak and his international team of authorities have accomplished this difficult task in *Fetal Brain Functioning*. This volume first describes the arduous journey from structure to function by professor Kurjak who has lived through and contributed to every step of this journey.

This is followed by international leaders from Greece, Japan, Poland, and Croatia who explain in clear text and beautiful images the function of the perinatal brain both before and after birth.

This superb volume is recommended for all sonologists and sonographers as it will give new insights and enable greater awareness of the beauty and precision of the function of the perinatal brain.

Frank A Chervenak MD MMM
Chair, Obstetrics and Gynecology
Lenox Hill Hospital
Chair, Obstetrics and Gynecology
Associate Dean for International Medicine
Zucker School of Medicine at Hofstra/Northwell
New York, USA

Contents

From Structure to Function: A Long Journey

Asim Kurjak, Milan Stanojević, Panagiotis Antsaklis

■ INTRODUCTION

For centuries understanding the structure and function of the fetal nervous system has been the dream of physicians. In the second part of the 20th century, this dream become a reality due to the pioneering efforts of Ian Donald in obstetric ultrasound. Early contribution of obstetric ultrasound focused on normal and abnormal structure. Initially, anencephaly was described and followed by increasingly subtle central nervous system (CNS) abnormalities like agenesis of the corpus callosum. For investigators in obstetric ultrasound there is a current and growing challenge to have similar success with the understanding of fetal neurological function. In many functional neurological abnormalities like cerebral palsy (CP) causes are poorly understood. There has also been noticed an escalating number of results which show that a large presence of neurological problems (like minimal brain dysfunction or attention deficit hyperactivity disorder, schizophrenia, epilepsy, or autism spectrum disorder), at least in part, come from prenatal neurodevelopmental problems. Clinical and epidemiological studies showed that CP most often results from prenatal rather than perinatal or postnatal causes.[1]

Although significant advances in prenatal and perinatal care are obvious, currently there is no mean to identify or expect the development of these disorders. Consequently, one of the most imperative tasks of contemporary perinatal medicine became the development of diagnostic strategies to avoid and condense the saddle of perinatal brain damage. Understanding of the prenatal neurodevelopmental events and possibly antenatal detection of CP and other neurological diseases might be improved by applying the new neurobehavioral test—Kurjak's antenatal neurobehavioral test (KANET).

■ STRUCTURAL AND FUNCTIONAL DEVELOPMENT OF CENTRAL NERVOUS SYSTEM

Structural Development of Central Nervous System

Pomeroy and Volpe[2] wrote that "the development of CNS begins around the end of gastrulation. The generation of the neuro-ectoderm from ectoderm during the third postconceptional week, results in formation of the neural plate. Thus, the neural epithelium of the embryo, which is a precursor of neurons and glia, is virtually the first part of organism that acquires the separate identity from other cells."[2]

The formation of the neural plate is succeeded by the folding of its edges and formation of a neural tube, whose further growth and reshaping results in formation of structures of CNS. According to O'Rahilly and Muller, forebrain (prosencephalon), midbrain (mesencephalon), and hindbrain (rhombencephalon) can be distinguished in the rostral portion of the unfused neural folds[3] earlier than it is usually referred to, approximately at 22nd postconceptional day. In the rapid succession, during the 4th postconceptional week, the forebrain components—diencephalon and telencephalon—can be detected. Three embryonic zones—ventricular, intermediary, and marginal zone (seen from ventricular to pial surface)—are present in all parts of neural tube, while telencephalon contains additional two zones, subventricular and subplate zone.[3] Ventricular and subventricular zones of telencephalon are the site of neurogenesis and all the future neurons and glia are born in these structures.[3] During migration toward the pial surface they form other transitional zones before reaching their genetically predetermined final destinations.[3] Those destinations are cortical plate or different nuclei in the brain stem, diencephalon, and basal forebrain.[1] One of the transitional structures, a subplate zone that is a site for transient synapses and neuronal interactions, can play a major role in the developmental plasticity following perinatal brain damage.[4] Early appearance of interneuronal connections, given in **Table 1**, implicates a possibility of an early functional development.[3,4] However, these first synapses exist only temporarily and disappear due to the normal reorganization processes. Most embryonic zones, types of neurons and glia, and early synapses, which play crucial role in certain periods of fetal brain development, eventually disappear, significantly changing structure and function of the brain.[4] Reorganization processes include apoptosis, disappearance of redundant synapses, axonal retraction and transposition, and transformation of the neurotransmitters phenotype.[4]

Table 1 lists a significant overlap of neurogenesis, migration, and synaptogenesis in the embryonic and fetal life. At the time of delivery the development of human brain is not completed.[3,4] In an infant born at term, characteristic cellular layers can be observed in motor, somatosensory, visual, and auditory cortical areas.[1]

While in a term infant proliferation and migration are completed, synaptogenesis and neuronal differentiation continue very intensively.[5] Brainstem demonstrates high level of maturity, whereas all histogenetic processes actively persist in cerebellum.[6] Therefore, only subcortical formations and the primary cortical areas are well developed in a newborn.[6] Associative cortex which is barely visible in a newborn, is poorly developed in a 6-month-old infant.[6] Postnatal formation of synapses in associative cortical areas, which intensifies between 8th month and 2nd year of life, precedes the onset of

TABLE 1: Dynamics of the most important progressive processes in the development of the human brain.[3,4]

	Beginning	Most intensive activity	Ending
Neurogenesis	Early embryonic period (4th week)	8th–12th week	Approximately 20 weeks
Migration	Simultaneously with proliferation	18th–24th week	38th week
Synaptogenesis	6–7th week—spinal cord 8th week—cortical plate	13th–18th week, after 24th week, 8th month to 2 year of postnatal life	Puberty

first cognitive functions, such as speech.[1,6] Following the second year of age, many redundant synapses are eliminated.[6] The elimination of synapses begins very rapidly, and continues slowly until the puberty, when the same number of synapses as seen in adults is reached.[6]

Functional Development of CNS and Role of Four-dimensional Ultrasound

The first synapses appear in the spinal cord at 6–7 postconceptional weeks[7] and in the cortical plate at 8 postconceptional weeks.[8] This is the phase when the first electrical bustle and conduction of information take places. The earliest spontaneous fetal movements can be observed at 7.5 postconceptional weeks. These movements which consist of slow flexion and extension of the fetal trunk being accompanied by the inactive displacement of arms and legs and emerging in asymmetrical sequences, have been described as "vermicular".[9,10] They are substituted by various general movements (GMs) consisting of head, trunk, and limb movements, such as "rippling" seen at week 8, "twitching" and "strong twitching" at weeks 9 and 9.5, respectively, and "floating", "swimming", and "jumping" at week 10.[11] Almost simultaneously with the GMs isolated limb movements emerge. At the same time with the beginning of spontaneous movements, at 7.5 postconceptional weeks, the initial motor reflex activity can be detected, permitting the hypothesis to be made of the existence of the first afferent-efferent circuits.[7] Head tilting following perioral stimulation was noted at that time.[7] The primary reflex movements are immense and signify a limited number of synapses in a reflex pathway.[7] During the 8th week of gestation, these substantial reflex movements are replaced with local movements, possibly due to an

increase in the number of axodendritic synapses.[7] Hands become susceptible at 10.5 weeks and lower limbs start to contribute in these reflexes at around week 14.[11,12] First sign of a supraspinal control on fetal motor activity is GMs.[9,10] Brainstem which consists of the medulla oblongata, pons, and midbrain, begins to develop and mature in a caudal to rostral direction approximately at the 7 postconceptional weeks.[6–8] As the medulla matures in advance of more rostral structures of brainstem, reflexive movements of the head, body, and extremities, as well as breathing movements and heart rate alterations, appear in advance of other functions.[12] The amount and incidence of movements increase since the 10th week onward.[12] Fetuses are highly active with the longest period between movements of only 5–6 minutes by 14–19 weeks.[9–11] Fifteen singular types of movements can be observed in the 15th week.[9–11] We can see general body movements and isolated limb movements, retroflexion, anteflexion, and rotation of the head.[13] Furthermore, face movements, such as mouthing, yawning, hiccups, sucking, and swallowing, can be included to an ample repertoire of fetal motor activity at this stage.[13] However, during the first half of pregnancy, a dynamic pattern of neuronal production and migration, as well as the immature cerebral circuits are considered too immature for cerebral involvement in the motor behavior.[4] Merely at the end of this period do a quantifiable number of synapses appear in the structures preceding the cerebral cortex, perhaps forming a substrate for the first cortical electric activity, noted at week 19.[4] At the 20th week, the spinothalamic tract is established and myelinized by 29 weeks of gestation while at 24–26 weeks the thalamo-cortical connections penetrate the cortical plate.[14] At the 29th week evoked potentials can be detected from the cortex, suggesting that the functional connection between periphery and cortex operates from that time onward.[14] In the second half of pregnancy, particularly during the last 10 weeks, the number of GMs gradually decreases.[15] This decrease was first explained as a result of the reduction in amniotic fluid volume; however, it is now believed to be a result of maturation processes in the brainstem.[12] An increase in facial movements, as well as opening or closing of the jaw, swallowing and chewing, can be observed simultaneously with the decline in the number of generalized movements.[15] These activities can be seen mainly in the periods of absence of GMs. This pattern is considered to be a manifestation of the normal neurological development of the fetus.[15] However, alterations not only in the number of movements, but also in their complexity, are revealed to be the result of cerebral maturation processes.[12] It is important to point out that subunits of the brainstem remain the main regulators of all fetal behavioral patterns until delivery.[12] Study of prenatal behavior is still in its infancy despite medical reports from 100 years ago and almost 40 years of systematic research initiated by Prechtl and colleagues.[9,16-18] One of the most promising progress in the field of ultrasonography was the new four-dimensional ultrasound (4D US) technology. Its advance has been achieved in the last years giving visualizations in almost real time.[19-22] In an extraordinary way the availability of new diagnostic data raised our knowledge about intrauterine life, substantially modifying some earlier interpretations.[23] With conventional two-dimensional ultrasound (2D US) first spontaneous fetal movements can be observed around 8th gestational week, while the newly developed 4D US enables the visualization of fetal motility 1 week earlier **(Table 2)**.[24]

TABLE 2: Developmental sequence of fetal behavioral patterns observed by four-dimensional ultrasound (4D US) in the first trimester of pregnancy.[24]

	Postconceptional weeks				
Type of movements	7	8	9	10	11
General movement	+	+	+	+	+
Startle			+	+	+	+
Stretching			+	+	+	+
Isolated arm movement			+	+	+	+
Isolated leg movement		+	+	+	+
Head rotation				+	+	+
Head anteflexion				+	+	+
Head retroflexion				+	+	+

General movements are the first complex fetal movement patterns observable by 2D US; however, assessment by 4D US is a considerable improvement. They can be recognized from the 8th to 9th week of pregnancy (**Figure 1** showed by 4D US) and continue to be present until 16–20 weeks after birth.[18]

According to Prechtl, "these are gross movements, involving the whole body. They wax and wane in intensity, force, and speed, and they have a gradual beginning and end."[13,18] The majority of sequences of extension and flexion of the legs and arms is complex, and may be better assessed with 4D US.[24] In the literature, there is a range between the 8th and 12th week regarding the first appearance of limb movements.[13,18,20,25] De Vries found isolated arm and leg movements at the 8th week of gestation.[13] With 4D US, limb movements were found at the 8th–9th week.[24] By 4D sonography, Kurjak et al. found that from 13th gestational week onward, a "goal orientation" of hand movements appears and a target point can be recognized for each hand movement.[19] It was noticed that more limb joints were active and moved simultaneously,

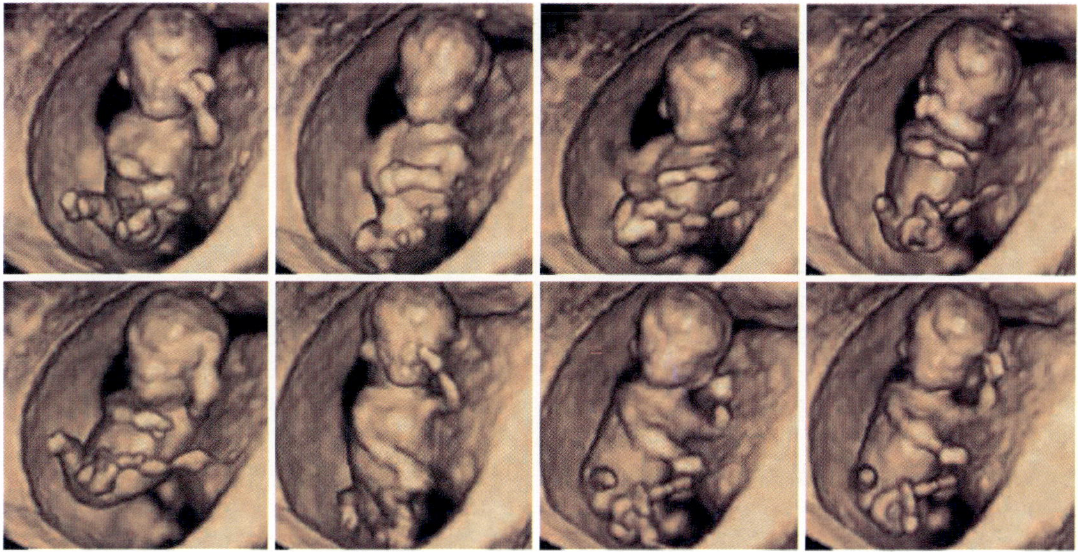

Fig. 1: Four-dimensional ultrasound (4D US) imaging demonstrated fetus at 13 weeks of gestation showing general movement pattern.

like extension or flexion in arm and elbow or hip and knee. Simultaneously, elevation of the hand, extension of the elbow joint, with a slight change in direction and rotation, could have been seen.[26] The isolated limb movements which were seen at the 9th week are followed by the appearance of the movements in the elbow joint at 10 week, changes in finger position in the 11th week, and by easily recognizable clenching and unclenching of the fist at the 12th–13th week.[26] Finally, isolated finger movements, as well as an increase in the activity and strength of movements of the hand or finger, can be seen at the 13th–14th week.[26] Recent examination of fetuses in the last trimester of gestation which were performed by 4D US, has discovered an even wider range of movements of hand and face than was formerly explained.[19] It has been also confirmed that the fetal movement patterns in the second half of pregnancy are about equal to those monitored after birth. However, the list of movements in the newborn consists of some patterns that cannot be observed in the fetus, such as the Moro reflex.[27] In addition, at around the 20th gestational week, study of anencephalic fetuses have presented clear evidence for the influence of supraspinal structures on motor behavior. In these fetuses the number of movements was normal or even increased, but the complexity of the movement patterns distorted radically and movements were stereotyped and simplified.[28]

The eminence of fetal movement patterns is distorted in fetuses undergoing intrauterine growth restriction (IUGR). The activities become monotonous and slower, similar to cramps, and we can see that their variability in force and amplitude is reduced.[29] These changes might designate the subsistence of brain lesions in growth-restricted and possibly hypoxic fetuses. Despite the premature postulations, the changes in the amplitude and complexity of movements in these fetuses do not show to be due to oligohydramnios. In cases of premature rupture of fetal membranes and a subsequently reduced volume of amniotic fluid, movements arise less frequently, but their complexity look likes that of movements achieved in the normal volume of amniotic fluid.[16] Qualitative including quantitative analysis of fetal movements divulged the consistency of the fetal nervous system, and can be applied for the recognition of different cerebral dysfunctions, and probably neuromuscular ailments.[28]

The new technology, 4D US, when applied in the examination of fetal facial movements, revealed existence of a full range of facial expressions including grimacing, tongue expulsion, and eye-lid movements **(Fig. 2)** similar to emotional expressions in adults.[27,30]

Possibility of studying such subtle movements could open a new area of investigation.[31]

During the first trimester, it was noticed a tendency toward increased frequency of fetal GMs with increasing gestational age **(Fig. 3A)**. While at the beginning of the second trimester, the fetuses began to display a tendency toward increased frequency of observed fetal facial expression up to the end of the second trimester. An oscillation and dispersion of the incidence of the facial expression as seen in the polynomial regression of isolated eye-blinking diagram is observable in **Figure 3B**.[30]

In the second trimester, the most frequent facial movement patterns were isolated

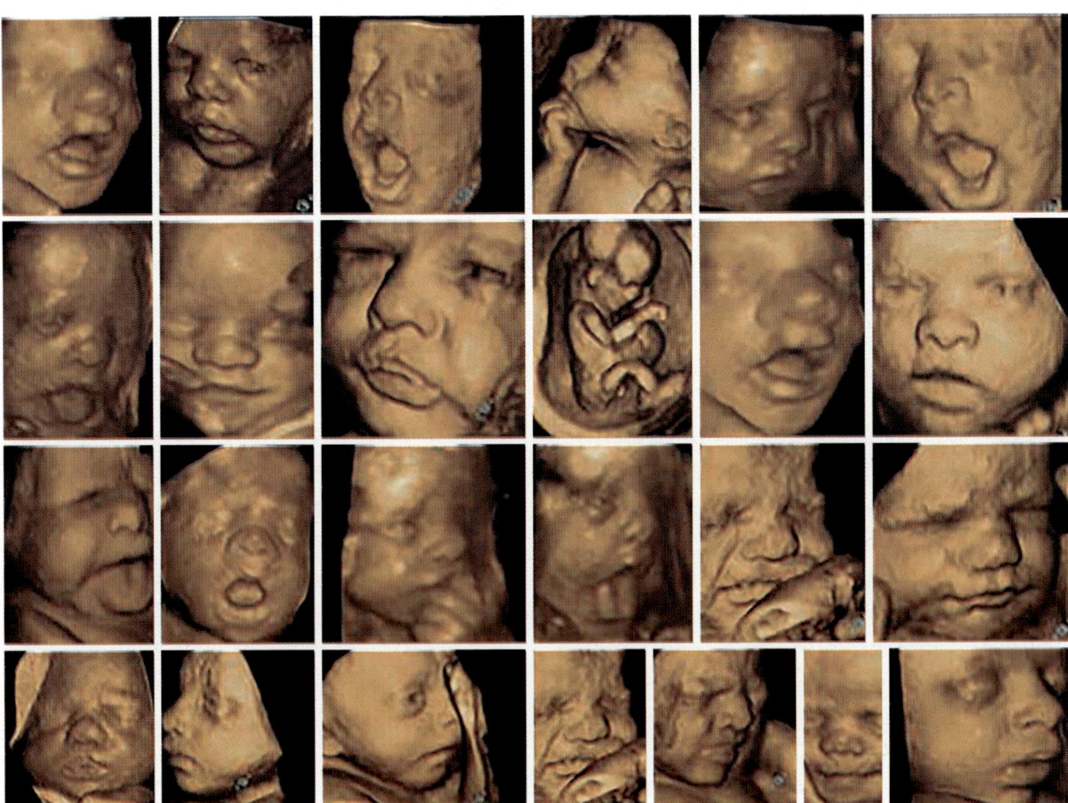

Fig. 2: Three-dimensional/four-dimensional ultrasound provides clear depiction of dynamic changes of fetal facial expression allowing study of fetal behavior during all trimesters of pregnancy.

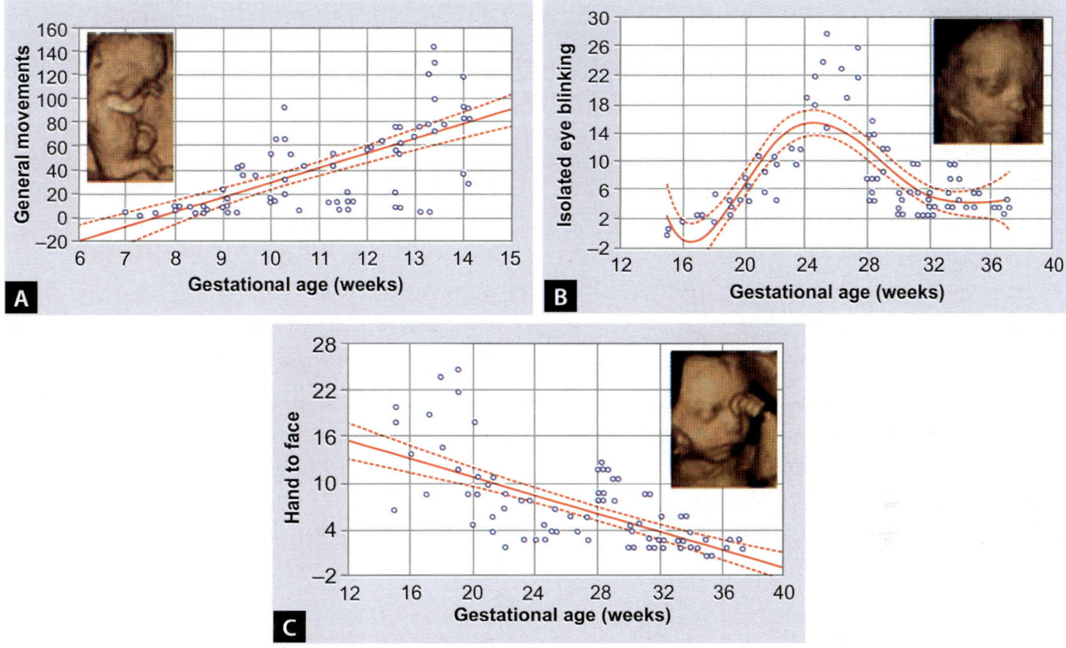

Figs. 3A to C: Quantitative analysis of normal fetal behavior patterns using four-dimensional ultrasound (4D US): (A) General movements; (B) Hand to face movement; (C) Isolated eye blinking.[30]

eye blinking, grimacing, suckling, and swallowing, while yawning, mouthing, tongue expulsion, and smiling could be observed less frequently.[25,30] The fetuses began to display decreasing or stagnant incidence of fetal facial expression during the third trimester. From the beginning of the second trimester to the end of the third trimester, all types of head movements and hand to body contact indicated a tendency to decrease frequency **(Fig. 3C)**.[30]

In this period, the investigations of fetal facial expressions established that all mechanisms of the fetal yawning pattern, prolonged jaw opening followed by a quick closure and accompanied by head flexion and elevation of arms, can easily be documented by 4D US **(Fig. 4)**.[32]

If we compared fetal yawning in the third trimester with the yawning in the neonates during the first week of life, no differences in the frequencies of this reaction were found.

It was noticed that the frequency of yawning steadily increased between 15th and 24th week, then from 24th to 26th week a short plateau was observed which was followed by a slight decrease toward the term.[30] A gestational age-related tendency in the frequency of yawning could be assumed as the maturation of the brainstem and probably the gaining of control of more cranial structures over yawning pattern. These results gave new data about the route of neurodevelopment of this fascinating, but poorly implicit reflex.[30] It still continues to be determined whether this is distorted in cases of neurodevelopmental disorders and whether such adaptations can give us impending into the function of fetal nervous system in high risk pregnancies. To what possibility are the facial motoric patterns related to the function and integrity of the CNS also stays to be determined. However, the fact that even in the embryonic stage, the identical inductive forces that

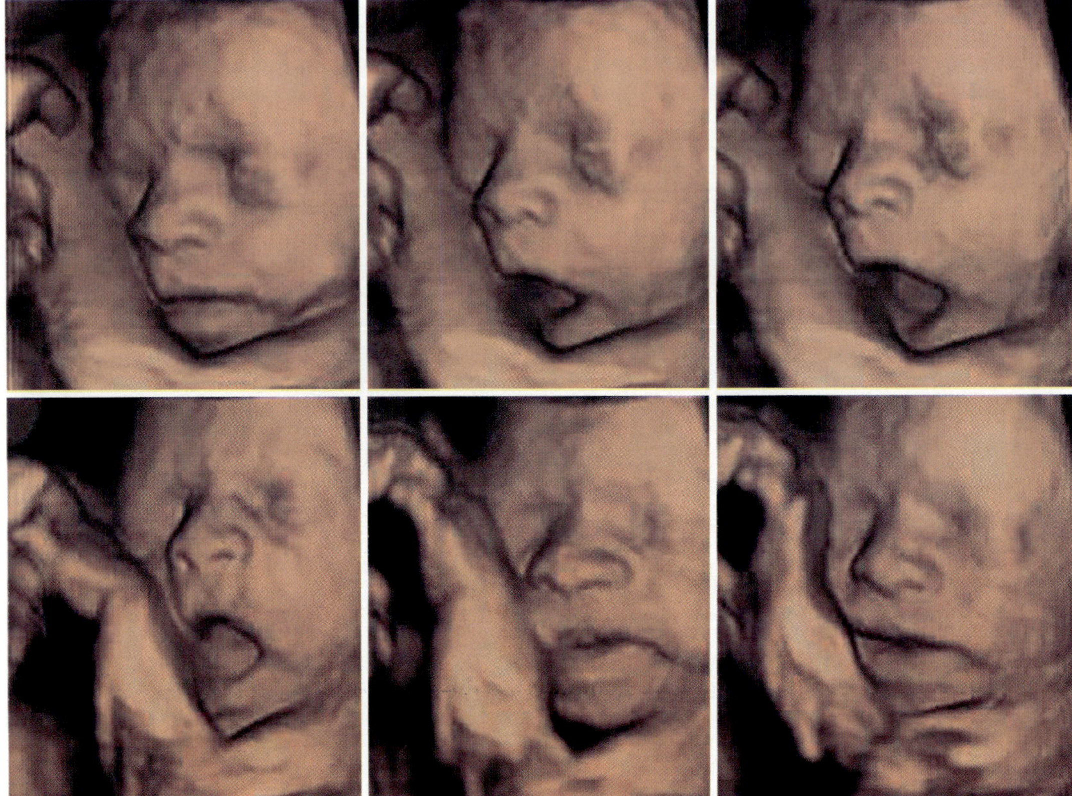

Fig. 4: Four-dimensional ultrasound (4D US) image sequences of facial expression characterized by stereotyped yawning opening.

cause growth and restyling of the neural tube influence the development of facial structures, and that many genetic disorders affecting the CNS are also described by dysmorphology and dysfunction of facial structures, underline the value of these studies.[2,30,31]

NEONATAL ASPECT OF FETAL NEUROLOGY

In our previous publications, we have extensively discussed obstetric aspects of fetal neurology.[19-25,27-31] In order to come to better understanding of fetal neurobehavioral patterns, we have learned a lot from basic studies of brain development and from clinical postnatal studies of neonates. Now, when we have reached the edge of fetal behavioral investigation by 4D US in normal fetuses, we intend to find some new ideas and ways of investigation presenting neonatal aspect of fetal neurology.

Cerebral palsy is an "umbrella" term for disorders of development, movement, and posture, resulting in limitations of activity due to nonprogressive impairment of developing brain.[33] The diagnosis of CP is retrospective and it is exceptionally made before the age of 6 months in only most severely affected infants, and the specificity of the diagnosis will improve as the child ages and the nature of the disability evolves.[34] CP does not result from a single event but rather there is a sequence of interdependent adverse events providing to the condition.[35]

We should take into account this time frame of evolving adverse events when considering the possibility of CP diagnosis in infants.[34,35] The understanding of the profile of a child's disability across multiple domains is an ongoing process which is necessary for proper treatment and future planning.[34] This theoretical statement is sometimes very difficult to be implemented in practice. In every patient an attempt to make early diagnosis of CP should be followed with factors related to pathogenesis, impairment, and functional limitations.[34] To identify pathogenesis of the process, neuroimaging methods should be used. In very low-birthweight premature infants and in term infants with encephalopathy, cranial ultrasound, magnetic resonance imaging (MRI), magnetic resonance (MR) spectroscopy, and diffusion-weighted imaging are the most frequently used.[34] Impairment of organs or systems by clinical assessment of muscle tone, strength, and control of voluntary movements for early detection of infants with the risk for CP is frustrating since 43% of 7-year-old children with CP had a normal newborn neurological examination.[34,36] Is it possible to change this discouraging fact resulting from our failure to diagnose neurological impairment early enough to intervene? Among ultrasonographers using 4D US interests in diagnosis of neurological impairment have been recently shifted toward prenatal period.[23,37] Question is whether there is any possibility to improve timing of postnatal diagnosis of neurologically disabled infant? It is probably easier to perform postnatal assessment than prenatal, by using a simple and suitable for everyday work screening clinical test with good reliability, specificity,

and sensitivity. Such tests are still not widely used. However, those complicated and time-consuming are used mostly for clinical research purposes. There is a possibility for the early and simple neurological assessment of the term and preterm newborns with the aim to detect associated risks and anticipate long-term outcome of the infant, and to establish a possible causative link between pregnancy course and neurodevelopmental outcome.[38] Since CP is a disorder of movement and postural control resulting in functional limitations, its diagnosis could help in detection of early impairment.[34] Clinical neurological assessment which was proposed and practiced by Amiel-Tison, could be very useful in the early detection of newborns at risk.[38] Development of CNS is a very complex and long-lasting process, therefore the assessment of its developmental optimality is something which should be assessed in order to investigate whether the infant is neurologically normal or damaged. Neurological assessment at term by Amiel-Tison (ATNAT) is taking into account neurological maturation exploring so called lower subcortical system developing earlier from the reticular formation, vestibular nuclei, and tectum and upper cortical system developing from the corticospinal pathways.[39] The role of lower system is to maintain posture against gravity, while the upper system is responsible for the control of erect posture and for the movements of the extremities.[39] At the corrected age of 40 gestational weeks optimality assessment consists of head circumference measurement, assessment of cranial sutures, visual pursuit, social interaction, sucking reflex, raise-to-sit and reverse, passive tone in the axis, passive tone in the limbs, finger movements and thumbs outside the fist, and autonomic control during assessment.[39] The ATNAT is increasing accuracy in assessing CNS function in the neonate by using simple scoring system, focusing on the most meaningful items, promoting a clinical synthesis at term, for term and preterm infants.[39] It was recognized that clinicoanatomic correlations using high-resolution neuroimaging techniques could be helpful in the neurological assessment of newborns, while the neurological examination and the functional assessment of the developing CNS are bringing a new perspective of CNS status in neonatal period.[40]

POSTNATAL ASSESSMENT OF GENERAL MOVEMENTS

In the last 30 years objective assessment of videotaped GMs by Prechtl's method has been shown to be predictive of later CP.[9,16,18,41] The quality of GMs at 2–4 months post-term (so-called fidgety GM age) has been found to have highest predictive value in the detection of the infants at risk for development of CP.[42] It seems that assessment of the quality of GM is a window for early detection of children at high risk for developmental disorders.[17,42] Method is simple and it is based on the so called Gestalt perception of GM complexity and variation.[17,41,42] Assessment of GMs at 2–4 months post-term at so called fidgety GM age has been found to have the highest predictive value for development of CP if abnormal.[17,41,42]

Heinz Prechtl's work enabled that spontaneous motility during human development has been brought into focus of interest of many perinatologists prenatally and developmental neurologists postnatally.[9,16,18,41,42] According to the research preceding Prechtl's ingenious idea, during the development of the individual the functional repertoire of the developing neural structure must meet the requirements of the organism and its environment.[41] This concept of ontogenetic adaptation fits excellently to the development of human organism, which is during each developmental stage adapted to the internal and external requirements.[41] Prechtl stated that spontaneous motility, as the expression of spontaneous neural activity, is a marker of brain proper or disturbed function.[41,42] The observation of unstimulated fetus or infant which is the result of spontaneous behavior without sensory stimulation is the best method to assess its CNS capacity.[41] All endogenously generated movement patterns from unstimulated CNS could be observed as early as from 7 to 8 weeks of postmenstrual age, with developing a reach repertoire of movements within the next two or three weeks, continuing to be present for 5–6 months postnatally.[13] This remarkable fact of the continuity of endogenously generated activity from prenatal to postnatal life is the great opportunity to find out those high-risk fetuses and infants in whom development of neurological impairment is emerging. The most important among those movements are GMs involving the whole body in a variable sequence of arm, leg, neck, and trunk movements, with gradual beginning and the end. They wax and wane in intensity, force, and speed being fluent and elegant with the impression of complexity and variability. GMs are called fetal or preterm from 28 to 36 to 38 weeks of postmenstrual age, while after that we have at least two types of movements: (1) writhing present to 46–52 weeks of postmenstrual age and (2) fidgety movements present till 54–58 weeks of postmenstrual age.[18,41,42] Main characteristics of mildly abnormal GMs are lack of fluency and existence of considerable variation and complexity.[43] We are dealing with definitely abnormal GMs when complexity, variation, and fluency are absent.[43]

The quality of each individual movement includes speed, amplitude, and force combined in one complex perception.[13,18,41-44] Investigation of normal and neurologically impaired preterm infants showed that except for higher incidence of clonuses in the abnormal group, there was no marked difference in the quantity of different motor patterns studied.[44,45] However, video analysis of another group of sick preterm infants revealed a "reduction of elegance and fluency as well as variability, fluctuation in intensity and speed rather than any change in incidence of distinct motor patterns."[44-46] Based on postnatal studies, it would be very important to seek for abnormal quantity and quality of prenatal movements in order to find fetuses neurologically at risk.[46]

Some facts are very important in the assessment of GMs. The first important fact is that evaluation of GMs should be based on the video-recorded movements either pre- or postnatally. The second fact is that when assessing GMs examiner should use so called "gestalt perception", which could be described as overall impression of GMs with standardized procedure.[41] During the perception one should recognize the movement patterns of GMs, than assess their complexity, variability, and fluency.[41,42] According to Hadders-Algra, GMs could be classified as (A) normal-optimal, (B) normal-suboptimal, (C) mildly abnormal, and (D) definitely abnormal.[42] This modality of GM assessment is important for the prenatal and postnatal observation of GMs. It is not so important to assess the quantity of GMs, while the assessment of their quality is of utmost importance in terms of the prognosis of neurodevelopmental outcome. They can better foresee neurodevelopmental outcome than classical neurologic examination alone.[47]

It can be concluded that prenatal and postnatal assessment of GMs according to Prechtl's method, gives quite new awareness on the function and development of CNS. We are aware that this important modality is time-consuming and requires some technology and expertise to be practiced; however, advantages of its application in prenatal and postnatal life are very promising and encouraging in terms of its prognostic value. Prenatal assessment of GMs is well developed and established. However, prenatal assessment needs sophisticated real-time 4D ultrasonographic or other technology in order to support more precise assessment of GM quality in fetuses.

CONTINUITY OF GENERAL MOVEMENTS FROM PRENATAL TO POSTNATAL LIFE

Postnatal studies of neonatal behavior have taught us that the assessment of behavior is a better predictor of neurodevelopment disability than neurological examinations.[46] It is important to mention that postnatal observation of movement patterns was launched by Prechtl and coworkers. They have been observing spontaneous movements of the infant using video typing and "off-line" analysis of quantity as well as quality of the movement.[17,48] They have shown that assessment of GMs in high-risk newborns has significantly higher predictive value for later neurological development than neurological examination.[46,47,49] Kurjak and coworkers performed a study by 4D US and were able to confirm earlier findings made by 2D US, that there is behavioral pattern continuity from prenatal to postnatal life.[27] Assessment of neonatal behavior has been shown a better method for early detection of CP than neurological examination alone.[50] It is being speculated that intrauterine detection of encephalopathy would improve the outcome. Many fetal behavioral studies have been conducted; however, it is still uncertain whether the assessment of continuity from fetal to neonatal behavior could improve our ability of early detection of brain pathology. Early detection could possibly rise an opportunity to intervene and even prevent the expected damage.

COULD SOME POSTNATAL SIGNS OF NEUROLOGICAL DISABILITY BE USED PRENATALLY?

Fact that ultrasonography is a powerful tool in the assessment of fetal behavior has been proven by 4D US-enabled visual observation of the fetus, particularly in two especially important domains: fetal finger movements and facial expressions.[19,51] This new technology is not only a tool of fetal observation but a very useful tool to evaluate the development of fetal CNS in normally developing fetuses and those at high risk. A basic understanding of fetal neurology includes: (1) defining of motor pathways involved, (2) chronology of their maturation, and (3) direction of myelination.[52,53] This information helps clinician to better interpret fetal movements. The experience acquired with the ATNAT helps us in interpretation of fetal movements.[39,54,55]

The domain of fetal neurology is already too extensive, but the focus of interest is mainly second trimester, despite the fact that spontaneous fetal mobility emerges and has already became differentiated at a very early age.[56] This means that we will take into a consideration period of pregnancy from 20 till 40 weeks of gestation, including the end of the neuronal migration and the postmigratory phase corresponding to the development of neocortex.[4,57]

As already mentioned, CP describes a group of disorders of the development of movement and posture, causing limitations in activity, which are attributed to nonprogressive disturbances occurring at the time of development of fetal brain.[58-65]

Motor disorders which occur in patients with CP are often accompanied by disturbances of sensation, cognition, communication, perception, behavior, and/or with seizure disorder.[58-65] "Disturbances" is a term which refers to events or processes influencing in some way the expected pattern of brain maturation.[55] Those events or processes are many, with consequences varying from very conspicuous to very subtle. We should always keep in mind what many neurologists emphasize that morphology does not always correspond to neurological outcome.[39,54,55] The opposite view is the one from pediatricians and neurophysiologists. They are involved in long-term follow-up studies, and they are certainly not that optimistic. It would be wise to consider long run prognosis, for each specific type of fetal brain damage and make appropriate decisions for conservative management.

Hopes have been headed toward MR, but in many cases brain changes cannot be detected as early as the first year of life, like for example, pathological gliosis which causes secondary hypomyelinization.

While examining the fetal head by 4D, sonographer should examine bony structures and fetal cranial sutures. If they are folding over one another, it is considered to be a bad sign as previously described by Amiel-Tison.[39,55] The same sign should be searched for postnatally, as a part of neurological examination.[62]

The majority of pediatricians believe that the main obstacle for early prediction of CP based on a functional observation of the fetus such as visual observation by 4D US, is due to the "precompetent" stage of most of the motor behavior observed in utero.[39,55] One of the possible signs detected could be high-arched palate, described by Amiel-Tison, in clinical assessment of the infant nervous system.[39,55] What was believed as undetectable became visible by 4D. Recently, the three-dimensional

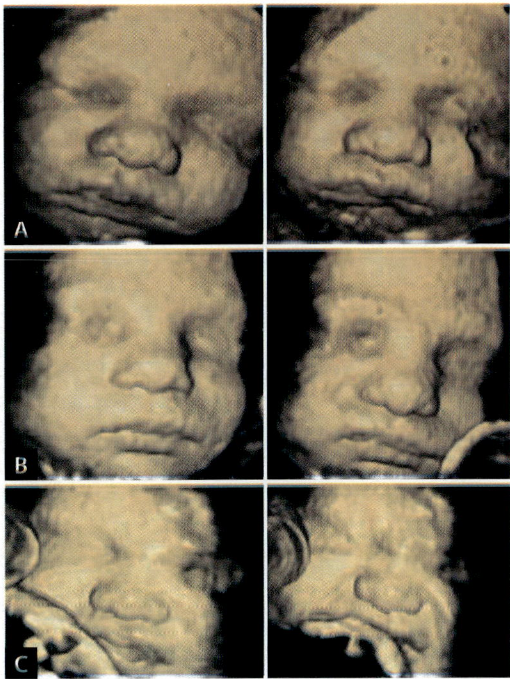

Figs. 6A to C: Face grimacing.

informative and important (the face is the mirror of the brain). Overall number of movements should be defined in very active or inactive fetuses and compared with normal values of previous studies **(Figs. 5 and 6)**.[25,30]

For the application of KANET test all the examiners should have extensive hands-on education, both in low- and high-risk pregnancies. Interobserver and intraobserver variability should be available. It is advisable to use 4D US machines, with frame rate of minimum 24 volumes/sec. KANET consists of eight parameters **(Table 3)**.[68]

A score range of 0–5 is characterized as abnormal, a score calculated from 6–13 is considered borderline, and a score range of 14–20 is normal **(Table 4)**.[1,21,68] After that neonates should be followed up postnatally for neurological development for a 2 years period.

The test evaluates quantitative as well as qualitative aspects of fetal motor behavioral patterns. The parameters examined by this test are a combination of GMs and parameters adopted from ATNAT.[70,71] It is believed that the criterion of quality and quantity of spontaneous GMs has excellent reliability in evaluating the integrity of fetal CNS.[72,73] Furthermore a continuity of behavioral patterns from prenatal to the postnatal period has been proven.[27,74,75] Both those facts support the choice of the parameters used in this test which make KANET theoretically appropriate for the assessment of fetal behavior. According to previous reports[28,29,76-79] KANET easily detects serious functional impairment associated with structural abnormalities. Studies have shown that application of KANET in both low- and high-risk populations has given good results. Especially in high-risk populations, KANET may provide useful information regarding the neurological outcome of these fetuses.[80] KANET is the first test which is based on 4D US, with an original scoring system and has been standardized. Therefore, it can be implemented in everyday practice, overcoming the difficulties and covering the gaps of methods that were used in the past for the evaluation of fetal behavior.[16,81,82] Studies show that KANET is easily applicable to most pregnancies. Furthermore, the learning curve is reasonable for physicians who already have training in obstetrical ultrasound. Actual duration of KANET ranges from 15 to 20 minutes.[83] All of these show strong evidence that it can be widely implemented in everyday clinical practice.[84]

Kurjak's Antenatal Neurobehavioral Test has been introduced in training and it has been calculated that the number of KANET tests needed to be performed by experienced ultrasound specialist in order to be familiar to assess a fetus with 4D US in 20 minutes is 80.[85] The success rate of the test ranges from 91 to 95%. Further study of each parameter revealed a success rate for the assessment of particular signs of 88% for isolated eye blinking and 100% for mouth opening and

TABLE 3: Proposal for the new Kurjak's antenatal neurobehavioral test (KANET) assessment tool consisting of eight parameters.[68,84]

Sign	Score			Sign score
	0	**1**	**2**	
Isolated head anteflexion	Abrupt	Small range (0–3 times of movements)	Variable in full range, many alteration (>3 times of movements)	
Cranial sutures and head circumference (HC)	Overlapping of cranial sutures	Normal cranial sutures with measurement of HC below or above the normal limit (–2 SD) according to GA	Normal cranial sutures with normal measurement of HC according to GA	
Isolated eye blinking	Not present	Not fluent (1–5 times of blinking)	Fluency (>5 times of blinking)	
Facial alteration (grimace or tongue expulsion) or Mouth opening (yawning or mouthing)	Not present	Not fluent (1–5 times of alteration)	Fluency (>5 times of alteration)	
Isolated leg movement	Cramped	Poor repertoire or small in range (0–5 times of movement)	Variable in full range, many alteration (>5 times of movements)	

Contd...

Contd...

Sign	Score			Sign score
	0	**1**	**2**	
Isolated hand movement				
or Hand to face movements	Cramped or abrupt	Poor repertoire or small in range (0–5 times of movement)	Variable in full range, many alteration (>5 times of movements)	
Fingers movements	Unilateral or bilateral clenched fist, (neurological thumb)	Cramped invariable finger movements	Smooth and complex variable finger movements	
Gestalt perception of GMs	Definitely abnormal	Borderline	Normal	
			Total score	

(GA: gestational age; GM: general movement; SD: standard deviation)

TABLE 4: Interpretation of Kurjak's antenatal neurobehavioral test (KANET) scores.[68,84]

Total score	Interpretation
0–5	Abnormal
6–9	Borderline
10–16	Normal

isolated leg movement.[85] KANET has almost 100% negative predictive value, interobserver variability was satisfactory with lowest being for the facial expression (K = 0.68) and highest for the finger movements (K = 0.84).[85]

WHAT HAVE STUDIES ABOUT KANET SHOWN SO FAR?

One of the first studies which used a preliminary form of the KANET scoring system was that by Andonotopo et al. in 2006. They aimed to assess fetal facial expression and quality of body movements and examine if they are of diagnostic value for brain impairment in fetuses with growth restriction. In that prospective study of 50 pregnancies with IUGR fetuses in the third trimester of pregnancy, there has been noted a tendency of less behavioral activity in IUGR than normal fetuses.[29] Future investigation of the use of 4D US for quantitative and qualitative assessment of fetal behavior as possible indicators of the neurological condition in IUGR fetuses was encouraged by the results of this study **(Figs. 7 to 10)**.[29]

In 2008, the Zagreb group were the first to introduce the KANET for the

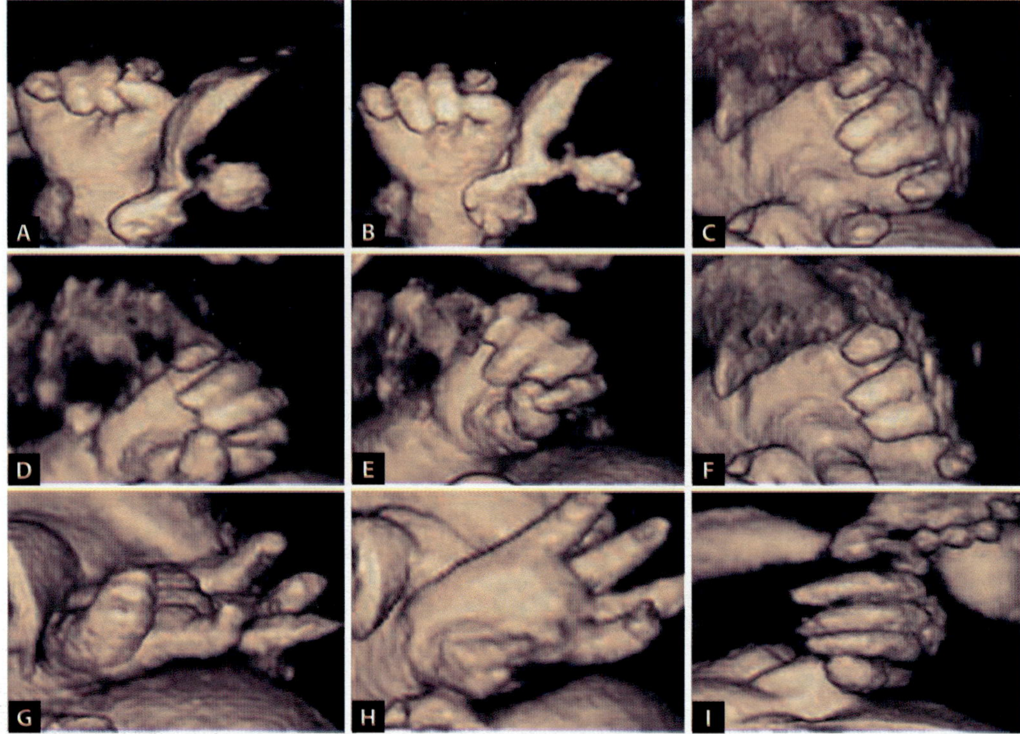

Figs. 7A to I: Hand and finger movement.

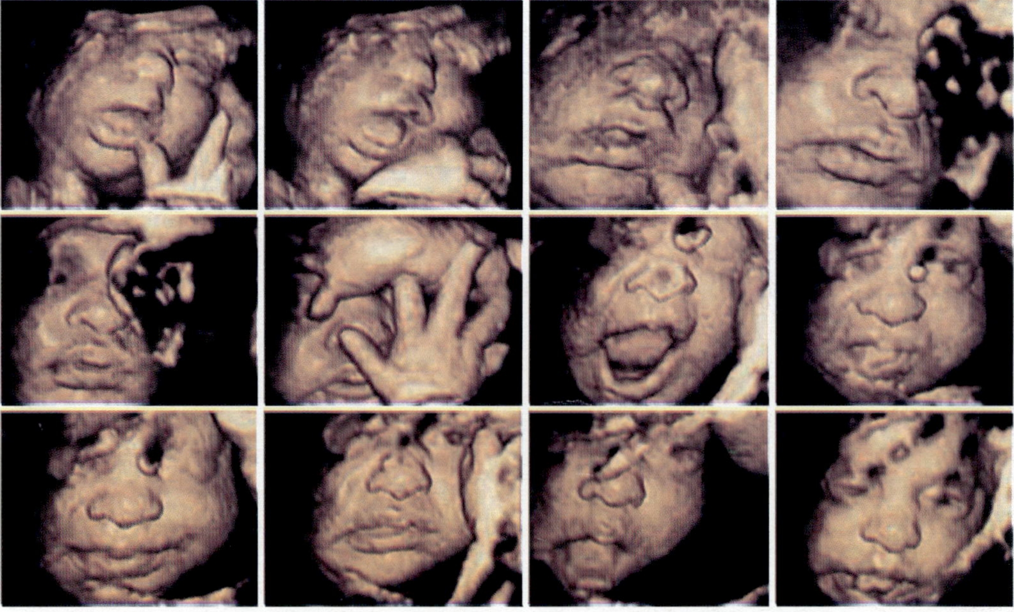

Fig. 8: Kurjak's antenatal neurobehavioral test (KANET)—facial alterations mouthing, eye blinking, and hand movement.

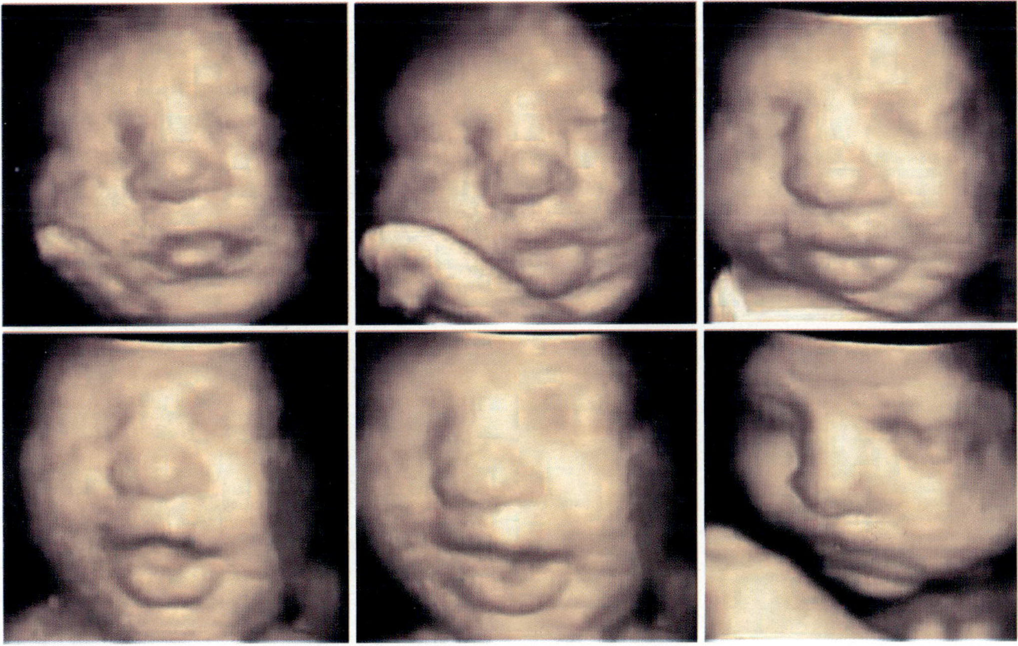

Fig. 9: Tongue expulsion and mouthing.

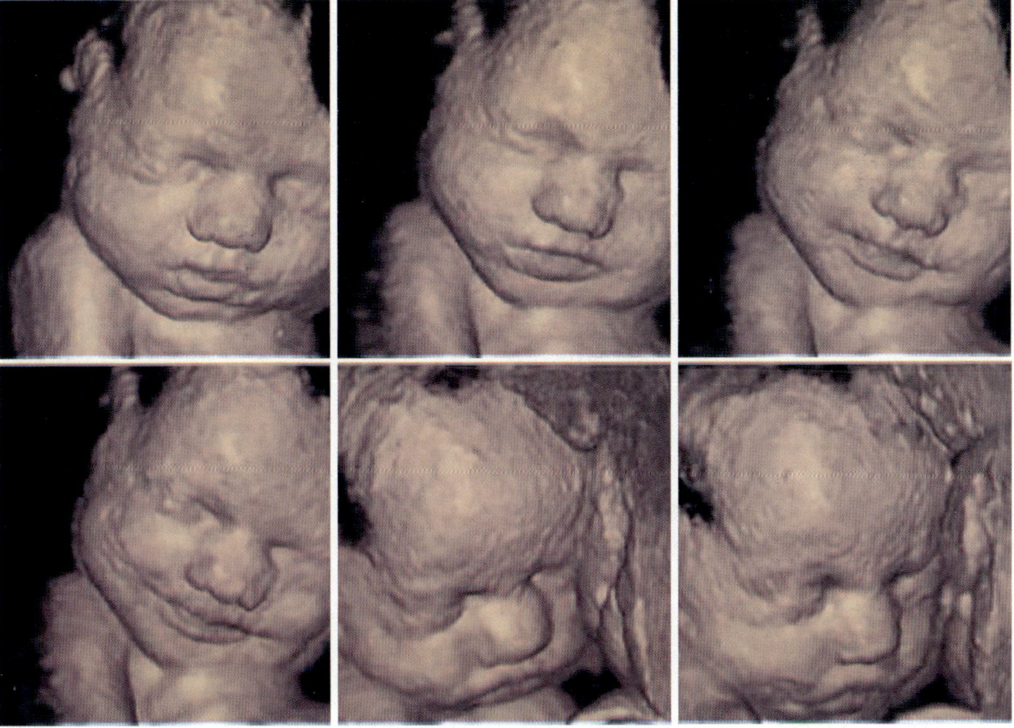

Fig. 10: Smiling.

assessment of neurological status of the fetus, aiming to the detection of fetal brain and neurodevelopmental alterations due to in utero brain impairment.[86,87] In order to develop the new scoring system they identified neonates with severe brain damage and neonates with good neurological condition and then compared the neonatal findings, with corresponding findings in utero.[86,87] In the group of 100 low-risk pregnancies they retrospectively applied KANET. After delivery, postnatal neurological assessment (ATNAT) was performed and all neonates assessed as normal reached a score between 14 and 20, assumed to be the score of optimal neurological development.[86,87] New scoring system was applied in the group of 120 high-risk pregnancies in which, based on postnatal neurological findings, three subgroups of newborns were identified: normal, mildly or moderately abnormal, and abnormal. Based on this, findings a neurological scoring system has been proposed.[86,87] All normal fetuses reached a score from 14 to 20. Ten fetuses who were postnatally described as mildly or moderately abnormal achieved a prenatal score of 5–13, while another 10 fetuses postnatally assigned as neurologically abnormal had a prenatal score 0–5.[86,87] Among this group, four had alobar holoprosencephaly, one had severe hypertensive hydrocephaly, one had thanatophoric dysplasia, and four fetuses had multiple malformations.[86,87] This study inspired a large series of multicenter studies **(Table 5)** that used the KANET in order to assess the usefulness of this promising new scoring system for the assessment of neurological status in fetuses and the recognition of signs of early brain impairment in utero.[86,87]

The first application of KANET was on growth-restricted fetuses,[29] where mainly facial expressions and body movements were studied. A decreased behavioral activity in the IUGR fetuses compared to normal growth cases was noticed.[29] The study that followed was the first with complete neurologic postnatal assessment for all studied fetuses. According to the used criteria neonates were divided into three groups: (1) normal, (2) mildly or moderately abnormal, and (3) abnormal.[29] Based on these groups, it was decided to form the first KANET scoring system which was as follows: 14–20 (normal), 5–13 (mildly or moderately abnormal), and 0–5 (abnormal). All the following studies were designed based on this scoring system.[84,86,87]

The first study which included a large number of high-risk pregnancies identified 32 fetuses at neurological risk: 7 cases with abnormal score were identified and 25 with a borderline KANET score.[88] There were also 11 cases which either died in utero or had a termination of pregnancy and all of these cases had an abnormal KANET score.[88] The seven remaining neonates with abnormal KANET were followed up postnatally at 10 weeks of neonatal life and three had confirmed pathological ATNAT score.[88] These three cases included a neonate with arthrogryposis, a neonate with cerebellar vermian complete aplasia, and one case with a history of CP in a previous pregnancy.[88] Among the parameters that KANET uses, facial expressions appeared to be most pathological—the fetal faces, due to lack of expressions on 4D US, were characterized by the authors as "masks."[88] The remaining four pathological KANET cases had normal postnatal assessment. However, these four cases had complications of pregnancy.[88] There was one case with ventriculomegaly, one case with pre-eclampsia, one case with maternal thrombophilia, and one case with oligohydramnios.[88] From 25 cases diagnosed with borderline KANET result, 22 neonates showed a borderline ATNAT score and were

TABLE 5: List of studies that have applied KANET test to different populations.

Author	Year	Study	Study design	Study population	Indication	No	GA (weeks)	Time (mins)	Result	Summary
Kurjak et al.[86,87]	2008	Cohort	Retrospective	High risk	Multiple	220	20–36	30	Positive	A new scoring system was proposed for the antenatal assessment of fetal neurological status
Kurjak et al.[88]	2010	Multi-center	Prospective	High risk	Multiple	288	20–38	30	Positive	KANET appeared to be prognostic of antenatal detection of serious neurological fetal problems. KANET also identified fetuses with severe structural abnormalities, especially associated with brain impairment
Miskovic et al.[89]	2010	Cohort	Prospective	High risk	Multiple	226	20–36	30	Positive	Correlation between antenatal (KANET) and postnatal (ATNAT) results was found. KANET showed differences of fetal behavior between high- and low-risk pregnancies
Talic et al.[90]	2011	Multi-center Cohort	Prospective	High risk	Multiple	620	26–38	15–20	Positive	KANET test had a prognostic value in discriminating normal from border-line and abnormal fetal behavior, in normal and in high-risk cases. Abnormal KANET scores were predictable of both intrauterine and postnatal death
Talic et al.[91]	2011	Multi-center Cohort	Prospective	High risk	Ventri-culomegaly	240	32–36	10–15	Positive	Statistically significant difference was identified in KANET scores between normal pregnancies and pregnancies with ventriculomegaly. Abnormal KANET scores and most of the borderline scores were noted in fetuses with severe ventriculo-megaly, especially associated with additional abnormalities

Contd...

Contd...

Author	Year	Study	Study design	Study population	Indication	No	GA (weeks)	Time (mins)	Result	Summary
Honemeyer et al.[92]	2011	Cohort	Prospective	Unselected	Unselected	100	28–38	N/A	Positive	Normal prenatal KANET scores had a significant predictive value of a normal postnatal neurological evaluation
Lebit et al.[93]	2011	Cohort	Prospective	Low risk	Normal 2D examination	144	7–38	15–20	Positive	A specific pattern of fetal neurobehavior corresponding to each trimester of pregnancy was identified
Abo-Yaqoub et al.[94]	2012	Cohort	Prospective	High risk	Multiple	80	20–38	15–20	Positive	Significant difference in KANET scores was noted. All antenatally abnormal KANET scores had also an abnormal postnatal neurological assessment
Vladareanu et al.[95]	2012	Cohort	Prospective	High risk	Multiple	196	24–38	N/A	Positive	Most fetuses with normal KANET → low-risk, those with borderline → IUGR fetuses with increased MCA RI and most fetuses with abnormal KANET → threatened PTD with PPROM. Difference in fetal movements was identified between the two groups. For normal pregnancies → 93.4% of fetuses achieved normal score, for high-risk pregnancies → 78.5% of fetuses had a normal score
Honemeyer et al.[96]	2012	Cohort	Prospective	High and low risk	Multiple	56	28–38	30 max	Positive	Introduction of the *average KANET* score → combination of the mean value of KANET scores throughout pregnancy. Revealed a relationship of fetal diurnal rhythm with the pregnancy risk

Contd...

Contd...

Author	Year	Study	Study design	Study population	Indication	No	GA (weeks)	Time (mins)	Result	Summary
Kurjak et al.[97]	2013	Cohort	Prospective	High and low risk	Multiple	869	28–38	20	Positive	Statistically significant differences in the distribution of normal, abnormal, and borderline KANET scores between low-risk and high-risk groups were found. Fetal behavior was significantly different between the normal group and the high-risk subgroups
Predojevic et al.[98]	2013	Case study	Prospective	High risk	IUGR	5	3139	30	Positive	KANET could recognize pathologic and borderline behavior in IUGR fetuses with or without blood flow redistribution. Combined assessment of hemodynamic and motoric parameters could enable in better diagnosis and consultation
Athanasiadis et al.[99]	2013	Cohort	Prospective	Unselected (High and low risk)	Multiple (IUGR, PET, GDM)	152	2nd and 3rd trimester	N/A	Positive	The neurodevelopmental score was statistically significant higher in the low-risk group compared to the high-risk group (p < 0.0004). The diabetes subgroup score was statistically significantly higher compared to the IUGR and the pre-eclampsia subgroup (p = 0.0001)

(KANET: Kurjak's antenatal neurological test; No: number of patients; IUGR: intrauterine growth restriction; MCA: middle cerebral artery; PTD: preterm delivery; PPROM: preterm premature rupture of membranes; PET: pre-eclampsia; GA: gestational age; GDM: gestational diabetes mellitus) followed up.[88] The three remaining cases showed normal ATNAT result.[88] There was an interesting paper which studied a case of a fetus with prenatally diagnosed acrania.[88] The authors studied the fetal behavior and managed to document how it altered from 20 weeks of gestation onward.[88] It was noticed that as pregnancy progressed and the control center of motoric activity shifted from the lower to the upper part, KANET score was decreasing respectively, suggesting that neurological damage in later pregnancy is possible.[88]

A study with 226 cases, including different study populations, identified three cases with pathological KANET score.[89] All three cases had chromosomal abnormalities and all three of them postnatally also had an abnormal ATNAT score.[89] Scores from antenatal KANET and postnatal ATNAT were compared between low- and high-risk groups, and they showed differences between them, for 8 out of the 10 parameters—these included: head anteflexion, eye blinking, facial expressions—grimacing, tongue expulsion, mouth movement such as yawning, jawing, swallowing—isolated hand movements, hand to face movements, fist and finger movements, and GMs.[89]

The comparison of the two tests revealed correlation between them and proved that the neonatal examination (ATNAT) was a satisfactory confirmation of the prenatal ultrasound examination (KANET), stating that KANET could offer useful information about the neurological status of the fetus and can be applied in clinical practice.[89]

One of the largest studies regarding KANET included 620 cases, of both low- and high-risk populations (100 low-risk and 520 high-risk cases) and it showed differences in the scores between the two groups.[90] The study showed interesting results that most

abnormal cases were noted from pregnancies with a previous history of CP (23.8%) and that most borderline scores were noted in cases with possible chorioamnionitis (56.4%).[90] There parameters of KANET that were more notably different between the two groups were: overlapping cranial sutures, head circumference, isolated eye blinking, facial expressions, mouth movements, isolated hand movements, isolated leg movements, hand to face movements, finger movements, and GMs.[90] This study confirmed the relationship of pathological KANET with increased risk of perinatal mortality and neurological impairment and showed that the results can be confirmed and are reproducible postnatally.[90]

A very interesting study which tried to shed some light on the clinical dilemmas caused by the prenatal diagnosis of ventriculomegaly, compared fetuses with ventriculomegaly[91] with apparently low-risk fetuses (normal CNS appearance on ultrasound examination). A significant difference was noted between the two groups, with the KANET score decreasing as the degree of ventriculomegaly was increasing.[91] For isolated cases of mild or moderate ventriculomegaly no pathological KANET scores were noted and postnatal evaluation confirmed the prenatal KANET, offering valuable information for the more complete assessment of these fetuses and better counseling regarding their prognosis.[91]

A recent study with a complete follow-up[92] postnatally up to 3 months of life, having complete postnatal documentation in all cases, showed that a normal KANET score is very reassuring of a good neonatal outcome, confirming the consistency of prenatal and postnatal assessment.[92] It was a great challenge to understand the evolution of fetal movements by 4D US throughout pregnancy, and how these movements reflect the development and integrity of fetal nervous system.[92] It was shown that during the first trimester of pregnancy the development of the frequency and the complexity of fetal movements is more important, while during the second trimester, the variation of fetal movements develop, with more detailed movements (facial expressions and eye blinking) appearing at the end of this trimester.[93] Finally at the end of third trimester, the number of fetal movements declines as a result of the increase of fetal rest periods, due to fetal cerebral maturation, and this is something that most pregnant women notice near term.[77–81]

Abo-Yaqoub et al.[94] aimed to study how practical is to apply 4D ultrasonography for the assessment of fetal neurobehavior and also how useful it is for the prediction of neurological impairment.[94] Their results showed agreement of prenatal scores with postnatal assessment. The parameters that were significantly different between the two groups were: isolated head anteflexion, isolated eye blinking, facial expressions, mouth movements, isolated hand movements, hand-to-face movements, finger movements, and GMs.[94] The difference was not statistically significant regarding isolated leg movements and cranial sutures.[94]

Vladareanu et al.[95] noted that the majority of normal KANET scores derived from low-risk populations that they studied, while the majority of cases with borderline or pathological KANET scores derived from the high-risk groups and in some cases were related to abnormal values of Doppler studies in IUGR fetuses.[95] The authors concluded that KANET can be useful for the detection of neurological impairment which could become obvious during the antenatal or postnatal period.[95]

The average KANET score was introduced for fetuses who had more than one assessments in order to have a more complete picture of the behavior of these fetuses.[96] The average KANET score derived from the mean calculation of KANET scores for each fetus throughout pregnancy, since these fetuses had more than one KANET assessments.[96] What was new from this study was the association of KANET score with fetal diurnal rhythm.[96] For the high-risk group 89% of the borderline scores were recorded at times that the mothers characterized them as active periods, compared with 33.3%, respectively in the low-risk pregnancies.[96]

Another important goal was to compare all parameters of KANET between high- and low-risk pregnancies and observe differences in fetal behavior between them. For pathological KANET score 5 out of 8 parameters were significant different: isolated head anteflexion, cranial sutures and head circumference, isolated hand movement or hand to face movements, isolated leg movement, and fingers movements.[97–99] Further results showed that only high-risk patients had abnormal scores (8.5%), while comparing high- and low-risk groups it was noticed that 80.6% of high-risk patients had borderline results while 85.3% of low-risk patients were normal, both being statistically significant.[97–99] For abnormal KANET results (score between 0 and 5), some were related to pregnancy complications (pre-eclampsia, threatened preterm labor, and drug abuse) and some were related to fetal condition (trisomy 13, 18, and 21 and IUGR).[97–99]

Other studies confirmed the feasibility of neurodevelopment assessment by 4D US and showed further evidence that KANET test is useful in early identification of fetuses prone to neurological impairment.[100,101]

When comparing Caucasian to Asian populations in order to check for ethnic differences, the total KANET score was normal in both populations, but there was a difference noted in total KANET scores between these two populations.[102] When individual KANET parameters were compared, significant differences were observed in four fetal movements: (1) isolated head anteflexion, (2) isolated eye blinking, (3) facial alteration or mouth opening, and (4) isolated leg movement.[102] No significant differences were noted in the four other parameters: (1) cranial suture and head circumference, (2) isolated hand movement or hand to face movements, (3) fingers movements, and (4) gestalt of GMs, showing that ethnicity is a parameter that should be considered when evaluating fetal behavior, especially during assessment of fetal facial expressions.[102] The authors concluded that although there was a difference in the total KANET score between Asian and Caucasian populations, all the scores in both groups were within normal range proving that ethnical differences in fetal behavior do not affect the total KANET score, but close follow-up should be continued in some borderline cases.[102]

Unpublished data from Greece collected from 655 singleton pregnancies, showed that KANET is a method which is feasible in everyday clinical practice, with a success rate of 95% and a very low negative predictive value. There were the cases where KANET could not be completed. The reason for that was severe oligohydramnios, fibroid uterus (difficult imaging), very high body mass index (BMI) and a case that due to vasovagal reaction-supine hypotensive syndrome ultrasound examination could not be completed. From the 655 cases, 1,712 KANET were performed from only two operators and the interobserver variability was calculated showing adequate results for all parameters, with the lowest being for facial alterations (K = 0.68) and the highest for finger movements (K = 0.84). This study was primarily designed to compare the neurological status of pregnancies complicated by diabetes, compared to low-risk pregnancies and it did show that there was a difference between the fetal neurobehavior of these two groups, with the diabetic pregnancies having lower scores.[103]

Figures 11 to 13 are illustrating important parameters of KANET depicted by high-definition (HD) 4D US.

Interpretation of KANET Test Research

Assessment of fetal neurobehavior and detection of fetal neurological impairment in utero is one of the greatest challenges in perinatal medicine. KANET is the first method that applied 4D US for the assessment of the fetus in the same way like a neonate is assessed neurologically after birth by neonatologists. It appears to be a powerful diagnostic method for the detection of neurological impairment and for the assessment of fetal neurobehavior, conditions that were not accessible with the traditional prenatal diagnostic methods which were used so far.[67] Studies have proved the validity of this method,[27,28,84] that it can be applied in everyday clinical practice, especially for high-risk cases, showed how and by whom it should be performed, what is the value of the result of KANET, and how it should be managed. It is very difficult to make diagnosis of neurological impairment prenatally and usually all these diagnosis are made postnatally, even months or years after delivery. Moreover, neurological conditions such as CP, are not adequately understood and they are falsely attributed to incidents during labor, although it has been proven that

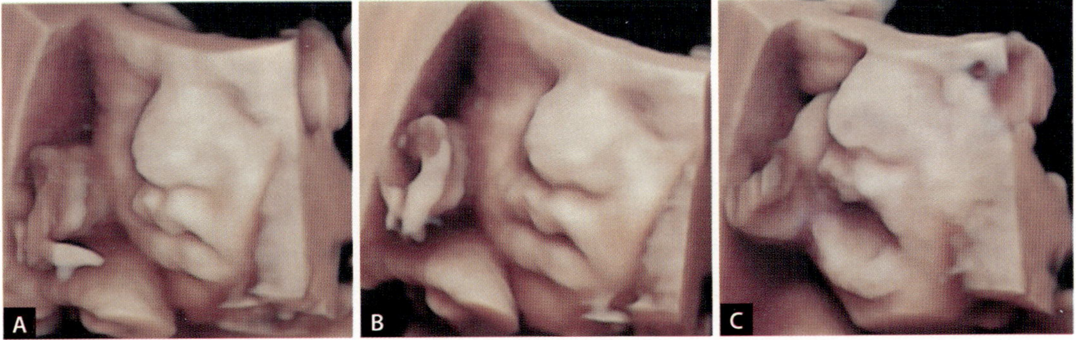

Figs. 11A to C: Mouthing as part of the assessment of fetal neurobehavior [high-definition four-dimensional ultrasound (4D US)].

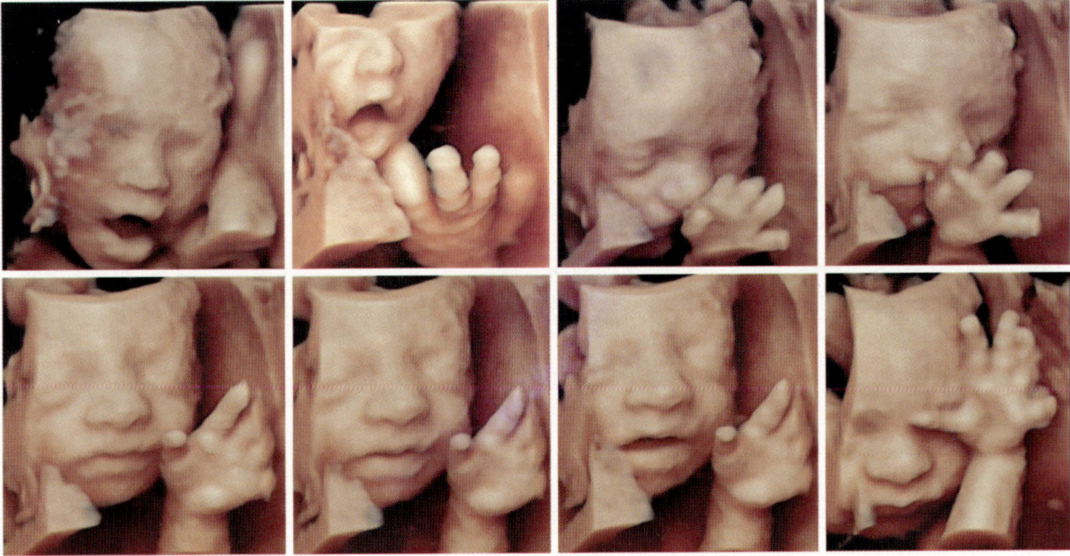

Fig. 12: Parameters of Kurjak's antenatal neurodevelopmental test (KANET): mouthing, yawning, and hand movements [high-definition four-dimensional ultrasound (4D US)].

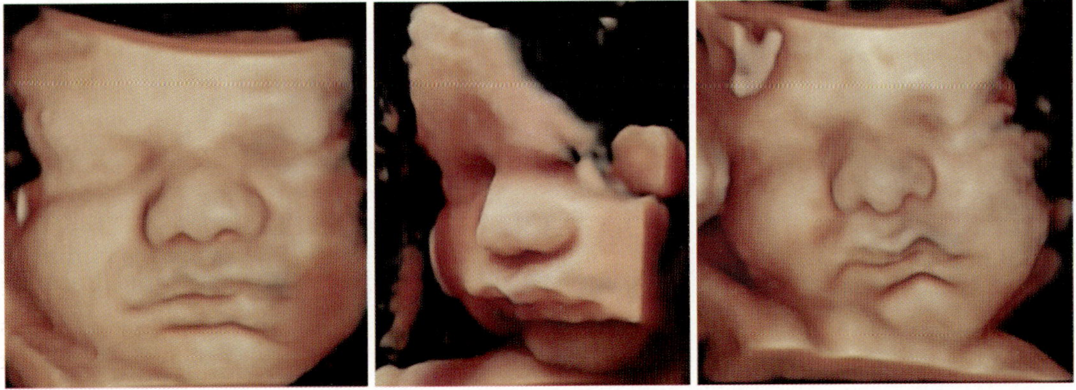

Fig. 13: Facial expression and grimacing [high-definition four-dimensional ultrasound (4D US)].

the majority of CP cases originate sometime during in utero life and are not related to intrapartum events. All these things lead to delayed diagnosis of neurological conditions. The later a neurological impairment is diagnosed the less is the possibility of an effective intervention. In order to increase a possibility of an effective intervention or even treatment, it would be extremely challenging to have a timely diagnosis of such conditions. KANET offers a possibility to detect prenatally fetuses at risk for neurological problems, offering a possibility of even an in utero intervention or at least an early postpartum intervention.[84] The earliest physiotherapy is commenced and intervention programs are applied in neonates that are born prematurely or with neurological problems the better the neurodevelopmental outcome of these neonates, with the cognitive benefits persisting into preschool age. KANET appears to be able to offer this advantage of early identification of these fetuses with neurological problems, so that they could be put under treatment as early as possible, aiming to a better outcome.[86,87,104,105]

Even more, the explicitly detailed pictures obtained by the new ultrasound machines but also the advanced techniques of molecular genetics, many times brings us, as ultrasound specialists, across findings (anatomical and chromosomal) of uncertain clinical significance and prognosis, especially regarding the neurological integrity of the fetus.[106,107] A method like KANET offers a more comprehensive diagnostic approach to such dilemmas and hopefully in the near future with more data we could form a complete neurosonobehavioral assessment of the fetus and a more complete counseling of these couples.[108]

Many centers for the assessment of fetal neurobehavior of not only high-risk pregnancies but also low-risk pregnancies have introduced KANET in everyday clinical practice.

Studies show that the sensitivity and specificity of the test are satisfactory, as are the positive and negative predictive values and the inter- and intraobserver variability of this method. The KANET has been introduced into systematical training and ultrasound specialists have already been certified to perform this examination. Hopefully, application of KANET on larger populations, both high- and low-risk, will give more knowledge regarding early detection of fetuses at risk for neurological impairment, in order to allow accurate diagnosis prenatally, and as a consequence prompt intervention that could possibly improve the outcome of some of these neonates.

The Most Recent Research Data on the KANET Test

The data of fetal prenatal neurological testing from nine centers by nine investigators from seven countries which were performed from May 2010 till April 2020, with the number of 25–1,344 fetuses from singleton pregnancies are presented.[109] Altogether there were 3,709 fetuses of whom 1,573 (42.4%) completed the pregnancy of which 1,556 were eligible for postnatal follow-up, while in 2,136 mostly low-risk pregnancies for 2,094 the data were missing while in 42 the pregnancies were still ongoing **(Table 6)**. From the group of 3,709 fetuses 3,206 (86.5%) had normal, 379 (10.2%) borderline, and 124 (3.3%) abnormal KANET scores, respectively, while in those after completed pregnancy 153 (9.7%) had borderline and 52 (3.3%) had abnormal KANET scores **(Tables 6 and 7)**.

The inter-rater reliability was substantial for low-risk pregnancies and moderate for

TABLE 6: The results of the KANET[+] test from nine centers: the date of the introduction of KANET, number of patients investigated, total number of borderline and abnormal scores, number with postnatal follow-up, number of borderline and abnormal cases in all fetuses, and those postnatally followed-up.[109]

| Name of the investigator/ country | Introduction of KANET[+] | Number of fetuses | All fetuses | | Number of children | Postnatal follow-up | |
| | | | KANET[+] scores | | | KANET[+] scores | |
			Borderline	Abnormal		Borderline	Abnormal
Lara Spalldi Barisic, Croatia*	May, 2010	1,344	98 (7.3%)	52 (3.9%)	482 (35.9%)	36 (7.5%)	19 (3.9%)
Panos Antsaklis, Greece[19]	January, 2012	1,180	105 (8.9%)	40 (3.4%)	520 (44.1%)	47 (9.0%)	19 (3.7%)
Raul Moreira Neto, Brazil[17]	November, 2014	631	115 (18.2%)	19 (3.0%)	212 (33.6%)	39 (18.2%)	6 (3.0%)
Suada Tinjić Tuzla, B and H[18]	May, 2015	141	38 (27.0%)	5 (3.5%)	60 (42.6%)	16 (27.0%)	2 (3.5%)
Sonal Panchal, India[33]	October, 2015	160	3 (1.9%)	0	145 (90.6%)	3 (1.9%)	0
Dorota Bomba Opon, Poland[18]	July, 2017	63	6 (9.5%)	3 (4.8%)	26 (41.3%)	2 (9.5%)	1 (4.8%)
Gigi Selvan, India*	July, 2018	64	0	1 (1.6%)	35 (54.7%)	0	1 (1.6%)
Sertac Esin, Turkey[18]	February, 2019	25	4 (16.0%)	1 (4.0%)	17 (68.0%)	3 (16.0%)	1 (4.0%)
Edin Medjedovic, B and H*	July, 2019	101	10 (9.9%)	3 (3.0)	76 (75.2%)	7 (9.2%)	3 (3.9%)
Total	May, 2010– July, 2019	3,709	379 (10.2%)	124 (3.3%)	1,573 (42.4%)	153 (9.7%)	52 (3.3%)

[+]KANET: Kurjak's Antenatal Neurodevelopmental Test
*Unpublished data
(B and H: Bosnia and Herzegovina)

high-risk pregnancies. There were 2,502 (67.5%) fetuses from low-risk pregnancies and 1,207 (32.5%) fetuses from high-risk pregnancies **(Table 7)**. Compared to the fetuses from low-risk pregnancies, fetuses from high-risk pregnancies had higher frequencies of borderline and abnormal KANET scores, which was statistically significant. We could speculate that a hostile intrauterine environment is affecting adversely fetal neurobehavior, which can be detected by the KANET test. Dropout rate in the investigation was high (47.6%), respectively, which is a severe constraint of the investigation. Most of the dropouts were from the low-risk pregnancies with low rates of borderline or abnormal KANET scores and high probability of normal postnatal development.

Out of 1,556 fetuses who were born after KANET testing the distribution based on age is presented in **Table 3**. Most of the children were older than 3 years (819 out of 1,556 or 52.6%). Most of the infants were developing normally (1,530 or 98.3%), 8 (0.5%) had

TABLE 7: The data on KANET[&] scores from low- and high-risk pregnancies shown as normal, borderline, and abnormal, comparing abnormal and borderline score prevalence depending on the pregnancy risk.[109]

Name of the investigator	Risk of the pregnancy	KANET score			Total number
		Normal	Borderline	Abnormal	
Lara Spalldi Barisic, N* = 1,344	Low	1,017	31	0	1,048
	High	177	67	52	296
Panos Antsaklis, N = 1,180	Low	772	23	0	795
	High	263	82	40	385
Raul Moreira Neto, N = 631	Low	348	58	0	406
	High	149	57	19	225
Suada Tinjic, N = 141	Low	96	33	0	129
	High	2	5	5	12
Sonal Panchal, N = 160	High	157	3	0	160
Dorota Bomba Opon, N = 63	Low	30	0	0	30
	High	24	6	3	33
Gigi Selvan, N = 64	Low	30	0	0	30
	High	33	0	1	34
Serac Esin, N = 25	High	20	4	1	25
Edin Medjedovic, N = 101	Low	64	0	0	64
	High	24	10	3	37
Subtotal low risk		2,357 (94.2%)	145 (5.8%)	0	2,502 (67.5%)
Subtotal high risk		849 (70.3%)	234 (19.4%)	124 (10.3%)	1,207 (32.5%)
Total		3,206 (86.5%)	379 (10.2%)	124 (3.3%)	3,709

$\chi^2 = 457.36$; d.f.[+] = 2; p < .01

[&]Kurjak's Antenatal Neurodevelopmental Test
*N = total number of pregnancies
[+]d.f. = degrees of freedom

slight and moderate developmental delay, while 18 (1.2%) had severe developmental delay. The severe and moderate developmental delay could develop more frequently in the group of infants who as fetuses had abnormal KANET scores which are presented in **Table 8**, which was statistically significant.

Most of the infants with abnormal KANET scores were from high-risk pregnancies, they had severe congenital malformations, often IUGR, and had more chance to die in utero. To investigate the validity of the KANET test for the prediction of developmental delay and CP, we made predictive value calculations from sensitivity, specificity, and prevalence for all age groups with developmental delay and only for the age group above 2 years for the CP and severe developmental delay. The calculations showed that the KANET test has low sensitivity for the detection CP, and

TABLE 8: Postnatal follow-up of infants who as fetuses had borderline and abnormal KANET[&] scores from low- and high-risk pregnancies including termination of pregnancy and postnatal death.[109]

Name of the investigator (N*)	KANET score (N*)	Postnatal developmental delay (N*)				Comment
		No	Slight	Moderate	Severe	
Lara Spalldi Barisic, N = 482	Borderline N = 36	33	0	0	2	1 IUD[+]
	Abnormal N = 19	15	0	0	4	All severe congenital malformations
Panos Antsaklis, N = 520	Borderline N = 47	45	0	0	1	1 IUD[+]
	Abnormal N = 19	7	0	0	1[++]	5 died 6 terminated
Raul Moreira Neto, N = 212	Borderline N = 39	39	0	0	0	-
	Abnormal N = 6	3	0	0	3	One case of trisomy 13, 18, and 21
Suada Tinjic, N = 60	Borderline N = 16	16	0	0	0	-
	Abnormal N = 2	1	1	0	0	IUGR** one with slight developmental delay
Sonal Panchal, N = 145	Borderline N = 3	0	0	2	1	-
	Abnormal N = 0	0	0	0	0	-
Dorota Bomba Opon, N = 26	Borderline N = 2	2	0	0	0	-
	Abnormal N = 1	0	0	0	1	One with severe delay Kagami Ogata syndrome
Gigi Selvan, N = 35	Borderline N = 0	0	0	0	0	-
	Abnormal N = 1	0	0	1	0	IUGR**
Serac Esin, N = 17	Borderline N = 3	3	0	0	0	-
	Abnormal N = 1	0	0	0	1	Trisomy 18, died in the first day of life
Edin Medjedovic, N = 76	Borderline N = 7	7	0	0	0	-
	Abnormal N = 3	3	0	0	3	Two severe congenital malformations and one IUGR**
Subtotal normal KANET	1,351 (86.8%)	1,348 (99.8)	0	2 (0.1%)	1 (0.1%)	One with severe delay Kagami Ogata syndrome
Subtotal borderline KANET	153 (9.8%)	145 (94.8%)	0	2 (1.3%)	4 (2.6%)	2 IUD (1.3%)
Subtotal abnormal KANET	52 (3.3%)	26 (50.0%)	1 (1.9%)	1 (1.9%)	13 (25.0%)	11 terminated or died (21.2%)
Total	1,556 (100.0%)	1,519 (97.6%)	1 (0.1%)	5 (0.3%)	18 (1.2%)	13 (0.8%)

$\chi^2 = 315.28$; d.f.[+++] = 6; p <0.01

[&]Kurjak's Antenatal Neurodevelopmental Test

*N: Number of infants

[+]IUD: Intrauterine death

[++]One infant with CP (with previous case of cerebral palsy in the family)

**IUGR: Intrauterine growth restriction

[+++]d.f. = Degrees of freedom

lower sensitivity for the detection of slight, moderate, and severe developmental delay, than for only severe developmental delay. Specificity was rather high for detection of CP, it was lower for the detection of developmental delay. In concordance, positive predictive value and the false positive rate were high. The negative predictive value was high and the false negative rate was low. If the KANET score is normal, then there is a huge probability of postnatal normal development, with a very small chance that it is false negative meaning that the probability of abnormal postnatal development is low if KANET was normal. There is a problem with the interpretation of abnormal and borderline KANET scores which appears to have very low sensitivity and positive predictive value and high false positive rate. This means that based on the borderline or abnormal KANET score one cannot predict the neurodevelopmental outcome, although there is a higher tendency of developmental disorders to occur in infants with abnormal KANET scores from high-risk pregnancies, however, it cannot be concluded concerning the type and severity of the disorder, especially not CP. As it has been pointed out many times in the papers published up to now by our team, the most important aim of KANET introduction was to early predict the development of CP in order to intervene early enough to decrease possible consequences of the condition on individual, family, societal, and public health level. We were aware that early diagnosis of CP was and is not easy even postnatally. There is a rule saying that making the diagnosis of CP is inversely proportional to the age, undermining confidence in diagnosing CP early. Possible barriers in postnatal early diagnosis could be[110-119]:

- There are no clinical signs on the clinical examination which can confirm or rule out the diagnosis.
- High probability of false positive diagnosis
- Lack of specific biomarkers, genetic, or other tests helpful in making the diagnosis
- Due to grief and the stigma of the family with the child diagnosed with CP, there is the desire of the healthcare providers to rule out every treatable condition first by wide differential diagnosis
- There are no curative treatments and evidence of the efficacy of the early intervention is scarce.

Another important recurrent discussion lasting for decades on CP is when the earliest diagnosis of CP could be made to avoid the development of deformities connected with the disease.[110-119] For many years from the 1970s, it is accepted that it is almost impossible to make the diagnosis of CP in infancy, and that acceptable age for the diagnosis is between 3 and 5 years.[110-119] It has been claimed that in a well-developed healthcare system the diagnosis of CP could be made in one of five children at the age of 6 months and in more than half of the cases after the first year of life.[117] There is a belief that CP is neurologically silent in the first few months of age and almost impossible to be diagnosed. This was the reason for the development of the concept of GMs by Prechtl et al. which enabled detection of neurological impairment by the recording of GMs by a camera and assessing them off-line. The assessment was time-consuming and not practical or clinically applicable for everyday clinical practice. However, in the recently published guidelines for the early diagnosis (by the age of 5 months in high-risk infants) of CP the following criteria have been mentioned[110-119]:

- General movements assessment {sensitivity 98% [95% confidence interval (CI) 74%–100%]; specificity 91% (95% CI 83%–93%)} at fidgety age[26]
- Magnetic resonance imaging at term equivalent age (sensitivity 86%–100%, specificity 89%–97%)
- Hammersmith Infant Neurological Examination (HINE) (sensitivity at 3 months 96%, specificity 85%, CI not reported).[119]

Mentioned criteria is aimed for high-risk infants, while infants with CP who do not have newborn detectable risks, and are seemingly healthy at birth, are less likely to be followed up, and there is a need for identifying these infants and administering best practice tools in order not to miss the diagnosis of CP, which is nowadays in low-risk population very often overlooked and missed.[110-119] For such term and high-risk preterm infants automated computer assisted/smartphone GMs assessment tool is under development,[119] which will make a time-consuming assessment of GMs more practical, standardized, and clinically applicable.

We are aware of weaknesses of our study: nine investigators included, high dropout rate, heterogeneity of the investigation group in terms of nationality and race, inhomogeneous groups of pregnant women in terms of risk of pregnancy, social status, age, parity, and many other characteristics. Although KANET was standardized and it was advised to be used in everyday clinical practice, it would be much better if all those weaknesses could have been avoided.[69,98]

The main weakness of the investigation is the postnatal follow-up of infants, which was dependent on local circumstances, and the information for infants who had developmental delays has been obtained from the parents and available medical charts. Such an approach may cause that some children with developmental delay may have been missed, without awareness of the investigator(s). That is why the results of the study should be taken with due caution.

Based on the results of the study we can conclude that if the KANET score is normal then there is a high probability that the development of the infant will be normal, with a very low probability that the child with developmental delay would have been missed. However, if the KANET score is borderline and especially if abnormal in high-risk pregnancy, postnatal development of the child may appear abnormal. Due to a high false-positive rate in those fetuses, thorough postnatal prospective neurodevelopmental follow-up especially in high-risk infants with a positive family history on CP should be advised.[110-119] To make an early diagnosis of CP in high-risk cases, the protocol proposed by Novak et al. should be followed,[117] while for low-risk infants with abnormal KANET scores the protocol should be individualized and follow-up established on a case by case basis. The future development of fetal neurology should be multidisciplinary with special emphasis on scrutinized postnatal follow-up of infants who had abnormal and borderline KANET scores and were born from high-risk pregnancies.

REFERENCES

1. Salihagic-Kadic A, Kurjak A, Medic M, Andonotopo W, Azumendi G. New data about embryonic and fetal neurodevelopment and behavior obtained by 3D and 4D sonography. J Perinat Med. 2005;33(6):478-90.
2. Pomeroy SL, Volpe JJ. Development of the nervous system. In: Polin RA, Fox, WW (Eds). Fetal and Neonatal Physiology. Philadelphia-London-Toronto-Montreal-Sydney-Tokyo: WB Saunders Company; 1992. pp. 1491-509.

3. O'Rahilly R, Muller F. Minireview: Summary of the initial development of the human nervous system. Teratology. 1999;60(1):39-41.

4. Kostovic I, Judas M, Petanjek Z, Simic G. Ontogenesis of goal-directed behavior: anatomo-functional considerations. Int J Psychophysiol. 1995;19(2):85-102.

5. Schaher S. Determination and differentiation in the development of the nervous system. In: Kandel ER, Schwartz JH (Eds). Principles of Neural Science, 2nd edition. New York: Elsevier Science Publishing; 1985. pp. 730-2.

6. Kostovic I. Prenatal development of nucleus basalis complex and related fiber systems in man: a histochemical study. Neuroscience. 1986;17(4):1047-77.

7. Okado N. Onset of synapse formation in the human spinal cord. J Comp Neurol. 1981; 201(2):211-9.

8. Kostovic I. Zentralnervensystem. In: Hinrichsen KV (Ed). Humanembryologie. Berlin: Springer-Verlag; 1990. pp. 381-448.

9. Prechtl HF. Ultrasound studies of human fetal behavior. Early Hum Dev. 1985;12(2):91-8.

10. Ianniruberto A, Tajani E. Ultrasonographic study of fetal movements. Semin Perinatol. 1981;5(2):175-81.

11. Goto S, Kato TK. Early movements are useful for estimating the gestational weeks in the first trimester of pregnancy. In: Levski RA, Morley P (Eds). Ultrasound '82. Oxford: Pergamon Press; 1983. pp. 577-82.

12. Joseph RG. Fetal brain behavior and cognitive development. Dev Rev. 2000;20(1):81-98.

13. de Vries JI, Visser GH, Prechtl HF. The emergence of fetal behavior. I. Qualitative aspects. Early Hum Dev. 1982;7(4):301-22.

14. Kostovic I, Rakic P. Development of prestriate visual projections in the monkey and human fetal cerebrum revealed by transient cholinesterase staining. J Neurosci. 1984;4(1):25-42.

15. D'Elia A, Pighetti M, Moccia G, Santangelo N. Spontaneous motor activity in normal fetuses. Early Hum Dev. 2001;65(2):139-47.

16. Prechtl HF, Einspieler C. Is neurological assessment of the fetus possible? Eur J Obstet Gynecol Reprod Biol. 1997;75(1):81-4.

17. Roodenburg PJ, Wladimiroff JW, van Es A, Prechtl HF. Classification and quantitative aspects of fetal movements during the second half of pregnancy. Early Hum Dev. 1991;25(1):19-35.

18. Prechtl HF. Qualitative changes of spontaneous movements in fetus and preterm infant are a marker of neurological dysfunction. Early Hum Dev. 1990;23(3):151-8.

19. Kurjak A, Azumendi G, Vecek N, Kupesic S, Solak M, Varga D, et al. Fetal hand movements and facial expression in normal pregnancy studied by four-dimensional sonography. J Perinat Med. 2003;31(6):496-508.

20. Andonotopo W, Stanojevic M, Kurjak A, Azumendi G, Carrera JM. Assessment of fetal behavior and general movements by four-dimensional sonography. Ultrasound Rev Obstet Gynecol. 2004;4(2):103-14.

21. Kurjak A, Stanojevic M, Azumendi G, Carrera JM. The potential of four-dimensional (4D) ultrasonography in the assessment of fetal awareness. J Perinat Med. 2005;33(1):46-53.

22. Kurjak A, Pooh RK, Merce LT, Carrera JM, Salihagic-Kadic A, Andonotopo W. Structural and functional early human development assessed by three-dimensional and four-dimensional sonography. Fertil Steril. 2005;84(5):1285-99.

23. Kurjak A, Miskovic B, Andonotopo W, Stanojevic M, Azumendi G, Vrcic H. How useful is 3D and 4D ultrasound in perinatal medicine? J Perinat Med. 2007;35(1):10-27.

24. Andonotopo W, Medic M, Salihagic-Kadic A, Milenkovic D, Maiz N, Scazzocchio E. The assessment of fetal behavior in early pregnancy: comparison between 2D and 4D sonographic scanning. J Perinat Med. 2005;33(5):406-14.

25. Kurjak A, Stanojevic M, Andonotopo W, Scazzocchio-Duenas E, Azumendi G, Carrera JM. Fetal behavior assessed in all three trimesters of normal pregnancy by four-dimensional ultrasonography. Croat Med J. 2005;46(5):772-80.

26. Pooh RK, Ogura T. Normal and abnormal fetal hand positioning and movement in early pregnancy detected by three- and

four-dimensional ultrasound. Ultrasound Rev Obset Gynecol. 2004;4(1):46-51.

27. Kurjak A, Stanojevic M, Andonotopo W, Salihagic-Kadic A, Azumendi G, Carrera JM. Behavioral pattern continuity from prenatal to postnatal life—a study by four-dimensional (4D) ultrasonography. J Perinat Med. 2004;32(4):346-53.

28. Andonotopo W, Kurjak A, Kosuta MI. Behavior of an anencephalic fetus studied by 4D sonography. J Matern Fetal Neonatal Med. 2005;17(2):165-8.

29. Andonopo W, Kurjak A. The assessment of fetal behavior of growth restricted fetuses by 4D sonography. J Perinat Med. 2006;34(6):471-8.

30. Kurjak A, Andonotopo W, Hafner T, Salihagic-Kadic A, Stanojevic M, Azumendi G, et al. Normal standards for fetal neurobehavioral developments—longitudinal quantification by four-dimensional sonography. J Perinat Med. 2006;34(1):56-65.

31. Kurjak A, Azumendi G, Andonotopo W, Salihagic-Kadic A. Three- and four-dimensional ultrasonography for the structural and functional evaluation of the fetal face. Am J Obstet Gynecol. 2007;196(1):16-28.

32. Walusinski O, Kurjak A, Andonotopo W, Azumendi G. Fetal yawning assessed by 3D and 4D sonography. Ultrasound Rev Obstet Gynecol. 2005;5:210-7.

33. Rosenbaum P, Paneth N, Leviton A, Goldstein M, Bax M, Damiano D, et al. A report: the definition and classification of cerebral palsy April 2006. Dev Med Child Neurol Suppl. 2007;109:8-14.

34. Palmer FB. Strategies for the early diagnosis of cerebral palsy. J Pediatr. 2004;145(2 Suppl): S8-S11.

35. Walstab JE, Bell RJ, Reddihough DS, Brennecke SP, Bessell CK, Beischer NA. Factors identified during the neonatal period associated with risk of cerebral palsy. Aust N Z J Obstet Gynecol. 2004;44(4):342-6.

36. Nelson KB, Ellenberg JH. Neonatal signs as predictors of cerebral palsy. Pediatrics. 1979;64(2):225-32.

37. Amiel-Tison C, Gosselin J, Kurjak A. Neurosonography in the second half of fetal life: a neonatologist's point of view. J Perinat Med. 2006;34(6):437-46.

38. Gosselin J, Gahagan S, Amiel-Tison C. The Amiel-Tison Neurological Assessment at Term: conceptual and methodological continuity in the course of follow-up. Ment Retard Dev Disabil Res Rev. 2005;11(1):34-51.

39. Amiel-Tison C. Update of the Amiel-Tison neurologic assessment for the term neonate or at 40 weeks corrected age. Pediatr Neurol. 2002;27(3):196-212.

40. Volpe JJ. Neurological examination: Normal and abnormal features. In: Volpe JJ (Ed). Neurology of the Newborn, 4th edition. Philadelphia: WB Saunders; 2001. p. 127.

41. Einspieler C, Prechtl HFR, Bos AF, Ferrari F, Cioni G. Prechtl's Method on the qualitative assessment of general movements in preterm, term and young infants. Mac Keith Press: Cambridge; 2004. p. 104.

42. Hadders-Algra M. General movements: a window for early identification of children at high risk for developmental disorders. J Pediatr. 2004;145(2 Suppl):S12-8.

43. Hadders-Algra M, den Niewcendijk A KV, Martijn A, van Eyken LA. Assessment of general movements: towards a better understanding of a sensitive method to evaluate brain function in young infants. Dev Med Child Neurol. 1997;39(2):89-98.

44. Bekedam DJ, Visser GH, de Vries JJ, Prechtl HF. Motor behavior in the growth retarded fetus. Early Hum Dev. 1985;12(2):155-65.

45. Cioni G, Prechtl HF. Preterm and early postterm motor behavior in low-risk premature infants. Early Hum Dev. 1990;23(3):159-91.

46. Seme-Ciglenečki P. Predictive value of assessment of general movements for neurological development of high-risk preterm infants: comparative study. Croat Med J. 2003;44(6):721-7.

47. Cioni G, Prechtl HF, Ferrari F, Paolicelli PB, Einspieler C, Roversi MF. Which better predicts later outcome in full-term infants: quality of general movements or

neurological examination? Early Hum Dev. 1997;50(1):71-85.

48. Einspieler C, Prechtl HF, Ferrari F, Cioni G, Bos AF. The qualitative assessment of general movements in preterm, term and young infants—review of the methodology. Early Hum Dev. 1997;50(1):47-60.

49. Ferrari F, Cioni G, Einspieler C, Roversi MF, Bos AF, Paolicelli PB, et al. Cramped synchronized general movements in preterm infants as an early marker for cerebral palsy. Arch Pediatr Adolesc Med. 2002;156(5):460-7.

50. Prechtl HF. State of the art of a new functional assessment of the young nervous system. An early predictor of cerebral palsy. Early Hum Dev. 1997;50(1):1-11.

51. Kurjak A, Jackson D (Eds). An Atlas of Three- and Four-Dimensional Sonography in Obstetrics and Gynecology. London: Taylor & Francis Group; 2004. p. 216.

52. Sarnat HB. Anatomic and physiologic correlates of neurologic development in prematurity. In: Sarnat HB (Ed). Topics in Neonatal Neurology. New York: Grune and Stratton; 1984. pp. 1-24.

53. Sarnat HB. Functions of the corticospinal and corticobulbar tracts in the human newborns. J Pediatr Neurol. 2003;1(1):3-8.

54. Amiel-Tison C. Clinical assessment of the infant nervous system. In: Levente MI, Chervenak FA, Whittle M (Eds). Fetal and Neonatal Neurology and Neurosurgery, 3rd edition. London: Churchill Livingstone; 2001. pp. 99-120.

55. Salisbury AL, Fallone MD, Lester B. Neurobehavioral Assessment from Fetus to Infant: The NICU Network Neurobehavioral Scale and the Fetal Neurobehavioral Coding Scale. Ment Retard Dev Disabil Res Rev. 2005;11(1):14-20.

56. de Vries JIP, Visser GHA, Prechtl HFR. Fetal motility in the first half of pregnancy. In: Prechtl HFR (Ed). Continuity of Neural Functions from Prenatal to Postnatal Life. Oxford: Blackwell; 1984. pp. 46-63.

57. Kostović I, Seress L, Mrzljak L, Judaš M. Early onset of synapse formation in the human hippocampus: a correlation with Nissl-Golgi architectonics in 15- and 16.5-week-old fetuses. Neuroscience. 1989;30(1):105-16.

58. Mutch L, Alberman E, Hagberg B, Kodama K, Perat MV. Cerebral palsy epidemiology: where are we now and where are we going? Dev Med Child Neurol. 1992;34(6):547-51.

59. Bax M, Goldstein M, Rosenbaum P, Leviton A, Paneth N, Dan B, et al; Executive Committee for the Definition of Cerebral Palsy. Proposed definition and classification of cerebral palsy, April 2005. Dev Med Child Neurol. 2005;47(8):571-6.

60. Sankar C, Mundkur N. Cerebral palsy-definition, classification, etiology and early diagnosis. Indian J Pediatr. 2005;72(10):865-8.

61. Shapiro BK. Cerebral palsy: a reconceptualization of the spectrum. J Pediatr. 2004;145(2 Suppl):S3-7.

62. Amiel-Tison C, Gosselin J, Infante-Rivard C. Head growth and cranial assessment at neurological examination in infancy. Dev Med Child Neurol. 2002;44(9):643-8.

63. Pooh RK, Pooh K, Nakagawa Y, Nishida S, Ohno Y. Clinical application of three-dimensional ultrasound in fetal brain assessment. Croat Med J. 2000;41(3):245-51.

64. Campbell S, Lees C, Moscoso G, Hall P. Ultrasound antenatal diagnosis of cleft palate by a new technique: the 3D "reverse face" view. Ultrasound Obstet Gynecol. 2005;25(1):12-8.

65. DiPietro JA. Neurobehavioral assessment before birth. Ment Retard Dev Disabil Res Rev. 2005;11(1):4-13.

66. Yigiter AB, Kavak ZN. Normal standards of fetal behavior assessed by four-dimensional sonography. J Matern Fetal Neonatal Med. 2006;19(11):707-21.

67. Rees S, Harding R. Brain development during fetal life: influences of the intra-uterine environment. Neurosci Lett. 2004;361(1-3): 111-4.

68. Kurjak A, Carrera JM, Stanojevic M, Andonotopo W, Azumendi G, Scazzocchio E, et al. The role of 4D sonography in the neurological assessment of early human development. Ultrasound Rev Obstet Gynecol. 2004;4(3):148-59.

69. Eidelman AI. The living fetus—dilemmas in treatment at the edge of viability. In: Blazer S, Zimmer EZ (Eds). The Embryo: Scientific Discovery and Medical Ethics. Basel: Karger; 2005. p. 351e70.

70. Stanojevic M, Zaputovic S, Bosnjak AP. Continuity between fetal and neonatal neurobehavior. Semin Fetal Neonatal Med. 2012;17(6):324-9.

71. Haak P, Lenski M, Hidecker MJC, Li M, Paneth N. Cerebral palsy and aging. Dev Med Child Neurol. 2009;51 (Suppl 4):16-23.

72. Einspieler C, Prechtl HFR. Prechtl's assessment of general movements: a diagnostic tool for the functional assessment of the young nervous system. Ment Retard Dev Disabil Res Rev. 2005;11(1):61-7.

73. Moster D, Wilcox AJ, Vollset SE, Markestad T, Lie RT. Cerebral palsy among term and postterm births. JAMA. 2010;304(9):976-82.

74. Almli CR, Ball RH, Wheeler ME. Human fetal and neonatal movement patterns: Gender differences and fetal-to-neonatal continuity. Dev Psychobiol. 2001;38(4):252-73.

75. DiPietro JA, Bronstein MH, Costigan KA, Pressmen EK, Hahn CS, Painter K, et al. What does fetal movement predict about behavior during the first two years of life? Dev Phychobiol. 2002;40(4):358-71.

76. DiPetro JA, Hodson DM, Costigan KA, Johnson TR. Fetal antecedents of infant temperament. Child Dev. 1996;67(5):2568-83.

77. DiPietro JA, Costigan KA, Pressman EK. Fetal state concordance predicts infant state regulation. Early Hum Dev. 2002;68(1):1-13.

78. Thoman EB, Denenberg VH, Sievel J, Zeidner LP, Becker P. State organization in neonates: developmental inconsistency indicates risk for developmental dysfunction. Neuropediatrics. 1981;12(1):45-54.

79. St James-Roberts I, Menon-Johansson P. Predicting infant crying from fetal movement data: an exploratory study. Early Hum Dev. 1999;54(1):55-62.

80. de Vries JI, Visser GH, Prechtl HF. The emergence of fetal behavior. II. Quantitative aspects. Early Hum Dev. 1985;12(2):99-120.

81. de Vries JI, Visser GH, Prechtl HF. The emergence of fetal behavior. III. Individual differences and consistencies. Early Hum Dev. 1988;16(1):85-103.

82. Nijhuis JG (Ed). Fetal Behavior: Developmental and Perinatal Aspects. Oxford: Oxford University Press; 1992.

83. Kurjak A, Antsaklis P, Stanojevic M, Porovic S. Fetal behavior assessed by four-dimensional sonography. Donald School J Ultrasound Obstet Gynecol. 2017;11(2):146-168.

84. Stanojevic M, Talic A, Miskovic B, Vasilj O, Shaddad AN, Ahmed B, et al. An Attempt to Standardize Kurjak's Antenatal Neuro-developmental Test: Osaka Consensus Statement. DSJUOG. 2011;5(4):317-29.

85. Kurjak A, Antsaklis P. 4D in functional studies of the fetus. Donald School J Ultrasound Obstet Gynecol. 2019;13(1):23-33.

86. Kurjak A, Tikvica A, Stanojevic M, Miskovic B, Ahmed B, Azumendi G, et al. The assessment of fetal neurobehavior by three-dimensional and four-dimensional ultrasound. J Matern Fetal Neonatal Med. 2008;21(10):675-84.

87. Kurjak A, Miskovic B, Stanojevic M, Amiel-Tison C, Ahmed B, Azumendi G, et al. New scoring system for fetal neurobehavior assessed by three- and four-dimensional sonography. J Perinat Med. 2008;36(1):73-81.

88. Kurjak A, Luetic AT. Fetal neurobehavior assessed by three-dimensional/four-dimensional sonography. Zdr Varst. 2010;79(11):790-9.

89. Miskovic B, Vasilj O, Stanojevic M, Ivanković D, Kerner M, Tikvica A. The comparison of fetal behavior in high risk and normal pregnancies assessed by four-dimensional ultrasound. J Matern Fetal Neonatal Med. 2010;23(12):1461-7.

90. Talic A, Kurjak A, Ahmed B, Stanojevic M, Predojevic M, Salihagic-Kadic A, et al. The potential of 4D sonography in the assessment of fetal behavior in high-risk pregnancies. J Matern Fetal Neonatal Med. 2011;24(7):948-54.

91. Talic A, Kurjak A, Stanojevic M, Honemeyer U, Badreldeen A, DiRenzo GC. The assessment of fetal brain function in fetuses with ventriculomegaly: the role of the KANET test. J Matern Fetal Neonatal Med. 2012;25(8):1267-72.

92. Honemeyer U, Kurjak A. The use of KANET test to assess fetal CNS function. First 100 cases. 10th World Congress of Perinatal Medicine 8-11 November 2011. Uruguay: Poster Presentation. p. 209.

93. Lebit FD, Vladareanu R. The role of 4D ultrasound in the assessment of fetal behavior. Maedica (Bucur). 2011;6(2):120-7.

94. Abo-Yaqoub S, Kurjak A, Mohammed AB, Shadad A, Abdel-Maaboud M. The role of 4-D ultrasonography in prenatal assessment of fetal neurobehavior and prediction of neurological outcome. J Matern Fetal Neonatal Med. 2012;25(3):231-6.

95. Vladareanu R, Lebit D, Constantinescu S. Ultrasound assessment of fetal neurobehavior in high-risk pregnancies. DSJUOG. 2012;6(2):132-47.

96. Honemeyer U, Talic A, Therwat A, Paulose L, Patidar R. The clinical value of KANET in studying fetal neurobehavior in normal and at-risk pregnancies. J Perinat Med. 2013;41(2):187-97.

97. Kurjak A, Talic A, Honemeyer U, Stanojevic M, Zalud I. Comparison between antenatal neurodevelopmental test and fetal Doppler in the assessment of fetal wellbeing. J Perinat Med. 2013;41(1):107-14.

98. Predojević M, Talić A, Stanojević M, Kurjak A, Salihagić-Kadić A. Assessment of motoric and hemodynamic parameters in growth restricted fetuses—case study. J Matern Fetal Neonatal Med. 2014;27(3):247-51.

99. Athanasiadis AP, Mikos T, Tambakoudis GP, Theodoridis TD, Papastergiou M, Assimakopoulos E, et al. Neurodevelopmental fetal assessment using KANET scoring system in low and high risk pregnancies. J Matern Fetal Neonatal Med. 2013;26(4):363-8.

100. Neto RM, Kurjak A. Recent results of the clinical application of KANET test. DSJUOG 2015 Oct-Dec;9(20):420-425. 78.

101. Neto RM. KANET in Brazil: first experience. Donald School J Ultrasound Obstet Gynecol 2015 Jan-Mar;9(1):1-5.

102. Hanaoka U, Hata T, Kananishi K, Mostafa AboEllail MA, Uematsu R, et al. Does ethnicity have an effect on fetal behavior? A comparison of Asian and Caucasian populations. J Perinat Med 2016 Mar;44(2):217-221. 79.

103. Antsaklis P, Porovic S, Daskalakis G, Kurjak A. 4D assessment of fetal brain function in diabetic patients. J Perinat Med. 2017;45(6):711-5.

104. Pooh RK, Pooh K. Assessment of fetal central nervous system. Donald School J Ultrasound Obstet Gynecol 2013;7(4):369-84.

105. Kurjak A, Ahmed B, Abo-Yaquab S, Younis M, Saleh H, Shaddad AN, et al. An attempt to introduce neurological test for fetus based on 3D and 4D sonography. DSJUOG. 2008;2(4):29-44.

106. Kuno A, Akiyama M, Yamashiro C, Tanaka H, Yanagihara T, Hata T. Three-dimensional sonographic assessment of fetal behavior in the early second trimester of pregnancy. J Ultrasound Med. 2001;20(12):1271-5.

107. Koyanagi T, Horimoto N, Maeda H, Kukita J, Minami T, Ueda K, et al. Abnormal behavioral patterns in the human fetus at term: correlation with lesion sites in the central nervous system after birth. J Child Neurol. 1993;8(1):19-26.

108. Kurjak A, Abo-Yaqoub S, Stanojevic M, Yigiter AB, Vasilj O, Lebit D, et al. The potential of 4D sonography in the assessment of fetal neurobehavior—multicentric study in high-risk pregnancies. J Perinat Med. 2010;38(1):77-82.

109. Stanojevic M, Antsaklis P, Panchal S, Porovic S, Salihagic-Kadic A, Barisic LS, et al. A critical appraisal of Kurjak Antenatal Neurodevelopmental Test: five years of wide clinical use. DSJUOG. 2021;14(4):304-10.

110. Hepper PG. Fetal behavior: who so sceptical? Ultrasound Obstet Gynecol. 1996:8(3):145-8.

111. Greenwood C, Newman S, Impey L, Johnson A. Cerebral palsy and clinical negligence litigation: a cohort study. BJOG. 2003;110(1): 6-11.

112. Strijbis EMM, Oudman I, van Essen P, MacLennan AH. Cerebral palsy and the application of the international criteria for acute intrapartum hypoxia. Obstet Gynecol. 2006;107(6):1357-65.

113. de Vries JIP, Fong BF. Changes in fetal motility as a result of congenital disorders: an overview. Ultrasound Obstet Gynecol. 2007;29(5):590-9.

114. de Vries JIP, Fong BF. Normal fetal motility: an overview. Ultrasound Obstet Gynecol. 2006;27(6):701-11.

115. Rosier-van Dunné FM, van Wezel-Meijler G, Bakker MP, de Groot L, Odendaal HJ, de Vries JI. General movements in the perinatal period and its relation to echogenicity changes in the brain. Early Hum Dev. 2010;86(2):83-6.

116. te Velde A, Morgan C, Novak I, Tantsis E, Badawi N. Early diagnosis and classification of cerebral palsy: an historical perspective and barriers to an early diagnosis. J Clin Med. 2019;8(10):1599.

117. Novak I, Morgan C, Adde L, Blackman J, Boyd RN, Brunstrom-Hernandez J, et al. Early, accurate diagnosis and early intervention in cerebral palsy: advances in diagnosis and treatment. JAMA Pediatr. 2017; 171(9):897-907.

118. Romeo DMM, Cioni M, Palermo F, Cilauro S, Romeo MG. Neurological assessment in infants discharged from a neonatal intensive care unit. Eur J Pediatr Neurol. 2013;17(2):192-8.

119. Kwong AK, Eeles AL, Olsen JE, Cheong JL, Doyle LW, Spittle AJ. The Baby Moves smartphone app for General Movements Assessment: Engagement amongst extremely preterm and term-born infants in a statewide geographical study. J Pediatr Child Health. 2019;55(5):548-54.

Morphological Approach to Cortical Formations

Ritsuko K Pooh

■ INTRODUCTION

The central nervous system (CNS) changes its morphology surprisingly from the time of embryonic development. In this rapid developmental change, various developmental disorders and events occur, resulting in different phenotypes of neurological deficits. Brain abnormalities occur due to disorders at each stage of changing neurodevelopment. The first stage is neurulation, which includes primary and secondary neurulation, followed by prosencephalic development. During the growth phase of neurons, more than twice as many of the 100 billion neurons inside the adult brain as the final active neurons are produced in the first and early second trimesters. The peak proliferation of neurons is third to fourth gestational month, and neurons are produced mainly in the ventricular zone (VZ) and subventricular zone (SVZ). The neurons then differentiate and travel to their final destination. After neuronal migration, organization and myelination occur and last even after birth. On the other hand, apoptosis (programed cell death) regulates the number of nerve cells **(Fig. 1 and Table 1)**.

During the developmental stage, the cerebral cortex is dramatically formed. The mature cerebral cortex has a layered structure consisting of six layers of nerve cells

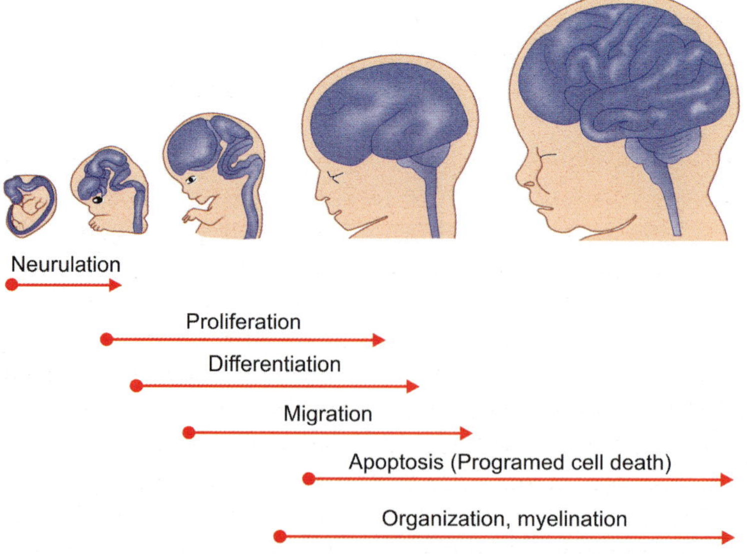

Fig. 1: The developmental stage of the developing nervous system.

TABLE 1: Representative disorders in each development stage.

Developmental stage	Representative cerebral disorders
Neurulation (3–4 weeks' gestation)	Cranial and spinal dysraphism (craniorachischisis totalis, anencephaly, encephalocele, myelomeningocele, myeloschisis)
Prosencephalic development (2–3 months' gestation)	Holoprosencephaly, the corpus callosum agenesis, the septum pellucidum agenesis
Neuronal proliferation (3–4 months' gestation)	Macrencephaly, micrencephaly
Neuronal migration (3–5 months' gestation)	Lissencephaly, pachygyria, focal cortical dysplasia, heterotopias (band heterotopias and periventricular nodular heterotopia), polymicrogyria, schizencephaly
Organization (5 months' gestation—years postnatal)	Mental retardation (idiopathic), learning disability, link to epilepsy and autism
Myelination (Birth—years postnatal)	Range of disorders including adrenoleukodystrophy

with different morphologies and functions. Still, these cells are not born in that place from the beginning. Still, the VZ facing the lateral ventricle (a proliferative layer called the VZ), neurons generated as a result of final division from neural progenitor cells migrate hundreds of times their cell length and reach the position of the cerebral cortex defined by a genetic program, and build a tightly controlled six-layer structure. Neurons start migrating from the VZ and SVZ, stay in the lower layer in the SP for early-born cells, and reach the upper layer in the cortical plate (CP) for late-born cells. This is called the "inside-out" principle. Excitatory neurons that make up the cerebral cortex undergo final division from neural stem cells or neural progenitor cells distributed in the VZ and SVZ during development and migrate radially toward the cortical surface and form a CP. SP neurons are born before these CP neurons, but their types and origins are not uniform. Neurons are roughly divided into excitatory and inhibitory, and the source of excitatory neurons includes the VZ and the rostral medial telencephalic wall. These excitatory neurons are born before CP neurons and form preplates with Cajal–Retzius cells located in the future marginal zone. In addition to these, some gamma-aminobutyric acid (GABAergic) inhibitory neurons born in the basal ganglionic eminence migrated tangentially and placed on the SP, as shown in **Figure 2**.

It is hard to depict cortical development and its disorder by ultrasonography during the fetal period. The phenotype of cortical development does not appear until 8 months of gestation when gyrus/sulcus formation becomes apparent. Early detection of impaired cell migration and cortical maldevelopment is a challenge in the field of prenatal fetal neuroimaging. The author believes that some sonographic features in the middle of gestation can predict future cortical maldevelopment. In this chapter, the author explains how cortical maldevelopment can be demonstrated by sonographic neuroimaging in an easy-to-understand manner.

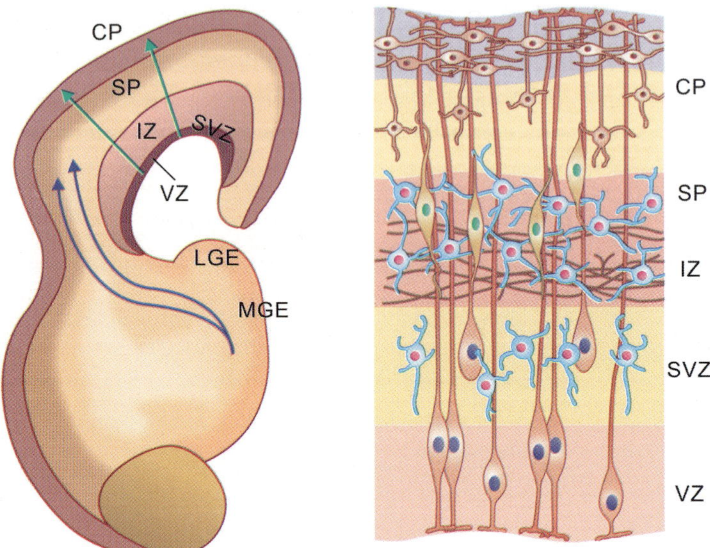

Fig. 2: Schematic illustration of neuronal cell migration. Neurons that have started migrating from the ventricular zone (VZ) stay in the lower layer in the cortical plate (CP) for early-born cells and reach the upper layer in the CP for late-born cells. This is called the "inside-out" principle. Excitatory neurons that make up the cerebral cortex undergo final division from neural stem cells or neural progenitor cells distributed in VZ/subventricular zone (SVZ) during development. They migrate radially toward the surface (green arrows) to form a CP. Subplate (SP) neurons are born before these CP neurons, but their types and origins are not uniform. Neurons are roughly divided into excitatory and inhibitory, and the origin of excitatory neurons includes the VZ and the rostral medial telencephalic wall. These excitatory neurons are born before CP neurons and form preplates with Cajal–Retzius cells located in the future marginal zone. In addition to these, some GABAergic inhibitory neurons born in the basal ganglionic eminence [lateral ganglionic eminence (LGE), medial ganglionic eminence (MGE)] migrated tangentially and placed on the SP (blue arrows). Intermediate zone (IZ) is between SVZ and SP.

◾ MALFORMATIONS OF CORTICAL DEVELOPMENT

Malformations of cortical development (MCD) are cortical disorders resulted from various causes such as single-gene mutations, fetal infections, vascular abnormalities, or metabolic abnormalities. MCD is associated with abnormal cortical structure, ectopic gray matter, odd brain size (microcephaly and macrocephaly).[1-3] MCD can cause severe morbidity at any age, with symptoms such as developmental delay, epilepsy, cerebral palsy, and intellectual disability. It is estimated that about half of drug-resistant epilepsy is caused by MCD.[4] The definitive diagnosis of MCD has been based on neuropathological evidence, and in practice, the clinical diagnosis will be based on neuroimaging findings. The relevant clinical phenotype and genetic results are significant. Despite the many literature reports related to MCD, the definition and classification of MCD are not clear cut, and the category of MCD can constantly be changing and becoming more difficult based on new genetic findings. The high pattern-specificity based on neuroimaging enables more targeted testing and discovery of new genotype-phenotype correlations, which may improve diagnostic rates. MCD results from disorders of one or more combined developmental steps. Developmental steps include neuronal proliferation, neuronal cell migration, organization, and neuronal maturation.[3,5,6]

Table 2 lists the details of MCDs in the three developmental phases. More than 100 genes were identified, being responsible for MCD. However, because MCD-related genes are involved in multiple developmental stages, it has been assumed that the tissues of proliferation, migration, and postmigration are genetically and functionally interdependent; it has turned out that it is challenging to classify MCDs into these three groups.[5,7]

■ PROLIFERATION DISORDERS

Microcephaly

Microcephaly is defined when a frontal occipital circumference (OFC) is below −2.0 standard deviations (SD).[8,9] An OFC of −2.0 to −3.0 SD is considered mild microcephaly.[9] The term "microcephaly" refers to a small head, but micrencephaly clinically indicates a small brain volume. Genetic disorders or in utero insults result in microbrain and microcephaly.[1] Therefore, microcephaly and micrencephaly are used interchangeably. Mutated genes responsible for microcephaly are microcephalin (*MCPH1*[10-13]), *ASPM*,[14] *CDK5RAP2*,[6,15] *CENPJ*,[6,15] *STIL*,[16] *WDR62*,[5,6,14,17] and *CEP152*[3,8] and others.

Prenatal images of cases with microcephaly are shown in **Figures 3A to F**. It is often quite difficult to observe brain structure by neurosonography in microcephalic fetuses due to narrow cranial fontanels and sutures, as shown in **Figure 3B**. Therefore, transfontanel neurosonography is often tricky.

Macrocephaly and Brain Overgrowth Spectrum

Macrocephaly is defined when an OFC +2.0 SD and over, and 2.0–3.0 SD is mild

macrocephaly. Macrocephaly has various causes, including ventriculomegaly, hydrocephalus ex vacuo, or several types of skeletal dysplasia.[18,19] In megalencephalic cases, brain overgrowth is bilateral, unilateral, or localized. Therefore, cases of megalencephaly do not always present with macrocephaly. Megalencephaly is a consequence of disrupted signaling pathways that regulate nerve cell proliferation, differentiation, cell cycle regulation, or survival, inborn metabolic errors, and leukodystrophy.[20-24] Megalencephaly is recognized as a spectrum of the impaired proliferation of the brain.[18,21,23,24] Complete hemimegalencephaly involving the entire hemisphere is synonymous with a classic hemimegalencephaly. Localized megalencephaly is primarily caused by somatic mosaic mutations affecting the focal brain area.[5] **Figures 4A and B** show the case of hemimegalencephaly due to somatic mutation of *AKT1*, with cortical maldevelopment, at 21 weeks of gestation.

Focal Cortical Dysplasia

The term "focal cortical dysplasia" (FCD) is defined as a spectrum of localized brain malformations characterized by disturbed cortical stacking, with or without abnormal neuron types. Magnetic resonance imaging (MRI) more easily demonstrates type II (a and b) FCDs and the presence of morphologically abnormal cell types, especially atypical neurons characterized by irregular shapes. It is characterized by significant destruction of the cortical layer. FCD type IIa has only atypical neurons, and FCD type IIb has atypical neurons and balloon cells.[22] Recent studies have reported that type II FCD has germline, somatic, or germline combined with somatic "two-hit" mutated genes relating to the mechanistic target of rapamycin (mTOR) pathway.[5,21] The tubers of

TABLE 2: Classification of malformations of cortical development.

Group	MCD type	Associated genes	Associated pathways and etiology	Imaging findings
Group I: Malformations secondary to abnormal cell *proliferation or apoptosis*	Microcephaly	*MCPH1, CENPJ, CDK5RAP2, WDR62, NDE1, ASPM, TUBA1A, TUBB2B, TUBB3, TUBGI, LIS1, DCX, DYNC1H, K1F5C*	Neurogenesis and cell replication, tubulin, and microtubule-associated proteins (MAP)	Small head size, small cerebellum, and pons and lissencephaly (with tubulin and MAP-associated genes)
	Megalencephaly spectrum	*AKT3, P1K3CA,* and *P1K3R2*	mTOR	Focal (localized), hemispheric or diffuse cortical enlargement, cerebellum and deep gray nuclei also enlarged, gray/white boundary blurring
	Focal cortical dysplasias (FCDs) type IIa	*MTOR, DEPDCS,* and *P1K3CA*	mTOR	Gray/white matter blurring with apparent cortical thickness
	Focal cortical dysplasias (FCDs) type IIb	*MTOR, DEPDC5, NPRL3*	mTOR	Cortical/sulcal T2 hyperintensity may extend to ventricular surface (transmantle sign)
Group II: Malformations secondary to *abnormal cell migration*	Tubulinopathies	*TUBA1A, TUBB2B, TUBB3. TUBG1, LIS1, DCX, DYNC1H, KIF5C, NDE1*	Microtubule structure and function	Microcephaly, lissencephaly, fused basal ganglia (BG), cortical dysgyria, callosal abnormalities, asymmetric brainstem, and small cerebellar vermis
	Variant lissencephalies	*ARX, DCX, RELN* and *VLDR*	Reelin	*ARX*—lissencephaly, callosal abnormalities, dysmorphic BG, hydrancephaly; *Reelin*—lissencephaly in anterior-posterior gradient, cortical thickening, small cerebellum, and vermis
	Gray matter heterotopia	*FLNA* and *ARFGEF2*	Neuroependyma/ neuroepithelium	Normal gray matter in abnormal locations
	Cobblestone malformations	*GPR56, LAMB1, LAMB2, LAMC3,* and *SRD5A3 Fukutin, POMGNT1*	Dystroglycanopathies affecting pial limiting membrane	Lissencephaly/pachygyria or polymicrogyria (PMG), possible cerebellar involvement, Fukuyama syndrome, muscle-eye-brain disease (MEB), Walker–Warburg syndrome, also called HARD(E) syndrome
Group III: Malformations secondary to *abnormal postmigrational development*	Polymicrogyria (PMG)	*lp36.3* and *22q11.2* mutations. *mTOR* genes	Etiology can be from prenatal ischemic, teratogenic or infectious brain injury	Perisylvian bilateral PMG (most common), associated with schizencephaly

(MCD: malformations of cortical development; mTOR: mechanistic target of rapamycin)
Source: Modified with permission from Desikan and Barkovich.[6]

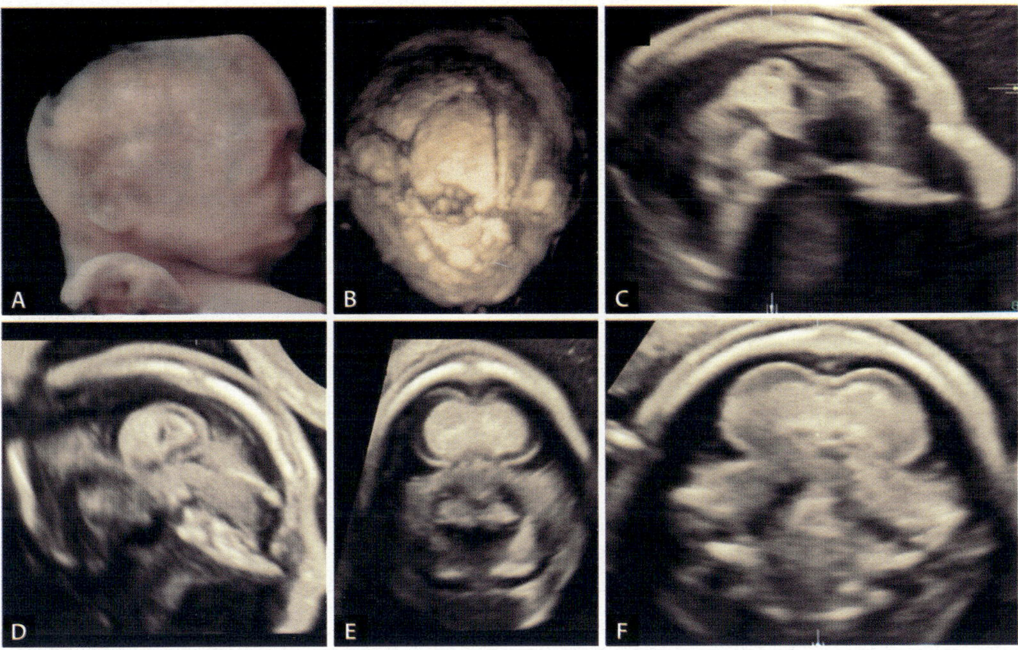

Figs. 3A to F: Microcephaly at 18 weeks of gestation. (A) Three-dimensional (3D) reconstructed image of fetal craniofacial appearance; (B) 3D image of craniofacial skeletal appearance. Note the narrow cranial sutures and fontanels because of microcephaly. In cases with microcephaly, transfontanel ultrasound becomes difficult because of narrow ultrasound windows; (C and D) Mid-sagittal and parasagittal sections demonstrating microbrain; (E and F) Coronal cutting sections of microbrain. Note the premature brain with prosencephalic and proliferation disorder.

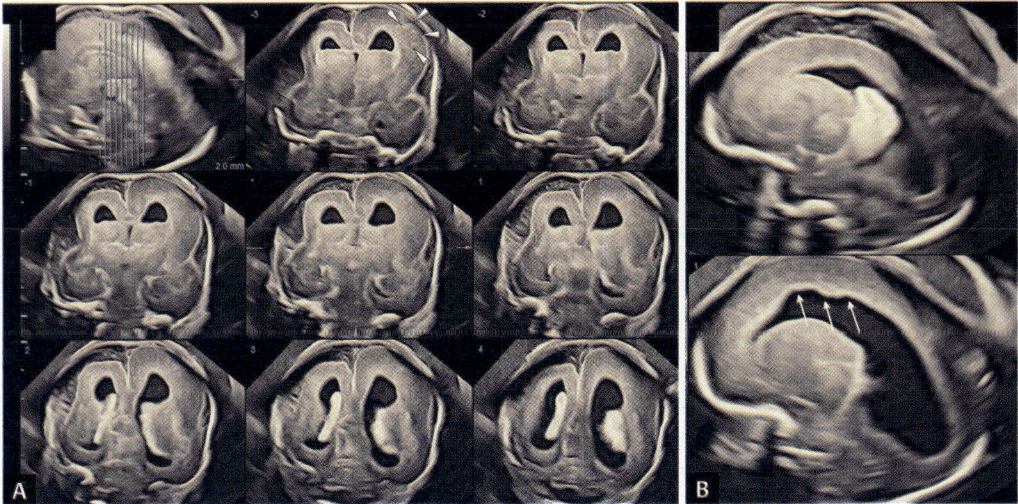

Figs. 4A and B: Neurosonographic images of hemimegalencephaly at 21 weeks of gestation. (A) Tomographic ultrasound image in the coronal section. Note a significant difference in cerebral size between the right and left hemispheres. The irregular border between SP and IZ (arrowheads); (B) Tomographic ultrasound image in the sagittal section. Note the irregular ventricular wall with hyperechogenicity of the ventricular/SVZs (arrows). In this case, the causal genetic factor was a somatic mutation of the *AKT1* gene.

the tuberous sclerosis complex (TSC) is considered as a subtype of type IIb FCD since histological findings and imaging are similar. It is considered for both to share the etiology of the mTOR pathway relating genes, *TSC1* and *TSC2*.[23]

■ MIGRATION DISORDERS

In the cerebral cortex, neurons are arranged in order, and a six-layered structure is formed. About 70–80% are excitatory neurons. They are produced in the VZ, which is facing the ventricle of the extravasation or in the SVZ, and travel toward the brain surface to their final destination by radial migration, as shown in **Figure 2**. Cortical neurons are produced in very early gestation. A CP is located between a marginal zone and an SP. CP neurons subsequently move sequentially toward the brain surface. They start to migrate and overtake nerves that have already finished to progress and reach just below the marginal zone and finish their movement. In the cerebral cortex, early-bone neurons are placed closer to the brain's inner side, and late-bone neurons are placed on the surface side (inside out). The CP becomes gray matter after birth.

As a result of neuronal cell migration, the brain matured with gyri and sulci from the second half of the 7th month of gestation. The fastest increase in the number of significant gyri occurs between 26 and 28 weeks. This additional gyral formation continues in the third trimester and after birth. Migration is controlled by a complex combination of chemical guides and signals. If these signals are absent or incorrect, neurons cannot reach where they should be. This can result in structurally abnormal or defective areas of any part of brain structure, such as the cerebri, cerebellum, brainstem, or hippocampus. Migration disorders include lissencephaly, pachygyria, agyria, micropolygyria, microgyria, band heterotopia, and periventricular nodular heterotopia. Neuronal migration disorder cause seizures and neurological deficits from the early period after birth. Gyri and sulci appear conspicuously in late gestation. Therefore, it seems to be impossible to detect migration disorder before the appearance of gyri. Toi et al.[24] reported a regular gyrus pattern, depicted by transabdominal sonography. During the latter half of the second trimester, the cortical structure macroscopically develops, and the most distinct morphological difference appears to be the different structures of Sylvian fissure. Thus, the Sylvian fissure is a landmark indicating cortical development by regular migration. According to cerebral development, changing the appearance of Sylvian fissure is well recognizable, and Poon et al.[25] proposed the Sylvian fissure angle (SFA) by three-dimensional (3D) transvaginal neurosonography and described the significant SFA decrease with gestation. Further, Pooh et al.[26] showed 22 cases with MCDs between 18 and 30 weeks of gestation and the delayed development of Sylvian fissure, as shown in **Figures 5A to F**.

Lissencephaly

The literal meaning of lissencephaly is a "smooth head" and is usually caused by neuronal migration disorders.[27] The characteristic features are a thickened cortex and a gyral/sulcal abnormality ranging from absent gyration (agyria) to reduced gyration (oligogyria). Conventionally lissencephaly was classified into two types: type I with a smooth brain surface and type II with a cobblestone appearance. After that, many responsible genes were identified, and classification has been changed by etiology, as given in **Table 3**. However, due to recent

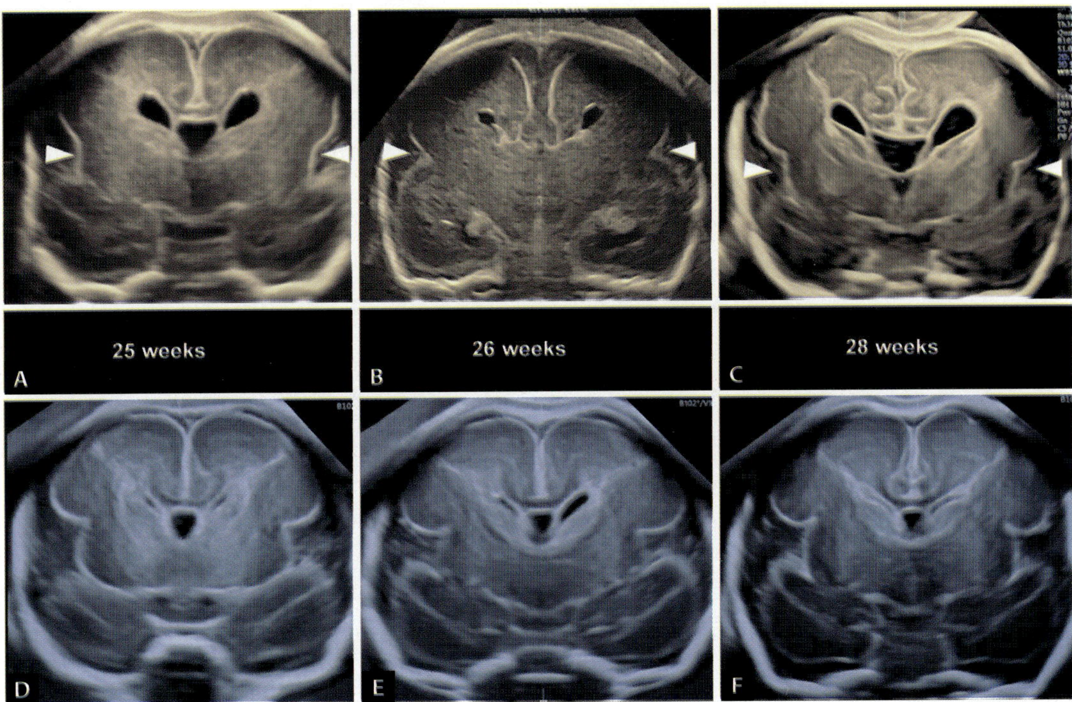

Figs. 5A to F: Abnormal Sylvian fissure development in cases of malformations of cortical development (upper figures), compared to normal cases (lower figures). (A) 25 weeks of gestation. Arrowheads indicate abnormal Sylvian fissures; (B) 26 weeks of gestation. The brain with abnormal Sylvian fissures (arrowheads) as well as agenesis of the corpus callosum; (C) 28 weeks of gestation; (D to F) are normal comparative images with matched gestational age to (A to C) respectively.

TABLE 3: Classification of lissencephaly.	
Category	*Types*
Classic lissencephaly	• *LIS1*[29-31] (17p13.3): *PAFAH1B1*[32] gene mutation Miller–Dieker syndrome • *DCX:*[5,6,31-33] Doublecortin mutation • Isolated lissencephaly
Cobblestone lissencephaly	• *POMGNT1:*[34-39] Muscle-eye-brain disease (MEB), Walker–Warburg syndrome • Fukutin:[37,39-41] Fukuyama disease
X-linked lissencephaly	• *ARX*[2,6,38] gene (Xq22.13) mutation
Lissencephaly with cerebellar hypoplasia	*Reelin* gene[3,42,43] (7q22.1): Norman–Roberts syndrome
Microlissencephaly	Lissencephaly associated with microcephaly

rapid genetic progress, a conventional category becomes insufficient to distinguish various lissencephaly. A new imaging-based classification system was proposed in 2017 to predict likely causative gene mutation.[28]

There are some publications reported on prenatal detection of lissencephaly.[17,41,44,45] It is quite difficult to reliably diagnose lissencephaly by the 26th–28th weeks of gestation in families with no history of affected siblings.

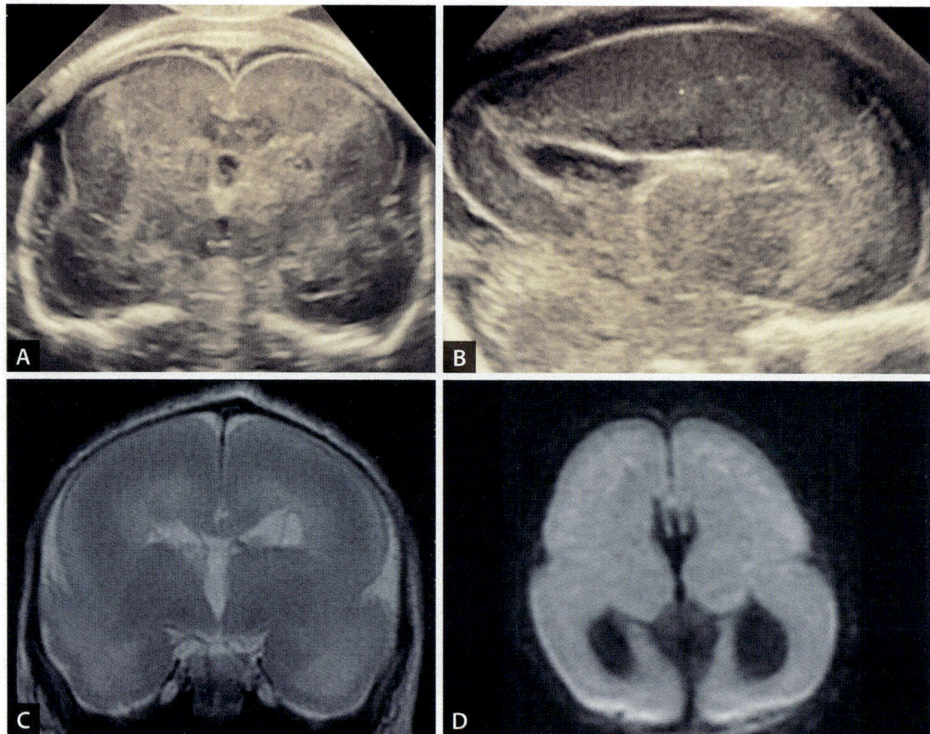

Figs. 6A to D: Microlissencephaly case at 25 and 30 weeks of gestation. (A) Coronal brain image at 25 weeks of gestation. Note the abnormal Sylvian fissure development compared to Figure D; (B) Parasagittal section image at 30 weeks of gestation, (C and D) Postnatal magnetic resonance images demonstrate an extremely pathological cortex. In this case, migration disorder was strongly suspected from 19 weeks of gestation, and a genetic examination revealed *TUBA1A* gene mutation.

However, recently, around 20 weeks of gestation, it has become possible to predict developmental brain abnormalities from abnormal patterns of brain morphology.[32] **Figures 6A to D** show ultrasound images of the microlissencephaly at 25 and 30 weeks gestation. In this example, abnormal brain morphology became noticeable from around the 20th week of pregnancy.

■ POSTMIGRATIONAL DISORDERS

Polymicrogyria

Polymicrogyria refers to the excessive presence of abnormally small gyrus.[46] The anatomical distribution of polymicrogyria can be localized, multiple, or diffuse. It can be unilateral or bilateral, and it can be bilaterally symmetric or bilaterally asymmetric.[47] Polymicrogyria is a heterogeneous cortical malformation due to genetic or nongenetic factors. The genetic causes include chromosomal microdeletions such as, 22q11 deletion and 1p36 monosomy, and mutated genes[17,46,48-53] such as, *COL4A1, COL4A2, RTTN, OCLN,* and *GRIN1.*[53] Nongenetic causes of polymicrogyria are in utero cytomegalovirus or Zika viral infection, trauma, teratogen exposure, ischemic infarction, twin-to-twin transfusion syndrome, and intrauterine fetal death (IUFD) of monochorionic twin.[1] Although any part of the cerebral cortex can be affected,[48,53] the most common location for polymicrogyria is in the area containing the Sylvian fissures in approximately 60–70% of cases.

Schizencephaly

Classically schizencephaly refers to a cleft lined by gray matter with polymicrogyria and heterotopia extending from ependyma to pial surface, and it is called a "pial ependymal seam".[1,49] The cause of schizencephaly may be an early focal insult of the germinal matrix or may result from insults in the immature cerebrum.[49] When the cleft is open, and the cerebrospinal fluid space is connected, it is called open-lip type, and when it is blocked by the marginal cortical layer, it is called closed-lip type.[50] Neuroimaging differentiation of schizencephaly from porencephaly is occasionally difficult but based on whether the cleft is lined by gray matter, not white matter with gliosis.[1]

Schizencephaly occurs unilaterally in 63% and bilatcrally 37%. Possiblc causal factors arc vascular disruption during early development, genetic factors, including *WDR62* gene mutation, which causes microcephaly and schizencephaly in some cases.[17,51] This fact indicates that there is a relation between the proliferation phase and the genesis of schizencephaly. *COL4A1* gene mutation is associated with schizencephaly as well as porencephaly after cerebral hemorrhage.[52-54] **Figures 7A to D** show neuroimages of schizencephaly at 25 and 27 weeks of gestation.

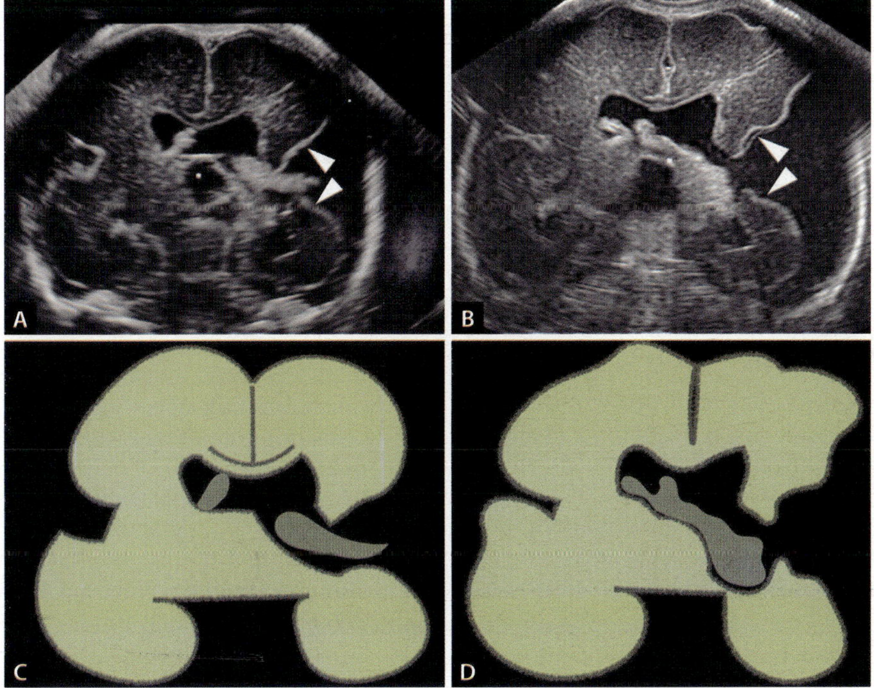

Figs. 7A to D: Schizencephaly at 25 and 27 weeks of gestation. (A) Coronal section of the fetal brain at 25 weeks. Arrowheads indicate congenital lined by gray matter, with communication between the subarachnoid space and ventricle. The choroid plexus (hyperechoic part) exists from intraventricular space to subarachnoid space; (B) Coronal section image at 27 weeks; (C) Illustration of Figure A; (D) Illustration of Figure B.

■ FUTURE PERSPECTIVE

Malformations of cortical developments are a significant cause of childhood epilepsy and frequently associate with cognitive deficits and behavioral alterations. Epileptogenicity of MCD determines the behavior and function of the brain and is characterized by many molecular, cellular, and structural changes that affect epileptic processes and epilepsy expression during early brain development. That is, it occurs during the fetal period. Fetal neuroimaging diagnosis of MCDs has not been established. However, as described and shown in this chapter, longitudinal neuroimaging throughout the embryological and fetal period, combined with the precise genetic investigation, fetal MCD has been diagnosed due to the development of neuroimaging and the remarkable development of the next-generation sequencing. Perhaps shortly, fetal MCD diagnosis will be possible more accurately and earlier. The combination of molecular genetics and detailed neuro-imaging has established "Neurosonogenetics", a new multidisciplinary field, for proper management, care, prevention, and treatment in the fetal and pediatric neurology.[55]

■ REFERENCES

1. Raybaud C, Widjaja E. Development and dysgenesis of the cerebral cortex: malformations of cortical development. Neuroimaging Clin N Am. 2011;21(3):483-543.
2. Guerrini R, Dobyns WB. Malformations of cortical development: clinical features and genetic causes. Lancet Neurol. 2014;13(7): 710-26.
3. Barkovich AJ, Guerrini R, Kuzniecky RI, Jackson GD, Dobyns WB. A developmental and genetic classification for malformations of cortical development: update 2012. Brain. 2012;135(5):1348-69.
4. Pasquier B, Péoc'h M, Fabre-Bocquentin B, Bensaadi L, Pasquier D, Hoffmann D, et al. Surgical pathology of drug-resistant partial epilepsy. A 10-year-experience with a series of 327 consecutive resections. Epileptic Disord. 2002;4(2):99-119.
5. Severino M, Geraldo AF, Utz N, Tortora D, Pogledic I, Klonowski W, et al. Definitions and classification of malformations of cortical development: practical guidelines. Brain. 2020;143(10):2874-94.
6. Desikan RS, Barkovich AJ. Malformations of cortical development. Ann Neurol. 2016;80(6):797-810.
7. Barkovich J. Complication begets clarification in classification. Brain. 2013;136(2):368-73.
8. Woods CG, Parker A. Investigating micro-cephaly. Arch Dis Child. 2013;98(9):707-13.
9. Ashwal S, Michelson D, Plawner L, Dobyns WB; Quality Standards Subcommittee of the American Academy of Neurology and the Practice Committee of the Child Neurology Society. Practice Parameter : Evaluation of the child with microcephaly (an evidence-based review): report of the Quality Standards Subcommittee of the American Academy of Neurology and the Practice Committee of the Child Neurology Society. Neurology. 2009;73(11):887-97.
10. Guernsey DL, Jiang H, Hussin J, Arnold M, Bouyakdan K, Perry S, et al. Mutations in centrosomal protein CEP152 in primary microcephaly families linked to MCPH4. Am J Hum Genet. 2010;87(1):40-51.
11. Manzini MC, Walsh CA. The genetics of brain malformations. In: Mitchell KJ (Ed). The Genetics of Neurodevelopmental Disorders. Hoboken, New Jersey: John Wiley & Sons, Inc; 2015.
12. Brunk K, Vernay B, Griffith E, Reynolds NL, Strutt D, Ingham PW, et al. Micro-cephalin coordinates mitosis in the syncytial Drosophila embryo. J Cell Sci. 2007;120(20): 3578-88.
13. Trimborn M, Bell SM, Felix C, Rashid Y, Jafri H, Griffiths PD, et al. Mutations in microcephalin cause aberrant regulation of chromosome condensation. Am J Hum Genet. 2004;75(2):261-6.
14. Edwards TJ, Sherr EH, Barkovich AJ, Richards LJ. Clinical, genetic and imaging

findings identify new causes for corpus callosum development syndromes. Brain. 2014;137(6):1579-613.

15. Bond J, Roberts E, Springell K, Lizarraga SB, Scott S, Higgins J, et al. A centrosomal mechanism involving CDK5RAP2 and CENPJ controls brain size. Nat Genet. 2005;37(4):353-5.

16. Kumar A, Girimaji SC, Duvvari MR, Blanton SH. Mutations in STIL, encoding a pericentriolar and centrosomal protein, cause primary microcephaly. Am J Hum Genet. 2009;84(2):286-90.

17. Squier W, Jansen A. Polymicrogyria: pathology, fetal origins and mechanisms. Acta Neuropathol Commun. 2014;2:80.

18. Mirzaa GM, Poduri A. Megalencephaly and hemimegalencephaly: breakthroughs in molecular etiology. Am J Med Genet C Semin Med Genet. 2014;166C(2):156-72.

19. Keppler-Noreuil KM, Rios JJ, Parker VER, Semple RK, Lindhurst MJ, Sapp JC, et al. PIK3CA-related overgrowth spectrum (PROS): diagnostic and testing eligibility criteria, differential diagnosis, and evaluation. Am J Med Genet A. 2015;167A(2):287-95.

20. Mirzaa GM, Rivière JB, Dobyns WB. Megalencephaly syndromes and activating mutations in the PI3K-AKT pathway: MPPH and MCAP. Am J Med Genet C Semin Med Genet. 2013;163C(2):122-30.

21. Jansen LA, Mirzaa GM, Ishak GE, O'Roak BJ, Hiatt JB, Roden WH, et al. PI3K/AKT pathway mutations cause a spectrum of brain malformations from megalencephaly to focal cortical dysplasia. Brain. 2015;138(6):1613-28.

22. Blümcke I, Thom M, Aronica E, Armstrong DD, Vinters HV, Palmini A, et al. The clinicopathologic spectrum of focal cortical dysplasias: a consensus classification proposed by an ad hoc Task Force of the ILAE Diagnostic Methods Commission. Epilepsia. 2011;52(1):158-74.

23. Northrup H, Krueger DA; International Tuberous Sclerosis Complex Consensus Group. Tuberous Sclerosis Complex Diagnostic Criteria Update: Recommendations of the 2012 International Tuberous Sclerosis Complex Consensus Conference. Pediatr Neurol. 2013;49(4):243-54.

24. Toi A, Lister WS, Fong KW. How early are fetal cerebral sulci visible at prenatal ultrasound and what is the normal pattern of early fetal sulcal development? Ultrasound Obstet Gynecol. 2004;24(7):706-15.

25. Poon LC, Sahota DS, Chaemsaithong P, Nakamura T, Machida M, Naruse K, et al. Transvaginal three-dimensional ultrasound assessment of Sylvian fissures at 18–30 weeks' gestation. Ultrasound Obstet Gynecol. 2019;54(2):190-8.

26. Pooh RK, Machida M, Nakamura T, Uenishi K, Chiyo H, Itoh K, et al. Increased Sylvian fissure angle as early sonographic sign of malformation of cortical development. Ultrasound Obstet Gynecol. 2019;54(2):199-206.

27. Dobyns WB. The clinical patterns and molecular genetics of lissencephaly and subcortical band heterotopia. Epilepsia. 2010;51(1):5-9.

28. Di Donato N, Chiari S, Mirzaa GM, Aldinger K, Parrini E, Olds C, et al. Lissencephaly: Expanded imaging and clinical classification. Am J Med Genet A. 2017;173(6):1473-88.

29. Parrini E, Conti V, Dobyns WB, Guerrini R. Genetic basis of brain malformations. Mol Syndromol. 2016;7(4):220-33.

30. Chen CP, Chang TY, Guo WY, Wu PC, Wang LK, Chern SR, et al. Chromosome 17p13.3 deletion syndrome: aCGH characterization, prenatal findings and diagnosis, and literature review. Gene. 2013;532(1):152-9.

31. Kato M. Genotype-phenotype correlation in neuronal migration disorders and cortical dysplasias. Front Neurosci. 2015;9:181.

32. Alford RE, Bailey AA, Twickler DM. Fetal central nervous system. MRI Fetal Matern Dis Pregnancy. 2016. pp. 91-118.

33. Cooper JA. Molecules and mechanisms that regulate multipolar migration in the intermediate zone. Front Cell Neurosci. 2014;8:386.

34. Hehr U, Uyanik G, Gross C, Walter MC, Bohring A, Cohen M, et al. Novel POMGnT1 mutations define broader phenotypic spectrum of muscle-eye-brain disease. Neurogenetics. 2007;8(4):279-88.

35. Vervoort VS, Holden KR, Ukadike KC, Collins JS, Saul RA, Srivastava AK. *POMGnT1* gene

alterations in a family with neurological abnormalities. Ann Neurol. 2004;56(1):143-8.

36. Biancheri R, Bertini E, Falace A, Pedemonte M, Rossi A, D'Amico A, et al. POMGnT1 Mutations in congenital muscular dystrophy: genotype-phenotype correlation and expanded clinical spectrum. Arch Neurol. 2006;63(10):1491-5.

37. Johnson K, Bertoli M, Phillips L, Töpf A, den Bergh PV, Vissing J, et al. Detection of variants in dystroglycanopathy-associated genes through the application of targeted whole-exome sequencing analysis to a large cohort of patients with unexplained limb-girdle muscle weakness. Skelet Muscle. 2018;8(1):23.

38. Aldinger KA, Doherty D. The genetics of cerebellar malformations. Semin Fetal Neonatal Med. 2016;21(5):321-32.

39. Kousi M, Katsanis N. The Genetic Basis of Hydrocephalus. Annu Rev Neurosci. 2016;39: 409-35.

40. Takeda S, Kondo M, Sasaki J, Kurahashi H, Kano H, Arai K, et al. Fukutin is required for maintenance of muscle integrity, cortical histiogenesis and normal eye development. Hum Mol Genet. 2003;12(12):1449-59.

41. Weisstanner C, Kasprian G, Gruber GM, Brugger PC, Prayer D. MRI of the fetal brain. Clin Neuroradiol. 2015;25(2):189-96.

42. Ventruti A, Kazdoba TM, Niu S, D'Arcangelo G. Reelin deficiency causes specific defects in the molecular composition of the synapses in the adult brain. Neuroscience. 2011;189:32-42.

43. Folsom TD, Fatemi SH. The involvement of Reelin in neurodevelopmental disorders. Neuropharmacology. 2013;68:122-35.

44. Van den Veyver IB. Prenatally diagnosed developmental abnormalities of the central nervous system and genetic syndromes: a practical review. Prenat Diagn. 2019;39(9): 666-78.

45. Chen X, Li SL, Luo GY, Norwitz ER, Ouyang SY, Wen HX, et al. Ultrasonographic characteristics of cortical sulcus development in the human fetus between 18 and 41 weeks of gestation. Chin Med J (Engl). 2017;130(8):920-8.

46. Stutterd CA, Leventer RJ. Polymicrogyria: a common and heterogeneous malformation of cortical development. Am J Med Genet C Semin Med Genet. 2014;166C(2):227-39.

47. Robson SC, Chitty LS, Morris S, Verhoef T, Ambler G, Wellesley DG, et al. Evaluation of array comparative genomic hybridization in prenatal diagnosis of fetal anomalies: a multicentre cohort study with cost analysis and assessment of patient, health professional and commissioner preferences for array comparative genomic hybridization. Effic Mech Eval. 2017;4(1):1-104.

48. Leventer RJ, Jansen A, Pilz DT, Stoodley N, Marini C, Dubeau F, et al. Clinical and imaging heterogeneity of polymicrogyria: a study of 328 patients. Brain. 2010;133(5):1415-27.

49. Yakovlev PI, Wadsworth RC. Schizencephalies; a study of the congenital clefts in the cerebral mantle; clefts with hydrocephalus and lips separated. J Neuropathol Exp Neurol. 1946;5(3):169-206.

50. Barkovich AJ, Kjos BO. Schizencephaly: correlation of clinical findings with MR characteristics. AJNR Am J Neuroradiol. 1992;13(1):85-94.

51. Bilgüvar K, Öztürk AK, Louvi A, Kwan KY, Choi M, Tatli B, et al. Whole-exome sequencing identifies recessive WDR62 mutations in severe brain malformations. Nature. 2010;467(7312):207-10.

52. Watanabe J, Okamoto K, Ohashi T, Natsumeda M, Hasegawa H, Oishi M, et al. Malignant hyperthermia and cerebral venous sinus thrombosis after ventriculo-peritoneal shunt in infant with schizencephaly and COL4A1 mutation. World Neurosurg. 2019;127:446-50.

53. Khalid R, Krishnan P, Andres K, Blaser S, Miller S, Moharir M, et al. COL4A1 and fetal vascular origins of schizencephaly. Neurologyogy. 2018;90(5):232-4.

54. Smigiel R, Cabala M, Jakubiak A, Kodera H, Sasiadek MJ, Matsumoto N, et al. Novel COL4A1 mutation in an infant with severe dysmorphic syndrome with schizencephaly, periventricular calcifications, and cataract resembling congenital infection. Birth Defects Res A Clin Mol Teratol. 2016;106(4):304-7.

55. Pooh RK. Sonogenetics in fetal neurology. Semin Fetal Neonatal Med. 2012;17(6):353-9.

Fetal Cognitive Functions

Aida Salihagić Kadić, Asim Kurjak, Anja Šurina, Oliver Vasilj

■ INTRODUCTION

Our brain is fantastically designed to execute cognitive functions, such as perception, action, attention, learning, thinking, speaking, reasoning, remembering, problem solving, decision making, etc. The modern imaging methods, such as three-dimensional/four-dimensional ultrasound (3D/4D US) and functional magnetic resonance imaging (fMRI) have indicated that some of the cognitive functions are being born in fetal life.[1] This chapter serves as a review of fetal neurodevelopment, fetal sensory and motor development, intrauterine behavior and activities, and development of fetal cognitive functions. New data about fetal sensory perception, motor action, emotions, as well as fetal learning, memory, and consequences of fetal stress response on cognitive functions have been presented in this chapter.

FETAL NEURODEVELOPMENT AND COGNITIVE FUNCTIONS

Prenatal and postnatal sensory and motor experience contours the structure and function of the cerebral cortex. It has been well known that >99% of the human neocortex is formed prenatally, resulting in amazing diversity of fetal abilities, including cognitive functions.[1] The maturation of the cerebral cortex is a very complex and dynamic process influenced by intrinsic and extrinsic factors, stimuli, and the environment.[2] Brain development is also very dynamic and it relies on interaction of genetic, systemic, and experiential factors. To unlock the mystery of neurocognitive development, understanding of how brain systems emerge through the interaction of all of these factors is essential.[3]

The central nervous system (CNS) begins its development in an early embryonic period from the ectodermal germinative layer, and its differentiation and maturation continue postnatally. The neural plate is formed at the beginning of the 3rd week as a precursor of the future brain and the spinal cord. Lateral edges of the neural plate elevate to form the neural folds which merge in the midline and create the neural tube. Fusion begins in the cervical region and proceeds in cephalic and caudal directions. The open ends of the neural tube form the cranial and caudal neuropores. Final closure of the cranial neuropore occurs at the 24th day while closure of the caudal neuropore occurs a few days later, on the 28th day. The process of neural tube formation is called "primary neurulation". Around the 22nd day of the embryonic life the forebrain (prosencephalon), midbrain (mesencephalon), and hindbrain (rhombencephalon) are distinguished in the rostral part of the neural tube as three primary brain vesicles. After the neural tube closes completely, cephalic flexure appears in the midbrain region and cervical flexure at the junction of the hindbrain and the spinal cord. Later on, the forebrain region is dividing into two parts: the diencephalon, characterized by outgrowing of the optic vesicles, and the telencephalon, basis for the future cerebral hemispheres. During the fetal life, the hemispheres continue to grow and develop into lobes, gyruses, and sulci. The rhombencephalon is the fundamental of the pons, cerebellum, and myelencephalon.[4] Caudal part of the neural tube, which is future spinal cord, develops in the process called "secondary neurulation".[5]

Histogenetic processes precede the growth of the neural tube and changes in shape and structure of its wall. Those are very complex overlapping processes divided into neurogenesis, migration, and cytodifferentiation. Production of neurons starts at the third gestational week (GW) with 125,000 and increases at the 7th week at a pace of 250,000/min.[6] Neurogenesis dominates in the embryonic and early fetal period, most intensively between the 8th and the 12th GW. Around the 20th GW neurogenesis is finished. Migration is accentuated in the middle of the gestation, from the 18th to the 24th GW, and cytodifferentiation at the end of the fetal period and postnatally. Migration finishes at the 38th GW. Synaptogenesis in the spinal cord begins at the 6/7th GW, it is very intensive in the middle of gestation, from the 8th to 18th GW and after the 24th GW. In the cortical plate, synaptogenesis starts at the 8th GW and it is most intensive after the 8th gestational month and it proceeds 2 years postnatally. It is important to note that by 20 weeks, the cortex has acquired its full complement of neurons. Cortical area differentiation begins between the 24th and the 34th GW and continues until the end of gestation.[7] Histologically, there are three zones of the neural tube. Those are ventricular, intermediary, and marginal zone. The telencephalon also has subventricular

and subplate zone. Neurogenesis is placed in the ventricular and subventricular zone of the telencephalon. The cortical plate, brainstem, diencephalon, and basal ganglia nuclei, which are final targets of the neurons and the glial cells, are genetically predisposed. Transitional zones are being created during their migration, representing temporary forms of the cerebral cortex organization. Hence, during the embryonic and fetal period, the brain is formed not only of adult structures but also of transitional structures which are not found in the adult human brain.[8]

The subplate zone is considered as a key zone for the development of the cerebral cortex since it is a place where early synaptogenesis, a creation of temporary synapses of afferent axons and neurons, is carried out. It is formed between the 13th and the 15th week of gestation when a number of cortical synapses grow. A six-layered lamination of cerebral cortex appears after the 32nd GW, proceeding the process of neuronal differentiation and laminar allocation of the thalamocortical axons. This, however, does not represent the end of the cerebral cortex development since it continues intensively even after the birth, especially in the association regions of the cortex.[7,8] Although the neurons and the pathways are present already at the neonates, their quantitative and qualitative features and their connections still need fine tuning. Therefore, in the permanent interaction with environment, the development continues during the postnatal life. Between 8 months and 2 years of life postnatal synapse generation is the most intensive, and it antecedes the development of more advanced cognitive functions such as speech.[9]

Cognitive functions are mediated by specialized areas of neocortex distributed across the cerebral hemisphere. Large areas of association cortex, which develop gradually during the fetal life, contribute to the cognition in particular ways. At the term, association areas display low activity, whereas high activity can be detected by fMRI in primary cortical areas. It is important to point out that deficits in the complex interneuronal connections can presage cognitive impairments.[10]

White matter myelination is a complex and long-lasting process. The development of the myelin sheath provides synchronized communication across the neural systems responsible for higher order cognitive functioning.[11] One of the fundamental parts of cerebral white matter—the corpus callosum—is formed around the 20th GW. It represents the major interhemispheric commissure and integrates sensory, motor, cognitive, and emotional functions from both cerebral hemispheres. Abnormalities of the corpus callosum include agenesis, partial agenesis, and thickness variations: hypoplasia and hyperplasia. In a large number of conditions that interfere with early cerebral development, these malformations are diagnosed. Different learning and behavioral difficulties, as well as speech and language delays, cognitive and motor impairments, including cerebral palsy have been associated with an abnormal volume of the corpus callosum.[11,12] There is also a correlation between splenial structure of corpus callosum and language skills. Impairment of visuospatial skills, attention, and motor coordination are results of over- or underdevelopment of the splenium. Furthermore, reduced posterior callosal connections have been linked with impaired social skills, diminished processing speed during complex tasks, and impairments in the excitatory interhemispheric transfer. Correlating the prenatal corpus callosum abnormalities with the known functions of its structures enables progressing into a more meaningful understanding of the prenatal neurological development of the white matter and postnatal neurological outcomes.[12]

PRENATAL MOTOR DEVELOPMENT AND FETAL ACTION

With the CNS development, the repertoire of fetal activities and functions during pregnancy increases. Fetal behavior, which is a product of the functioning CNS, embodies all the activities of the fetus which can be observed or recorded by US or other imaging techniques. Fetal behavioral patterns and their variations during the gestational period match to the development and maturity of the fetal CNS. Aberrations from the normal fetal behavior in certain gestational period can refer to the presence of neurological disorders as well as other organ system abnormalities.[9]

The synapses, interneuronal connections, and innervated muscle fibers are prerequisites for fetal mobility which plays an important role in the development of the fetus. Between the 6th and the 7th GW the earliest synapses in the spinal cord are detected.[13] The first movements that can be seen are vermicular movements at 7–7.5 weeks, and they are a result of the neural activity of spinal motoneurons.[14] The earliest motor reflex activity appears simultaneously with the onset of spontaneous movements, indicating the existence of the first afferent-efferent circuits in the spinal cord.[15] General movements, which arise between the 8th and the 9th GW, are the earliest complex and well-organized movement pattern. Those movements include the head, trunk, and limbs **(Figs. 1A to L)** and express a supraspinal control on motor activity.[16,17]

The brainstem consisting of the medulla oblongata, pons, and midbrain is fashioned

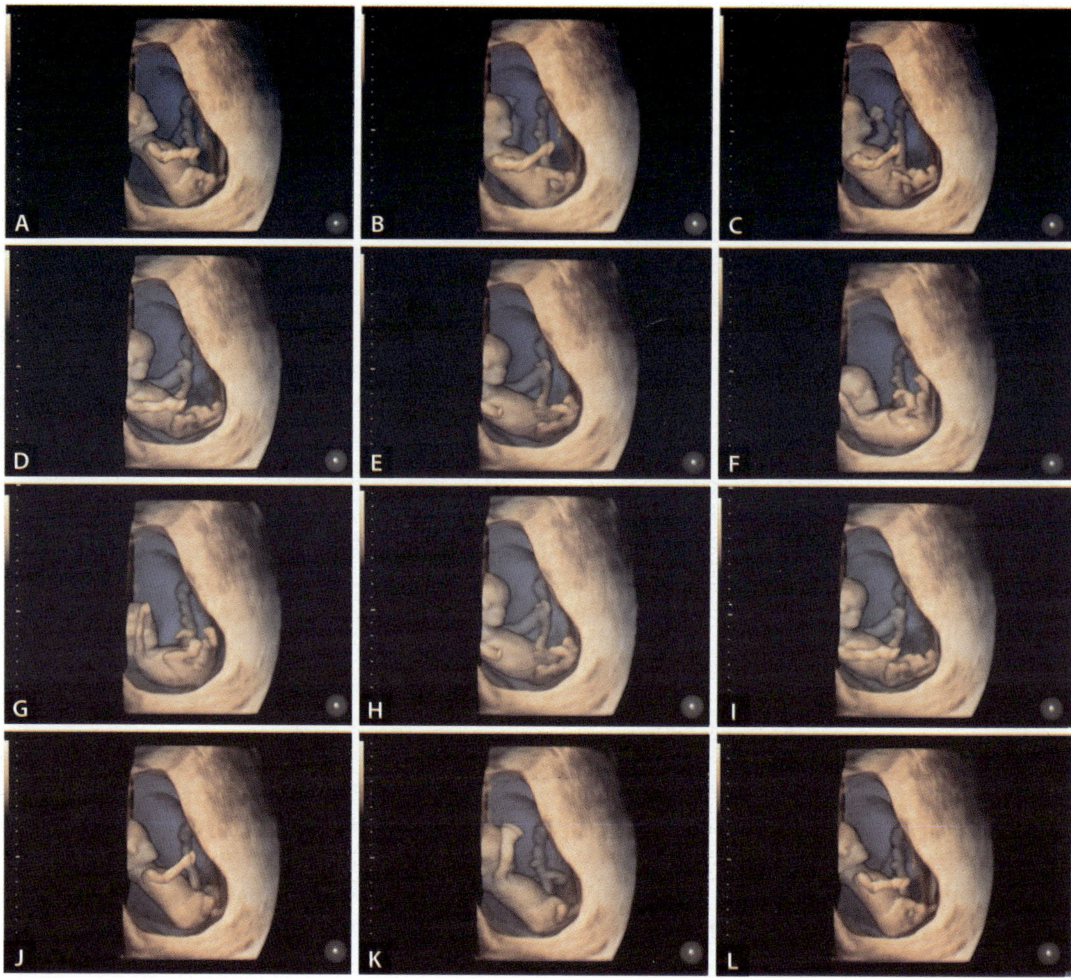

Figs. 1A to L: Series of three-dimensional ultrasonography (3D US) images of fetal general movements (11^{+1} weeks of gestation). The movements are of large amplitude and cause a shift in fetal position during this age period.

around 7th GW while by the end of the 8th GW the diencephalon and main parts of the cerebral hemispheres are formed.[18,19] Since the medulla matures earlier than other brainstem structures, activities under its control such as breathing-like movements, heart rate alternations, and reflexive movements of the head, trunk, and limbs appear prior to other functions. Around the 10–11th GW, facial movements, also controlled by cranial nerves V and VII, emerge.[18] Number, frequency, and diversity of fetal movements increase after 10 weeks. General movements, which used to be slow and of limited amplitude, become more pronounced.[20] From the 10th GW, when the fetus starts demonstrating signs of lateralized behavior, earliest signs of right- or left-"handedness" are present. Stimulation of the brain is known to influence the brain organization. It is considered that fetal motor activity may eventually stimulate the brain to develop lateralization of function.[10] From GW 13 onward, a "goal-orientation" of hand movements appears and a target point can be recognized for each hand movement.[21]

The most frequent movement pattern in the first trimester of pregnancy are general movements, which are always graceful in character.[22] These big (see Figs. 1A to L) and slow movements last from a few seconds to 1 minute. Their intensity, force, and velocity vary, and sequence of the head, neck, trunk, and extremities movements are undefined. Those characteristics are analyzed after the US recording when their qualitative aspects: complexity, variations, and fluency are being described. It appears that predictive value of general movements is important for detection of neurodevelopmental disorders, such as cerebral palsy.[23]

In the second trimester, fetal motor activity and fetal behavior are very diverse as a consequence of the development of neural connections, axons, synaptogenesis, and dendrite proliferation. Structures of the brainstem continue to mature, causing an increase in the complexity of fetal behavioral patterns and activities. Also, the second half of pregnancy is characterized by a gradual organization of fetal movement patterns.[9] The periods of fetal quiescence begin to increase, and the rest-activity cycles become recognizable. However, cerebral pathways are still not mature enough and the cerebral cortex cannot be considered responsible for motor activity and behavioral patterns.[7] On the other side, the brainstem gradually matures and starts to take over control of fetal movements and behavioral patterns.[18] During the second trimester a wide repertoire of fetal activity has been observed. This includes general movements, isolated movements of the extremities, head retroflexion, anteflexion, rotation as well as movements of the face,

such as yawning, hiccupping, thumb sucking, swallowing, and mouthing.[16] Between the 16th and the 18th week, there appear sporadic eye movements as a result of the midbrain maturation. Structures important for eye movement control—cranial nerves III, IV, and V and medial longitudinal fasciculus—are situated in the midbrain.[18] 4D US imaging in the second and third trimester of pregnancy shows that fetuses change facial expressions like smiling, grimacing, and crying.[24] The fetal face reflects the brain development very well and it represents a diagnostic window for fetal diseases and syndromes.

It is fascinating that fetal movements serve not only to express different orientations, but also emotional states and manifestations of intentions.[25] Moreover, a kinematic study has revealed a presence of a recognizable form of intentional fetal hand movements which can be detected by 22 weeks of gestation, with kinematic patterns that depend on the goal of the action. This suggests that there is a surprisingly advanced level of fetal action planning.[26] Fetal hand movements toward the face, complex individual finger movements, and different facial movements in the second trimester are presented in Figures 2A to L.

In the third trimester of pregnancy, the CNS continues its development. The pons and mesencephalon proceed their developmental pathways. The spinothalamic tract ends it myelination at the 29th GW.[18] Regarding the motor development, there is a decrease in a number of fetal facial movements, general movements, and the head and arm movements. On the other hand, those movements become more and more complex.[9] Smaller volume of amniotic fluid, thus less space for the bigger fetus to move, was thought to be the reason for this decrease in fetal movement number. Now, we know that this is a consequence of the maturation

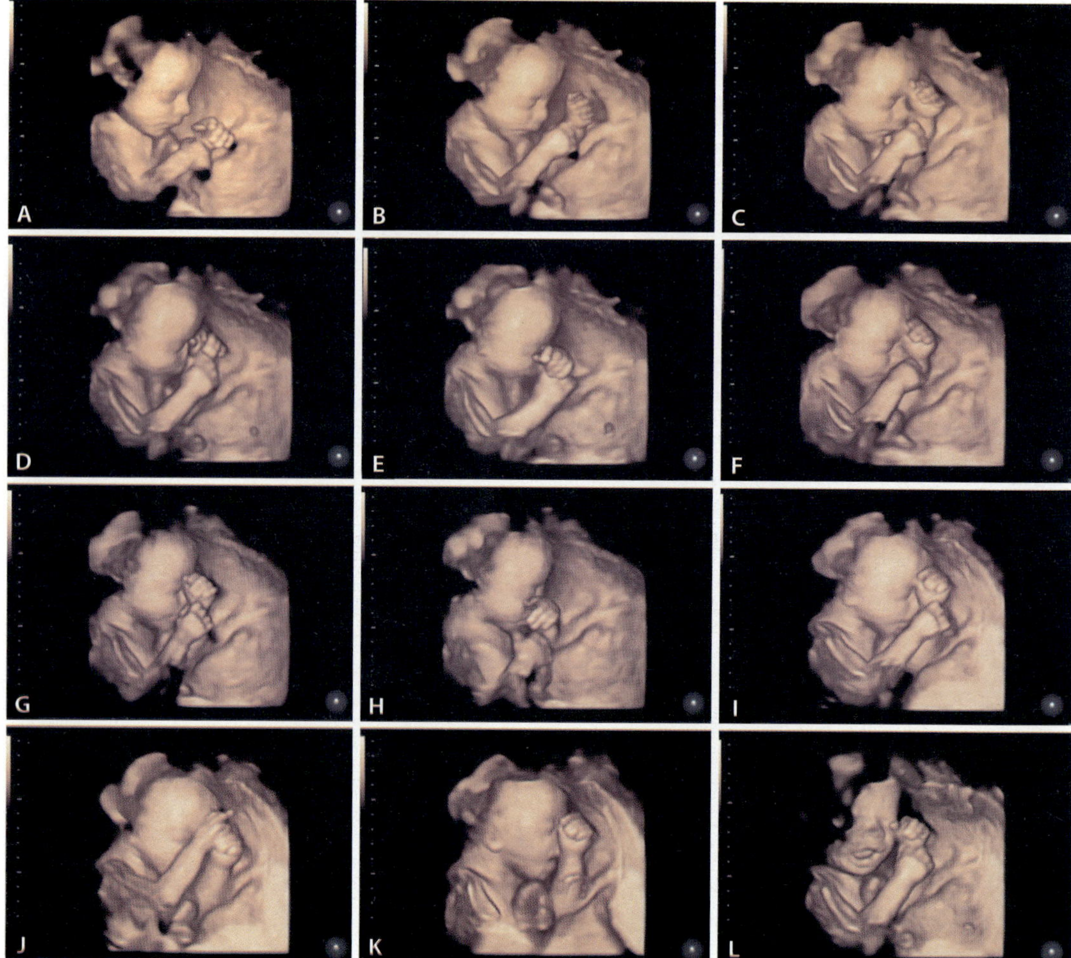

Figs. 2A to L: Series of three-dimensional ultrasonography (3D US) images of fetal hand movements toward fetal face (the second trimester). The movements are complex with variety of rotations, extensions, and flexions. This figure also shows complex individual finger movements accompanied with fetal head movements and different facial expressions.

of the medulla oblongata and more stable intrinsic activity of the brainstem, which includes control of the spontaneous fetal movements. At the 28th GW, eye-blinking movement pattern is at its peak frequency, while more complex eye movement occurs between the 33rd and 38th GW. It is important to stress that until delivery, the subunits of the brainstem remain the main regulator of all fetal behavior patterns.[18] However, developmental trends in fetal motor patterns may indicate the establishment of control of more cranial brain structures.[1]

It is unclear whether infants remember the movements they produced in utero. However, it has been found that fetal experiences, for example, exposure to sounds and language, are remembered postnatally.[27] Nevertheless, fetal movements provide the brain with sensory input that spurs its development.[1]

PRENATAL SENSORY DEVELOPMENT AND FETAL PERCEPTION OF STIMULI

Information enters the neural system by means of sensory receptors which register sensory stimuli, such as sound, light, touch, pain, cold, heat, etc. Sensory information from the somatic body segments enters into the spinal cord through the dorsal roots of spinal nerves. Then they travel up to the CNS through dorsal column of the medial lemniscus and anterolateral tract, the thalamus to the somatosensory part of the cerebral cortex.[28] The fetus is able to process tactile, vestibular, taste, olfactory, auditory, and visual sensations. When the thalamocortical connections are generated, which occur between the 24th and the 26th GW, sensory information can be processed at the cortical level.[8] A minimum level of consciousness emerges after the 25th GW.[29]

The first senses that develop in utero are touch and pain. The beginning of their development is at the 7th GW. Perioral region is touch-sensitive from the middle of the 7th GW. That is the time after which the fetus gives the earliest response to pain, a motor reflex, which can be induced in various ways. In the early phase of development, there is no perception or processing of the pain in the higher parts of the brain.[30] Studies on twin pregnancies were useful in research of the touch and pain. It was detected that after the 10th GW monochorionic twins react by moving when stimulated by touch. On the other side, dichorionic twins react to touch after the 12th GW.[31,32] All parts of the fetal body, with exception of the back and scalp, are sensitive to touch at the 14th GW.[33]

Fetal pain is a neural process and a sense having an important effect on the CNS development because of the possible long-term cognitive, emotional, and behavioral consequences.[34] The fetus responds to painful stimuli with a wide spectrum of reactions **(Table 1)**, which include the neuroendocrine answer, activation of hypothalamus-hypophysis-adrenal axis, and autonomic nervous system.[9] However, it is necessary to emphasize that these responses do not reach the cerebral cortex. The ability to sense pain requires developed neural pain system, from nociceptors to sensory areas in the cerebral cortex. The fetus has the necessary connections to sense pain after 24–26th GW.[8]

To prevent fetal pain during invasive intrauterine procedures, it is necessary to remember the knowledge about fetal pain and the effects of fetal stress response. It is still uncertain if the fetus is fully aware of the pain and if there is any memory of fetal pain.[35] The fetus cannot experience pain prior to reaching of connections from the periphery to the cortex. From about 25 weeks the cortical pain response has been recorded by near-infrared spectroscopy. Pain-like facial expressions have been observed in preterm infants after 25 weeks and these

TABLE 1: Fetal response to painful stimuli.

Weeks	Response
7, 5	Motor reflex
16–18	Increase in fetal cerebral blood flow
18–23	Elevation of noradrenaline, cortisol, and β-endorphin plasma levels
25	The cortical pain response
>25	Facial expressions are similar to those of adults experiencing pain
>28	Shifts in sleep/wake state Changes of the heart rate and blood oxygen saturation

Source: Modified according to Salihagić Kadić A et al.[9]

infants are probably conscious of pain. On the other hand, there is an opinion that the fetus may not be conscious of pain even after the 25th GW due to high endogenous sedatory and analgesic substances.[1] The fetus incorporates subconsciously pain experience into neurological development and plasticity. It has been shown that fetuses during fetal surgery can respond with bradycardia. This might be useful to assess fetal pain in the future.[36,37] According to the latest results of investigations, the fetus should be provided with analgesics directly during surgical interventions, in addition to doses administered to the mother, proving that fetal pain is evident in the second half of the pregnancy. Drugs used for maternal analgesia cross the placenta only partially and safety guidelines are given for fetal direct analgesia.[38]

The intrauterine environment is not deprived of the light and sound. Furthermore, for the development of fetal visual and auditory system, auditory and light stimulations are necessary.[39] Postnatal stimulation is also very important since the development of the visual system lasts until the 8th month after delivery.[40]

Studies revealed the developmental processes of the eye and their timeline. Visual connections between the retina, lateral geniculate nucleus, and visual cortex begin its development in the midgestation. Between the 23rd and the 27th GW, the thalamic projections reach the visual cortex. After the 36th GW, the maturation of visual cortex can be registered by surface positive evoked potentials. The amplitude of visually evoked potentials can be used in the assessment of fetal habituation to light stimuli.[41] Fetal eye motility is very important in retinal (neuronal) cell differentiation and in the eye functional maturation.[42] Stimulative intrauterine environment, as well as postnatal environmental enrichments, fosters the development of the optic system on the molecular, physiological, and behavioral level.[40,43]

The fetus lives not only in stimulating matrix of the tactile and motor information, but also the acoustic stimuli. The fetus reacts to exogenous acoustic stimulation and as the pregnancy progresses, fetal response to these stimuli changes.[44] Between the 22nd and the 25th GW, the cochlear function is developed and its maturation continues in the first 6 months postnatally. Neural structures which are important for auditory system development are cochlear nuclei in the medulla oblongata and pons, auditory follicles in the mesencephalon, and primary auditory cortex. The pons and mesencephalon are later to mature in comparison with the structures of the medulla oblongata. For this reason the selective answer to sound and vibration arises later. The fetus responds to strong sound stimuli delivered to the maternal abdomen by reflexive rotation of the trunk, head, and with lateral eye movements. Fetal reactions to very loud sounds have been registered at 26 weeks while in the third trimester progressive development of hearing has been observed.[18] At around 33 weeks of gestation, there is a change in the processing of complex sounds, such as music. In the younger fetuses, the response is limited to the acoustic properties of music. On the other hand, in older fetuses it seems that attention plays a role.[45] By the end of gestation, due to tonotopic organization of cochlear nuclei and maturation of the brainstem, the fetus is capable to distinguish different sounds. Moreover, the existence of preference to mother's voice and other familiar voices has been proved. Repeated sound stimulus, or lack of it, forms neural networks and tracts in the medulla oblongata. After that, these structures selectively react to the same stimulus that formed them. This indicates that the brainstem already at that time possesses the activity connected with learning, and the brainstem nuclei and auditory pathways show synaptic plasticity and sensitivity to exogenous stimuli.[18] Neuroprocessing mechanisms of music during fetal and neonatal development seem to have an important role in neuroplasticity and neurodevelopment, as human neural processing of music involves a complex bilateral network of the cortical and sub-cortical areas and integrates several auditory, cognitive, sensory, motor, and emotional functions.[46,47] Therefore, music could be integrated in the neonatal intensive care units. Improvement of environment increases positive experiences for a neonate.[47]

There are some factors that are known to affect the development of the auditory system. These are smoking,[48] intrauterine growth restriction (IUGR),[49] and hypertension in pregnancy.[50] Further, neonates of mothers who suffer from speech and hearing impairments, interestingly, may have delayed development of the auditory system.[51]

LEARNING AND MEMORY IN FETAL LIFE

Fetal learning and memory have been assessed by habituation methods, classical conditioning, and exposure learning. The possibilities of fetal learning and memory are astonishing. It should be emphasized that memory acquired prenatally lasts longer than it was initially considered.[52]

Habituation is a decline in response following repetition of the same stimulus from the 22nd GW onward.[53] This phenomenon is one of the most well documented and fundamental forms of nervous system plasticity. A major role of habituation is to limit the utilization of attentional resources for stimuli that are no longer salient.[54] We can distinguish habituation from adaptation of receptor as it requires an immediate recovery of the response on presentation of a different stimulus as well as faster response decrement upon representation of the original stimulus.[55,56] In 1925, the first study of fetal habituation was reported. Subsequent studies showed that, if fetuses repeatedly stimulated with the same stimulus, it resulted in a decrement of their response,[57,58] which was assessed by fetal heart rate alternations or fetal movements.[59] It has been noticed that younger fetuses require more exposure to the stimulus than older ones to register developmental trends. We need to mention that the presence of maternal stress and depression can affect in a negative way fetal habituation. This can cause developmental delays linked to the impaired function of the cerebral cortex.[60]

Classical conditioning involves the pairing of two stimuli: a conditioned and an unconditioned stimulus. When conditioned stimulus is presented alone it does not elicit response, while unconditioned stimulus elicits one. After repeated paired exposure to these two stimuli, the conditioned stimulus also elicits a response named a "conditioned response". This method of fetal learning has been demonstrated in 32–39 weeks old fetuses.[61] However, it could also be demonstrated on anencephalic fetuses. In studies conducted on chimpanzees, it was shown that fetuses can learn and retain obtained information for at least 2 months after birth.[62]

Exposure learning is done in a way that the fetus, after a number of exposures, is re-exposed to a stimulus, and then this response is compared to the "unfamiliar" stimulus or to the response of an unexposed fetus to the same stimulus. Exposure learning confirmed that fetuses can hear and learn the voice of the mother before birth, and this gave insight to the fetal preference of the mother's voice over an unacquainted one as well as mother's voice in utero over her voice after delivery.[63] Selective fetal cortical processing for the mother's voice over an unfamiliar voice has been reported at 34 weeks of gestation.[64] The fetus is able to learn and remember familiar auditory stimuli and retain this information over the birth period.[65] Rudimentary capacity for retention of information exists very early, at 30 weeks of gestation, while prenatally acquired auditory memory can last even 6 weeks. The long-term auditory memory might have a role in the developmental psychobiology of attention and perception as well as early speech perception.[52]

Other aspects of fetal learning and memory have been investigated as well. The fetus is able to distinguish pleasant from an unpleasant taste of amniotic fluid, and it seems that sweet taste is preferred. Furthermore, during fetal life the preference for a certain food may be acquired.[66,67] The fetus also learns through smell. In preterm infants, behavioral responses to pleasant and unpleasant smells can be observed from about the 29th week.[68]

It might be that fetal learning and memory have a role in the development of maternal recognition, attachment, establishment of breastfeeding, social recognition, and language acquisition.[61,69] When the fetus starts discriminating different speeches in utero, the process of prenatal language acquiring may be possible.[63] There was a study performed on 93 pregnant women to assess fetal learning and memory, based on habituation to repeated vibroacoustic stimulation of fetuses of 30–38 weeks of gestational age. Fetal learning and short-term

(10 min) memory is found at 30th GW. Also, there is evidence that at the 34th GW fetuses are able to store information and retrieve it 4 weeks later.[70]

The fetus can detect, respond as well as remember for a relatively long time the stimuli which it experienced during the prenatal period. Recent study has shown a remarkable experience-dependent plasticity in the primary auditory cortex even before the brain has reached full-term maturation. Namely, extremely premature infants exposed to maternal sounds had significantly larger auditory cortex compared with control infants receiving standard care.[71]

EMOTIONAL DEVELOPMENT OF THE FETUS

As mentioned before, fetal movements express not only different orientations but also emotional states.[25] Facial expressions are one of the external signs of emotion. It is possible that fetal facial movements demonstrate endogenously generated physiologic reflex patterns. Actually, smiling as well as crying can be induced by the brainstem stimulation even with complete forebrain transection or destruction.[18] A full range of different fetal facial expressions, similar to emotional facial expressions in children and adults, has been revealed during the second and the third trimester of pregnancy by the use of 4D US.[24,72,73] With the progress of pregnancy, fetal facial expressions become more complex **(Figs. 3A to O)** and some of them such as facial expressions of pain or distress, are considered to be an adaptive process which might be useful postnatally.[74] "Cry-face gestalt" or "laughter-face gestalt" appear in the third trimester. It might be beneficial for fetal and maternal communication and bonding in postnatal life, as well as for the regulation of

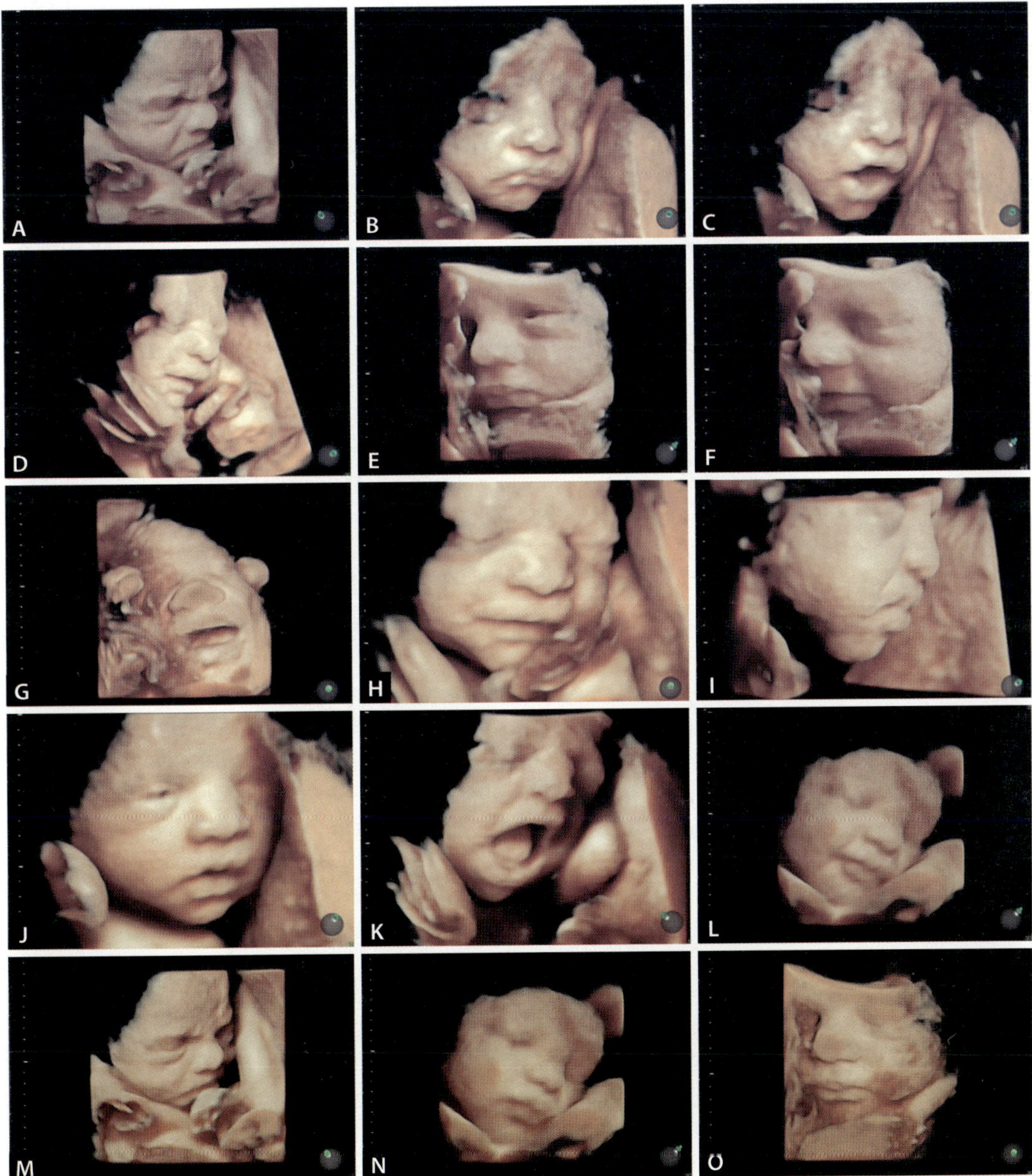

Figs. 3A to O: Series of three-dimensional ultrasonography (3D US) images of complex fetal facial expressions ranging from grimacing, sad, happy, expression of pain, calm fetal face, angry fetal face, facial expression of surprise, yawning, and smiling (36–39 weeks of gestation).

parental care.[75] It has been suggested that the facial expressions and emotion-like behaviors represent some kind of fetal emotion and awareness.[73]

The limbic system, and the amygdala in particular, is responsible for the experience and the expression of emotions. It is known that the amygdala begins its development in early embryonic life while during the first postnatal year it reaches an advanced stage of maturity.[76] It has an important and significant role in the mediation of emotional memory, attention, arousal, and the experience of love, fear, pleasure, and joy. It contains facial recognition neurons which discern the emotional significance of different facial expressions. The evaluation of faces in social processing is an area of cognition specific to the amygdala.[76] The amygdala is vital in evaluating the biological relevance of sensory information and for initiating behavioral responses based on the initial assessment of the presented stimulus. Facial expressions represent biologically important visual stimuli, and the amygdala neurons are very responsive to them.[54]

FETAL STRESS AND COGNITIVE DEVELOPMENT

Particularly important role in fetal growth and development has physiological condition in the intrauterine environment. It is necessary that the fetus is protected in an environment which gives optimal condition for growth and development. The stress has primarily protective role inducing different adaptations of the organism and allowing survival, however, fetal stress can have negative consequences on the structure and function of the organism, particularly the nervous system. There are several most important stressful factors which are: malnutrition of the mother, IUGR, fetal painful stimuli, and severe maternal emotional stress as well as stressful life events.[77]

Fetal hypothalamic-pituitary-adrenal response to stress is independent of mother's.[78] Moreover, it has been found that between the 18th and the 23rd GW the fetus secretes noradrenaline, cortisol, and beta-endorphin in response to painful stimuli

(see Table 1). Adaptation of the fetus to stress includes accelerated maturation, notably the maturation of the lungs and the brain. Unfortunately, even though this is a protective adaptation, interfering with the normal development of the CNS and other organ systems, it can leave long-term adverse sequels.[9,77] Cortisol, on one hand, initiates accelerated maturation of the brain and the lungs, but also, it has negative effects on growth of the fetal organism in a whole, as well as on the brain development. The hippocampus is the brain structure that contributes greatly to learning and memory. The hippocampus and parahippocampal region contain a large concentration of cortisol and the corticotropin-releasing hormone (CRH) receptors. Consequently, these regions are vulnerable to accelerated brain maturation, which can therefore cause different structural changes in the developing brain. Apart from structural changes, behavioral changes have been noticed as well. Stress-induced changes of the hippocampus include: decreased number of neurons and corticosteroid receptors, decreased level of serotonin, and decreased synaptic density on distinct hippocampal regions. These changes are later in life associated with memory impairment and learning disabilities. Hyperalertness and impaired fetal responsiveness to novel stimuli are behavioral changes associated with accelerated brain development. A cause of irritability and diminished attention may be fetal adrenocorticotropic hormone (ACTH) as well. Additionally, ACTH affects movement coordination and muscle tonus, which can be damaged due to great exposure to this hormone. Fetal CRH influences the timing of the birth, which means that the fetus has an active role in the initiation of the delivery. A high serum level of cortisol and CRH is correlated to pregnancies complicated with IUGR, preeclampsia, infectious diseases, diabetes, and twin pregnancies.[77]

Many neuropsychiatric disorders and diseases such as attention-deficit hyperactivity disorder (ADHD), disturbances in sleep, unsociable and inconsiderate behavior, schizophrenia, depressive, and neurotic symptoms, drug abuse, as well as anxiety, are considered as potential neurodevelopmental consequences of prenatal stress exposure.[77] Increased maternal stress during pregnancy can influence temperament and cognitive functions of an infant.[79,80] It may also leave adverse effects on learning and memory of a child at the age of 6.[81] It is, however, important to point out that cognitive development of an infant can be enormously moderated by increased mother's care and developed emotional mother-infant attachment.[82] Current neurobiological evidence suggests that targeted early intervention has the potential to mitigate the long-term negative outcomes related to adverse early experiences.[83] A recent study discussed an interesting connection between early secure attachment and cognitive decline later in life. It shows an enormous importance of early supportive and responsive social environment which creates a secure attachment profile. All these favor neurological and cognitive development and provide more reserve to compensate for neurodegeneration which makes us less vulnerable to cognitive decline and dementia.[84]

Fetal stress might have different effects on female and male fetuses.[85,86] Prenatal exposure to stress can create a greater risk of depressive symptoms, schizophrenia, and ADHD in boys than in girls.[87] On the other side, high levels of maternal cortisol in early pregnancy are associated with more affective problems in girls. This was linked with larger right amygdala volume measured by MRI.[88]

■ CONCLUSION

There are still many unanswered questions in the field of fetal cognitive functions but future advances in the application of new imaging methods will enable a better understanding of the cognitive abilities and functions of the fetus. New advanced techniques, such as 3D/4D HD live and silhouette mode, improved prenatal assessment of fetal structural, functional, behavioral development and assist in puzzle solving of fetal cognitive development.[1,89] Furthermore, the prenatal neurological scoring test, named KANET (Kurjak antenatal neurodevelopmental test) has proved its usefulness in prenatal assessment by 4D US of the neurological outcome. This test has been used to assess almost 2,000 fetuses and the results indicate that KANET has the ability to recognize normal, borderline, and abnormal behavior in fetuses from normal and pathological pregnancies.[90,91]

Prenatal period is annotated with an opportunity for prosperous development of the fetus, including fetal cognitive development, but also it is fragile period of great vulnerability to environmental effects. The fetus is exposed to numerous stimuli (e.g., tactile, chemical, auditory, etc.) which differently shape the brain structure and guide the brain's functional development. They provide very stimulative environment for the development of the fetus and higher order sensory perception begins in fetal life. It is astonishing that as early as the second trimester fetal action planning and motor learning occur. Primary cortical areas and subcortical formations are fully developed and highly active in a newborn; thus, cognitive functions at the end of the gestation rely on them. However, it should be emphasized that at term, there is also low activity in the association cortical areas.

Today, we know that possibilities of fetal learning and fetal memory are impressive. We also know that roots of emotions appear in the intrauterine life. Moreover, emotional and cognitive impairments and deficits in childhood and adulthood (impaired learning and memory, delayed language development, intellectual disabilities, attention deficits, etc.) may also originate in the prenatal life.[1] But it is important to implement the knowledge we have into bettering the prenatal, neonatal, and early childhood care. From clinical perspective, data on cognitive functions of the fetus could be important for the management of fetal pain, treatment of preterm infants, and improvement of the neurological outcome of the fetuses from high-risk pregnancies. Finally, it is of great importance to emphasize again that infant cognitive development can be moderated enormously by increased mother's care and developed emotional mother-infant attachment as well as by enrichment of positive environmental inputs (e.g., music). Secure attachment profile enhances further neurological and cognitive development.

◼ REFERENCES

1. Kadic AS, Kurjak A. Cognitive functions of the fetus. Ultraschall Med. 2018;39(2):181-9.
2. Huttenlocher P. Synaptogenesis in human cerebral cortex. In: Dawson G, Fisher KW, Coch D (Eds). Human Behavior and the Developing Brain. New York: Guilford Publications; 1994. pp. 137-52.
3. Stiles J, Brown TT, Haist F, Jernigan TL. Brain and cognitive development. In: Lerner M (Ed). Handbook of Child Psychology and Developmental Science, 7th edition. New York: John Wiley and Sons, Inc.; 2015. pp. 1-54.
4. Sadler T. Central Nervous System. In: Sadler T (Ed). Langman's Medical Embryology, 9th edition. Philadelphia: Lippincott Williams & Wilkins; 2004. pp. 433-80.
5. Saitsu H, Yamada S, Uwabe C, Ishibashi M, Shiota K. Development of the posterior neural tube in human embryos. Anat Embryol (Berl). 2004;209(2):107-17.
6. Nelson C. Neural development and lifelong plasticity. In: Keating DP (Ed). Nature and Nurture in Early Child Development. Cambridge: Cambridge University Press; 2010. pp. 45-69.
7. Kostović I, Judaš M, Petanjek Z, Šimić G. Ontogenesis of goal-directed behavior: anatomo-functional considerations. Int J Psychophysiol. 1995;19(2):85-102.
8. Kostovic I, Judas M. The development of the subplate and thalamocortical connections in the human foetal brain. Acta Paediatr. 2010;99(8):1119-27.
9. Kadic AS, Predojevic M, Kurjak A. Advances in fetal neurophysiology. In: Pooh RK, Kurjak A (Eds). Fetal Neurology. New Delhi: Jaypee Brothers Medical Publishers (P) Ltd; 2009. pp. 160-204.
10. Kurjak A, Vasilj O, Tomasović S, Kadiæ AS, Šurina A. Fetal cognitive functions and 3D/4D ultrasound. Donald Sch J Ultrasound Obstet Gynecol. 2019;13(1):41-53.
11. Qui A, Mori S, Miller MI. Diffusion tensor imaging for understanding brain development in early life. Annu Rev Psychol. 2015;66:853-76.
12. Pashaj S, Merz E. Detection of fetal corpus callosum abnormalities by means of 3D ultrasound. Ultraschall Med. 2016;37(2):185-94.
13. Okado N, Kakimi S, Kojima T. Synaptogenesis in the cervical cord of the human embryo: sequence of synapse formation in a spinal reflex pathway. J Comp Neurol. 1979;184(3):491-518.
14. Okado N, Kojima T. Ontogeny of the central nervous system: neurogenesis, fibre connection, synaptogenesis and myelination in the spinal cord. In: Prechtl HF (Ed). Continuity of Neural Functions from Prenatal to Postnatal Life. Oxford: Blackwell science; 1984. pp. 31-5.
15. Okado N. Onset of synapse formation in the human spinal cord. J Comp Neurol. 1981;201(2):211-9.

16. de Vries JI, Visser GH, Prechtl HF. The emergence of fetal behaviour. I. Qualitative aspects. Early Hum Dev. 1982;7(4):301-22.

17. Einspieler C, Prechtl HF. Prechtl's assessment of general movements: a diagnostic tool for the functional assessment of the young nervous system. Ment Retard Dev Disabil Res Rev. 2005;11(1):61-7.

18. Joseph RG. Fetal brain behavior and cognitive development. Dev Rev. 2000;20(1):81-98.

19. Pomeroy S, Volpe J. Development of the nervous system. In: Polin R, Fox W (Eds). Fetal and Neonatal Physiology. Phyladelphia-London-Toronto-Montreal-Sydney-Tokyo: WB Saunders Company; 1992. pp. 1491-509.

20. Lüchinger AB, Hadders-Algra M, van Kan CM, de Vries JIP. Fetal onset of general movements. Pediatr Res. 2008;63(2):191-5.

21. Kurjak A, Azumendi G, Veček N, Kupesic S, Solak M, Varga D, et al. Fetal hand movements and facial expression in normal pregnancy studied by four-dimensional sonography. J Perinat Med. 2003;31(6):496-508.

22. Andonotopo W, Medic M, Salihagic-Kadic A, Milenkovic D, Maiz N, Scazzocchio E. The assessment of fetal behavior in early pregnancy: comparison between 2D and 4D sonographic scanning. J Perinat Med. 2005;33(5):406-14.

23. Einspieler C, Prechtl HF, Ferrari F, Cioni G, Bos AF. The qualitative assessment of general movements in preterm, term and young infants—review of the methodology. Early Hum Dev. 1997;50(1):47-60.

24. Kurjak A, Azumendi G, Andonotopo W, Salihagic-Kadic A. Three- and four-dimensional ultrasonography for the structural and functional evaluation of the fetal face. Am J Obstet Gynecol. 2007;196(1):16-28.

25. Delafield-butt J, Trevarthen C. Theories of the development of human communication. Theories and Models of Communication. In: Cobley P, Schultz PJ (Eds). Handbook of Communication Science. Berlin: De Gruyeter Mouton; 2013. pp. 199-221.

26. Zoia S, Blason L, D'Ottavio G, Bulgheroni M, Pezzetta E, Scabar A, et al. Evidence of early development of action planning in the human foetus: a kinematic study. Exp Brain Res. 2007;176(2):217-26.

27. Kisilevsky BS, Hains SMJ, Lee K, Xie X, Huang H, Ye HH, et al. Effects of experience on fetal voice recognition. Psychol Sci. 2003;14(3):220-4.

28. Hall JE (Ed). Guyton and Hall Textbook of Medical Physiology, 13th edition. Philadelphia: Elsevier; 2016. pp. 577-688.

29. Lagercrantz H. The emergence of the mind: a borderline of human viability? Acta Paediatr. 2007;96(3):327-8.

30. Vanhatalo S, van Nieuwenhuizen O. Fetal pain? Brain Dev. 2000;22(3):145-50.

31. Arabin B, Bos R, Rijlaarsdam R, Mohnhaupt A, van Eyck J. The onset of inter-human contacts: longitudinal ultrasound observations in early twin pregnancies. Ultrasound Obstet Gynecol. 1996;8(3):166-73.

32. Piontelli A, Bocconi L, Kustermann A, Tassis B, Zoppini C, Nicolini U. Patterns of evoked behaviour in twin pregnancies during the first 22 weeks of gestation. Early Hum Dev. 1997;50(1):39-45.

33. Hepper P. Prenatal development. In: Slater A, Lewis M (Eds). Introduction to Infant Development. New York: Oxford University Press; 2007. pp. 39-101.

34. Gupta A, Giordano J. On the nature, assessment, and treatment of fetal pain: neurobiological bases, pragmatic issues, and ethical concerns. Pain Physician. 2007;10(4):525-32.

35. White MC, Wolf AR. Pain and stress in the human fetus. Best Pract Res Clin Anaesthesiol. 2004;18(2):205-20.

36. Lowery CL, Hardman MP, Manning N, Hall RW, Anand KJS, Clancy B. Neurodevelopmental changes of fetal pain. Semin Perinatol. 2007;31(5):275-82.

37. Mayorga-Buiz MJ, Marquez-Rivas J, Gomez-Gonzales E. Can fetus feel pain in the second trimester? Lessons learned from a sentinel event. Childs Nerv Syst. 2018;34(2):195-6.

38. Bellieni CV. Analgesia for fetal pain during prenatal surgery: 10 years of progress. Pediatr Res. 2021;89(7):1612-8.

39. Magoon EH, Robb RM. Development of myelin in human optic nerve and tract.

A light and electron microscopic study. Arch Ophthalmol. 1981;99(4):655-9.

40. Sale A, Cenni MC, Ciucci F, Putignano E, Chierzi S, Maffei L. Maternal enrichment during pregnancy accelerates retinal development of the fetus. PLoS One. 2007; 2(11):e1160.

41. Sheridan CJ, Preissl H, Siegel ER, Murphy P, Ware M, Lowery CL, et al. Neonatal and fetal response decrement of evoked responses: a MEG study. Clin Neurophysiol. 2008;119(4): 796-804.

42. Baguma-Nibasheka M, Reddy T, Abbas-Butt A, Kablar B. Fetal ocular movements and retinal cell differentiation: analysis employing DNA microarrays. Histol Histopathol. 2006;21(12):1331-7.

43. Landi S, Sale A, Berardi N, Viegi A, Maffei L, Cenni MC. Retinal functional development is sensitive to environmental enrichment: a role for BDNF. FASEB J. 2007;21(1):130-9.

44. Hepper PG, Shahidullah BS. Development of fetal hearing. Arch Dis Child Fetal Neonatal Ed. 1994;71(2):F81-7.

45. Kisilevsky S, Hains SMJ, Jacquet AY, Granier-Deferre C, Lecanuet JP. Maturation of fetal response to music. Dev Sci. 2004;7(5):550-9.

46. Koelsch S. Toward a neural basis of music perception - a review and updated model. Front Psychol. 2011;2:110.

47. Chorna O, Filippa M, Sa De Almeida J, Lordier L, Monaci MG, Hüppi P, et al. Neuroprocessing mechanisms of music during fetal and neonatal development: a role in neuroplasticity and neurodevelopment. Neural Plast. 2019;2019:3972918.

48. Cowperthwaite B, Hains SMJ, Kisilevsky BS. Fetal behavior in smoking compared to non-smoking pregnant women. Infant Behav Dev. 2007;30(3):422-30.

49. Kisilevsky BS, Davies GAL. Auditory processing deficits in growth restricted fetuses affect later language development. Med Hypotheses. 2007;68(3):620-8.

50. Lee CT, Brown CA, Hains SMJ, Kisilevsky BS. Fetal development: voice processing in normotensive and hypertensive pregnancies. Biol Res Nurs. 2007;8(4):272-82.

51. Marshall J. Infant neurosensory development: considerations for infant child care. Early Child Educ J 2011;39(3): 175-81.

52. Granier-Deferre C, Bassereau S, Ribeiro A, Jacquet AY, Decasper AJ. A melodic contour repeatedly experienced by human near-term fetuses elicits a profound cardiac reaction one month after birth. PLoS One. 2011;6(2):e17304.

53. Yamaguchi S, Hale LA, D'Esposito M, Knight RT. Rapid prefrontal-hippocampal habituation to novel events. J Neurosci. 2004;24(23):5356-63.

54. Wright CI, Fischer H, Whalen PJ, McInerney SC, Shin LM, Rauch SL. Differential prefrontal cortex and amygdala habituation to repeatedly presented emotional stimuli. Neuroreport. 2001;12(2):379-83.

55. Jeffrey WE, Cohen LS. Habituation in the human infant. Adv Child Dev Behav. 1971;6:63-97.

56. Thompson RF, Spencer WA. Habituation: a model phenomenon for the study of neuronal substrates of behavior. Psychol Rev. 1966;73(1):16-43.

57. van Heteren CF, Boekkooi PF, Jongsma HW, Nijhuis JG. Fetal learning and memory. Lancet. 2000;356(9236):1169-70.

58. Shalev E, Weiner E, Serr DM. Fetal habituation to sound stimulus in various behavioral states. Gynecol Obstet Invest. 1990;29(2):115-7.

59. Gagnon R, Hunse C, Carmichael L, Fellows F, Patrick J. Human fetal responses to vibratory acoustic stimulation from twenty-six weeks to term. Am J Obstet Gynecol. 1987;157(6): 1375-81.

60. Morokuma S, Fukushima K, Kawai N, Tomonaga M, Satoh S, Nakano H. Fetal habituation correlates with functional brain development. Behav Brain Res. 2004;153(2): 459-63.

61. Hepper PG. Fetal memory: does it exist? What does it do? Acta Paediatr Suppl. 1996;416: 16-20.

62. Kawai N, Morokuma S, Tomonaga M, Horimoto N, Tanaka M. Associative learning and memory in a chimpanzee fetus: learning

and long-lasting memory before birth. Dev Psychobiol. 2004;44(2):116-22.

63. Hepper PG, Scott D, Shahidullah S. Newborn and fetal response to maternal voice. J Reprod Infant Psychol. 1993;11(3):147-53.

64. Jardri R, Houfflin-Debarge V, Delion P, Pruvo JP, Thomas P, Pins D. Assessing fetal response to maternal speech using a noninvasive functional brain imaging technique. Int J Dev Neurosci. 2012;30(2):159-61.

65. Hepper PG. Fetal "soap" addiction. Lancet. 1988;1(8598):1347-8.

66. Mennella JA, Jagnow CP, Beauchamp GK. Prenatal and postnatal flavor learning by human infants. Pediatrics [Internet]. 2001;107(6):E88.

67. Salihagić Kadić A, Predojević M. Fetal neurophysiology according to gestational age. Semin Fetal Neonatal Med. 2012;17(5):256-60.

68. Lagercrantz H. The emergence of consciousness: Science and ethics. Semin Fetal Neonatal Med. 2014;19(5):300-5.

69. Partanen E, Kujala T, Näätänen R, Liitola A, Sambeth A, Huotilainen M. Learning-induced neural plasticity of speech processing before birth. Proc Natl Acad Sci U S A. 2013;110(37):15145-50.

70. Dirix CEH, Nijhuis JG, Jongsma HW, Hornstra G. Aspects of fetal learning and memory. Child Dev. 2009;80(4):1251-8.

71. Webb AR, Heller HT, Benon CB, Lahav A. Mother's voice and heartbeat sounds elicit auditory plasticity in the human brain before full gestation. Proc Natl Acad Sci USA. 2015;112(10):3152-7.

72. Merz E, Pashaj S. Fetal Facial Expressions: Demonstration of the smiling, the sad and the scowling fetus with 4D-ultrasound. Ultraschall Med. 2015;36(1):1-2.

73. Hata T, Kenenishi K, AboEllail MAM, Marumo G. Fetal Consciousness: Four-dimensional Ultrasound Study. Donald Sch J Ultrasound Obstet Gynecol. 2015;9(4):471-4.

74. Reissland N, Francis B, Mason J. Can healthy fetuses show facial expressions of "pain" or "distress"? PLoS One. 2013;8(6):e65530.

75. Reissland N, Francis B, Mason J, Lincoln K. Do facial expressions develop before birth? PLoS One. 2011;6(8):e24081.

76. Joseph R. Environmental influences on neural plasticity, the limbic system, emotional development and attachment: a review. Child Psychiatry Hum Dev. 1999; 29(3):189-208.

77. Salihagić Kadić A. Fetal neurology: The role of fetal stress. Donald Sch J Ultrasound Obstet Gynecol. 2015;9(1):30-9.

78. Gitau R, Fisk NM, Teixeira JM, Cameron A, Glover V. Fetal hypothalamic-pituitary-adrenal stress responses to invasive procedures are independent of maternal responses. J Clin Endocrinol Metab. 2001; 86(1):104-9.

79. Buitelaar JK, Huizink AC, Mulder EJ, de Medina PGR, Visser GHA. Prenatal stress and cognitive development and temperament in infants. Neurobiol Aging. 2003;24(Suppl 1):S53-60.

80. Davis EP, Glynn LM, Schetter CD, Hobel C, Chicz-Demet A, Sandman CA. Prenatal exposure to maternal depression and cortisol influences infant temperament. J Am Acad Child Adolesc Psychiatry. 2007;46(6):737-46.

81. Gutteling BM, de Weerth C, Zandbelt N, Mulder EJH, Visser GHA, Buitelaar JK. Does maternal prenatal stress adversely affect the child's learning and memory at age six? J Abnorm Child Psychol. 2006;34(6):789-98.

82. Bergman K, Sarkar P, Glover V, O'Connor TG. Maternal prenatal cortisol and infant cognitive development: moderation by infant-mother attachment. Biol Psychiatry. 2010;67(11):1026-32.

83. Newman L, Sivaratnam C, Komiti A. Attachment and early brain development—neuroprotective interventions in infant-caregiver therapy. Transl Dev Psyc. 2015;(3): 28647.

84. Walsh E, Blake Y, Donati A, Stoop R, von Gunten A. Early secure attachment as a protective factor against later cognitive decline and dementia. Front Aging Neurosci. 2019;11:161.

85. Cottrell EC, Seckl JR, Holmes MC, Wyrwoll CS. Foetal and placental 11beta-HSD2: a hub for developmental programming. Acta Physiol (Oxf). 2014;210(2):288-95.

86. Aiken CE, Ozanne SE. Sex differences in developmental programming models. Reproduction. 2013;145(1):R1-13.

87. Reynolds RM. Glucocorticoid excess and the developmental origins of disease: two decades of testing the hypothesis—2012 Curt Richter Award Winner. Psychoneuro-endocrinology. 2013;38(1):1-11.

88. Buss C, Davis EP, Shahbaba B, Pruessner JC, Head K, Sandman CA. Maternal cortisol over the course of pregnancy and subsequent child amygdala and hippocampus volumes and affective problems. Proc Natl Acad Sci USA. 2012;109(20):E1312-9.

89. Kurjak A, Barisic LS, Stanojevic M, Salihagić Kadić A, Porovic S. Are we ready to investigate cognitive function of fetal brain? The role of advanced four-dimensional sonography. Donald Sch J Ultrasound Obstet Gynecol. 2016;10(2):116-24.

90. Kurjak A, Miskovic B, Stanojevic M, Amiel-Tison C, Ahmed B, Azumendi G, et al. New scoring system for fetal neurobehavior assessed by three- and four-dimensional sonography. J Perinat Med. 2008;36(1):73-81.

91. Salihagić Kadić A, Stanojević M, Predojević M. Assessment of the Fetal Neuromotor Development with the New KANET Test. In: Reissland N, Kisilevsky BS (Eds). Fetal Development: Research on Brain and Behavior, Environmental Influences, and Emerging Technologies. Heidelberg, New York, Dordrecht, London, Switzerland: Springer International Publishing; 2016. pp. 177-89.

Evolution of Assessment of Fetal Brain Function

Panagiotis Antsaklis, Maria Papamichail, Marianna Theodora, George Daskalakis, Asim Kurjak

■ INTRODUCTION

Detailed examination of the nervous system of the fetus both in anatomical and functional way has been a great area of research for many years with still many unanswered questions. Advances of ultrasound techniques and especially the evolution of three-dimensional (3D) and four-dimensional (4D) techniques made reality the evaluation of fetal anatomy and activity in real time.[1] Development of human nervous system remains very complicated and timely process, evolving by strict and precise developmental steps, starting from the early first trimester and carries on for years throughout postnatal life.[2] The growth and maturation of central nervous system (CNS) are reflected by a specific behavioral pattern which undergoes changes and progress reciprocal to each week of gestation.[2] Corresponding to its complexity, human brain is extremely fragile and can be affected by numerous stimuli during any of the phases of in utero and ex utero life affecting brain function and development. Some of these factors are genetic factors or defects, epigenetic factors from the environment or from the human body which are at the vast majority of the cases unable to be assessed and obstetricians cannot evaluate the degree of their consequences.[1] Therefore, neurological impairment is one of the most feared perinatal complications and as data proved that cerebral palsy (CP) most often is the result of prenatal than perinatal or postnatal events,[3] the antenatal diagnosis of neurological impairment and evaluation of fetal nervous system integrity have been the dream of obstetricians.[4,5]

The first steps to make this dream reality have been made from Kurjak and his team. They realized that in order to evaluate and define neurological defects prenatally is more than important to comprehend firstly normal fetal behavior. Many scientists also noticed that neonatal behavior is not much different from fetal behavior.[4] A pioneer test introduced by Kurjak; Kurjak antenatal neurodevelopmental test (KANET) uses 4D ultrasound to assess fetal behavior and movements in a simulative way of neonatal assessment postnatally (ATNAT test–the Amiel-Tison Neurological Assessment At Term).[6] Many multicenter studies have been published since then, proving that the test has the potential to identify fetuses in risk for neurodevelopment impairment and it can be used in everyday clinical practice.[6]

■ FETAL CENTRAL NERVOUS SYSTEM: STAGES OF DEVELOPMENT

Behavioral patterns and motoric function of the fetus have to be assessed by comprehending the development of fetus' motor and sensory pathways, by understanding the maturational steps and myelination stages, as

TABLE 1: The most important progressive steps and landmarks of human brain development.

	Start	Active period	End
Formation of neurons	At 4 weeks	8–12 weeks	Approximately at 20 weeks
Migration	At the same time with proliferation	18–24 weeks	38 weeks
Formation of synapses	Spinal cord: 6th–7th week Cortical plate: 8th week	13th week to 2 years of postnatal life	Puberty

Source: Modified from Kurjak et al.[14]

fetal cerebral growth and maturation are in accordance with fetal motility.[7]

During third postconceptional week, neural plate is formed by the generation of the neuroectoderm from ectoderm.[8] The neural plate then gives rise to the neural tube, which will eventually lead to the formation of all the parts of the nervous system. The fetal brain starts developing as early as the 4th week of fetal life, and at that time the main parts of the brain can be identified.[9] Moreover, at 19th week of gestation, in the subplate zone the earliest cortical electric activity takes place. Interestingly, between weeks 13 and 25 of gestation, subplate zone inhabits in nearly half of the hemisphere.

The first signs of neurologic function can be noted with the appearance of connections between neurons, which are not permanent and disappear later as other early structured take part in this strict developmental process of fetal brain development. **Tables 1 and 2** list all these complicated and overlapping stages and processes that take part in the development of fetal nervous system.

By the first 20 weeks of pregnancy, a significant amount of synapses have already developed forming the right environment for the final stages of the formation of the fetal brain including not only the anatomical part but also the functional part.[9] As the fetus grows, neuronal paths develop and processes

TABLE 2: Major events in neural development.

Developmental event	Peak time of occurrence
Early formation of neurons	3–4 weeks
Prosencephalic formation	5–6 weeks
Cerebral neural formation	8–14 weeks
Cerebellar neural proliferation	2–10 months after delivery
Cerebral neural migration	14–26 weeks
Cerebellar neural migration	14–40 weeks
Neuronal differentiation (axon growth)	14 weeks—delivery
Neuronal differentiation	28 weeks—12 months after delivery
Organization of synapses	From delivery and on
Myelination	From delivery and on

Source: Modified by Kurjak et al.[2]

of myelination are completed until the 29th week of gestation, while final connections between the thalamus and the cortex are also completed by that time, playing a major role to the cortical processing of sensory information and mental processes.[10] Moreover, final myelination and connections from the cortex can be verified by evoked potentials from 29 weeks of gestation onward. At the third trimester, the formation of synapses could reach the speed of 40,000 synapses/min.

After the 32nd gestational week, the final neocortex appearance of six-layered lamination can be observed. Also, after 34th week of gestation the subplate zone disappears.[10] Finally, neocortex remains one of the parts of the brain that is not fully developed until delivery and many of its functions are taken over by parts of the brainstem.

For an overview, first and second trimester of pregnancy are the most critical periods for cortical development, as proliferation, neuronal migration, organization, and connection take place. At third trimester, growth and differentiation are the predominant events and continue after birth.[11] For neonates that are born at term the processes of proliferation and migration have finalized, there are still other processes that continue really intensively and these are mainly processes that have to do with differentiation of the neurons.[12,13]

FETAL MOVEMENTS EVALUATED BY ULTRASONOGRAPHY

Evolution of Four-dimensional Sonography Enables Fetal Movements Assessment

The primary assessment of fetal well-being was maternal registration of fetal movements. Nowadays, there is no doubt that the development of 4D ultrasound technology played a crucial role to in-utero functional study and movement patterns. Andonotopo et al.[15] showed that when 4D ultrasound is used, from 7th gestational week movements of the fetal parts can be seen, while the conventional two-dimensional (2D) ultrasound can detect fetal motility a week later. Importantly, the evolution of ultrasound technology allowed depiction in extreme detail of fetal movements of the face, even the most detailed ones,[16,17] as spatial recognition of facial details and visualizations of small structures are possible due to 4D sonography. Furthermore, 4D technology can define the characteristics of isolated limb movements, upper extremity movements, and target of the fingers.[18] The opportunity to visualize these detailed fetal characteristics opened a new window on how to assess fetal brain function and to form a method and standards of neurodevelopment.[19]

Fetal Movements throughout Pregnancy

Fetal behavior in utero should be evaluated as a whole due to the fact that the different movement patterns of each week could define normal and abnormal neurodevelopment.[6] According to Nijhuis and Arabin et al., fetal behavior can be the reaction of the fetus to stimuli reflecting CNS integrity and early neuromuscular development.[20,21]

At the first trimester, as fetal brain develops and matures fetal movement patterns are increasing.[18] As **Tables 1 and 2** list, spinal cord synapses appear between 6th and 7th week and during the 8th week in the cortical plate. At that time electrical synapses develop, and the time when the earliest spontaneous fetal movements make their appearance.[14] These movements have been described as "vermicular", as they consist of asymmetrical movements of the trunk and extremities.[22,23] Development of brainstem starts around 7th week, and is responsible for head, trunk movements, and movements of hands and feet, but also for the control of respiratory movements and fetal heart rate rhythm.[24]

General movements (GMs) are controlled by supraspinal centers and they consist of movements of the head, the body, and the extremities, including the subtle movements that are seen in the first week of pregnancy, until 10 weeks.[25] As pregnancy advances even from 8 weeks the movements become more detailed as a result of the increased synapses. Nevertheless, during the first 20 weeks of pregnancy the fetal brain has not developed substantially and does not yet control the motoric function of the fetus.[9] After the first 10 weeks, the fetal movements become more increased and organized, showing more skilled movements such as movements of the head such as rotational movements. Additionally, the first eye movements and mouth opening make their appearance at week 10, when in 12th week swallowing reflex is present. The most frequent movements after the 10th week are movements of the upper extremities while around the 12th week repetitive movements like jumping can be noticed more often.[26]

During the second trimester fetal activity increases and the longest period without observation of any movement is only 5–6 minutes. Furthermore, this period is characterized by increased complexity of movements. Zagreb group proved that as early as at the 13th gestational week, hand movements can be seen.[18] These fetal motility could be characterized further according to where the hand is directed.[18] As we reach the middle of the pregnancy period and around the 16th week, already 13 different types of movements have developed, and every week new movements make their debut. Therefore, during the period starting from 13th to 16th gestational week, there are prolonged episodes of position alterations, while after 17th week flexion and extension movements or even body movements accompany the isolated limb movements. Movements of the head and trunk are still present and harmonized. Additionally, facial expressions make their first appearance at 16th–18th gestational week and they are now part of the repertoire of fetal motor activity, mouthing,

yawning, hiccups, sucking, and swallowing.[14] By 28 weeks, movements and expressions of the face are seen with the exception of eyes opening and closing which begins to consolidate from 24 weeks of gestation.[27]

During second half of pregnancy and for the last 10 weeks,[28] number and frequency of fetal activity declines while resting periods are longer. This decrease was first attributed to the decrease of amniotic fluid, but studies show that is related to the increased maturation of brainstem during these last weeks.[24] At the same time that the fetal activity decreases, there is an increase in facial expressions and facial movements with tongue expulsion being the more frequently noticed facial movement. Interestingly, according to Patrick et al.[29] starting from the 30 gestational weeks, fetuses begin to stretch and roll. This is part of a normal fetal neurological development and is more obvious when the GM are not so prominent.[24]

To sum up, fetal movements have their debut in the embryonic life, even before they can be identified by the pregnant woman. They start general and synchronized fetal actions that include the trunk and at term near delivery fetal activity changes from random movements to well-organized and detailed behavioral patterns, accompanied by harmonized facial expressions.[30]

General Movements

General movements have to be discussed further, as they reflect directly brain function.[31] These movements are smooth and complex with fluctuation on their amplitude, involving head, trunk, arms, and limbs[32] lasting from a few seconds to a minute. Changes of their fluency, elegance, variability, fluctuation of intensity, and speed being monotonous and chaotic are signs of brain activity impairment and one initial sign of cortical influence of the fetal motoric activity.[31] Additionally, the quality of GM at 2–4 months postnatally is very sensitive for diagnosing neonates that have higher possibility regarding CP and other neurodevelopmental disorders.[7]

FROM FETUS TO NEONATE: THE PROGRESS OF NEUROBEHAVIOR

As it is mentioned several times above, synaptogenesis, neural differentiation, myelination, and the dynamic connection between neurons is a life-long procedure, continuing throughout pregnancy, birth, and adult life.[33] Hence, it is logical to be a progressive change of neurobehavior from antenatal to postnatal life.[34] Although fetal activity can be identified from early pregnancy even after 6th week, fetal movement behavior after second half of pregnancy should be taken into consideration when fetal behavior is compared to the neonatal, as during this period neuronal migration and development of the neocortex is complete.[14]

According to Stanojevic et al.,[4] all neonatal movements are also present in utero, and these are all the detailed movements that are described later in the so-called KANET test.[16] Concerning GM, their amplitude and pattern remain identical until the 2nd month after birth.[35] There is only one reflex that cannot be assessed on fetuses: the Moro reflex. This differentiation has been attributed to different environmental and epigenetic factors to which they are exposed in utero and also the first days of extrauterine life: during in utero life, the fetus lives in so-called "microgravity" and after birth, neonate meets the "tyranny of gravity". This statement has been doubted by many scientists, it cannot be proven that the fetus develops in gravity-free environment at least not for the entire gestational period.[36] Nevertheless, to the longest part of gestation, the fetus can move freely and away from the uterine walls, simulating a microgravity environment.[37] However, gravity forces have a significant role in normal musculoskeletal development of the fetus and neonate and the appearance of the earliest antigravity movements takes place within the first month of life. There is no doubt that "the fetus evolves to be a neonate so it is the same living human being under different environmental state".[4]

INTRODUCTION OF KURJAK'S ANTENATAL NEURODEVELOPMENTAL TEST

The stages of CNS development and mainly the stages of human brain maturation are reflected to the movements and overall neurobehavior during in utero life.[3,38] Additionally, many studies present data proving that the fetal activity, that is the type of movements in terms of frequency and which parts are involved mirror the neurological maturation of fetal brain.[39] Therefore, identification of activity models during in utero life and for different trimesters or weeks could make possible the formation of normal neurobehavior, which when are not identified could lead to the suspicion or diagnosis of pathological conditions[40-43] and more importantly to facilitate prompt identification of a wide variety of neurological abnormalities.[27] Moreover, postnatal studies evaluating neonatal behavior proved that it has higher sensitivity for detection of neurodevelopmental impairment than the traditional clinical examination.[44] Finally, this progressive formation of nervous system that is reflected by the behavioral patterns from in utero to postnatal life is established.[14]

Neurodevelopmental defects and especially CP are one of the most feared perinatal complications. A main reason for this concern is the delay on its diagnosis and because neurological deficits and their effects accompany both the patients and their environment for a lifetime. Additionally, the high prevalence of CP, the lack of an effective treatment, and its doubtful cause are the factors that made CP a great field for clinical research. CP is a multifactorial neurological condition with variable expressions, reasons, and time of diagnosis. Therefore, nowadays the term "cerebral palsy spectrum" (CPS) is recommended. Interestingly, although cesarean section rates have been launched during the 21st century, CP incidence did not change the last 50 years, with its prevalence staying stable at 2–2.5/1,000 births.[45] Therefore, it is obvious that CP is not related with the mode of delivery.

Considering the parameters above, Kurjak and his team introduced a renovating test for the examination of neurobehavior during in-utero life, by applying ultrasound techniques, mainly real time 4D ultrasound. The primary goal of this new test is the determination of normality as far as it concerns neurologic development and, hence, identify behaviors that are far from the so-called normality in utero, by examining fetal motoric activity and through that, fetal neurodevelopment. The so-called KANET consists of parameters regarding fetal behavioral patterns in terms of GM and aspects of postnatal Amiel-Tison postnatal test (ATNAT) **(Figs. 1A to H)**.[46]

Kurjak's antenatal neurodevelopmental test includes the following parameters: isolated head anteflexion, overlapping cranial sutures, head circumference, isolated eye blinking, facial alterations, mouth opening (yawning or mouthing), isolated hand and leg movements and thumb position, and gestalt perception of GM **(Table 3)**. Three of the parameters KANET evaluates (neurological thumb, overlapping sutures, and small head circumference) are also postnatal signs of

neurological impairment.[35] Special attention has to be taken to facial expressions, as "the face is the mirror of the brain". When the score is between 10 and 16 the test considers as normal, between 6 and 9 borderline, and between 0 and 5 abnormal **(Table 4)**.

Kurjak's antenatal neurodevelopmental test has been standardized through the first and second consensus in Osaka and Bucharest respectively and over the years has undergone simplified modifications. Its value in application of every day routine has been established as a powerful tool for early diagnosis of neurological impairment. The test has been designed for the last one-third of pregnancy, that is after 28 weeks and only while the fetus is active, and not in a sleeping period. If the fetus is not in an awake mode the test should be repeated after about 30 minutes or if that is not possible it could be transferred to the following day (after 14–16 hours). The test is calculated to take around 15–20 minutes. If the result of the case is pathological or borderline, then the protocol says to follow-up the fetus twice weekly to the delivery time and continue postnatal follow-up.[35] Furthermore, fetuses that have undergone KANET assessment should be followed up for 2 years so that the results are objective and conclusive.

Good reproducibility of the test has been verified.[4] Finger movements had the highest interobserver agreement (K = 0.84), while facial expressions had the lowest (K = 0.68). The teaching method has been standardized as well and a KANET diploma of training has been established. In addition, it has been calculated that the examiner has to perform 80 KANET tests in order to get acquainted to the test method, a number which is comparable with other prenatal US tests. KANET test presents extremely high negative predicting

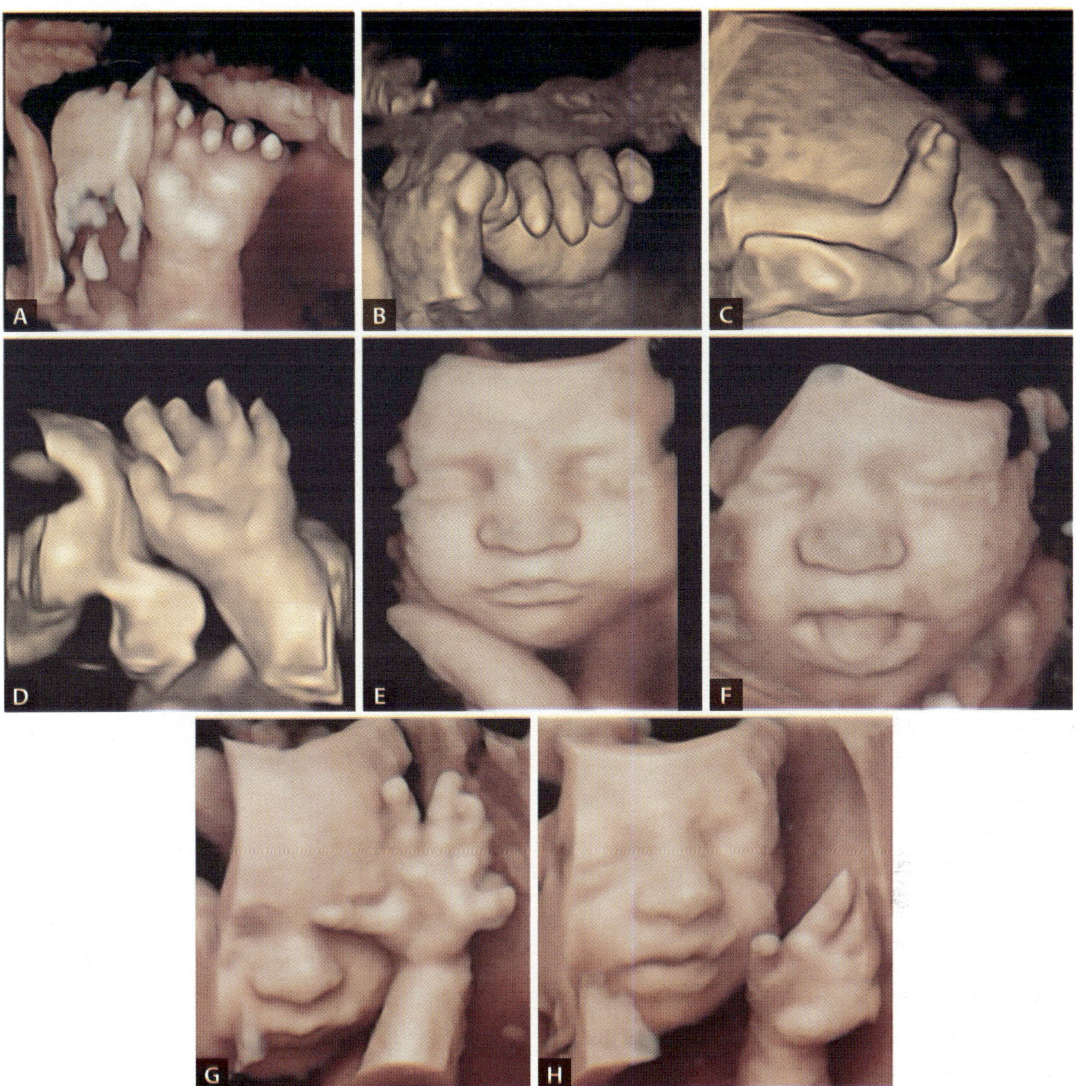

Figs. 1A to H: Kurjak's antenatal neurodevelopmental test (KANET) examines the fetal face and fetal extremities and evolution of technology reveals the potential of this test.

value (100%) and acceptable sensitivity and specificity.[11]

Studies regarding CP and other neurological disorders such as schizophrenia, epilepsy, and autism have their origin in fetal life.[35] Also, Palmer et al.[47] claimed that among 7-year-old children with CP, neonatal neurological examination was normal. Introduction of KANET test and its capability to diagnose in-utero neurological impairment carries significant advantages. The most important is that as this test has the potential of the very early detection of the fetuses in-risk for neurodevelopmental defects, intervention can occur much earlier resulting in a better outcome.[4] For example, early physiotherapy has been proved that has a great role and improves significantly the prognosis of infants

TABLE 3: KANET (Kurjak's antenatal neurodevelopmental test) parameters (Standardized by Bucharest Consensus).

Sign	Score 1	Score 2	Score 3
Isolated head anteflexion	Abrupt	Small range (0–3 times of movements)	Variable in full range, many alteration (>3 times of movements)
Cranial sutures and head circumferences	Overlapping cranial sutures	Normal cranial sutures with measurement of HC below or above the normal limit (–2 SD) according to GA	Normal cranial sutures with normal measurement of HC according to GA
Isolated eye blinking	Not present	Not fluent (1–5 times of blinking)	Fluency (>5 times of blinking)
Facial alteration (grimace or tongue expulsion) or *Mouth opening (yawning or mouthing)* **(Figs. 2 and 3)**	Not present	Not fluent (1–5 times of alteration)	Fluency (>5 times of alteration)
Isolated led movements	Cramped	Poor repertoire or small in range (0–5 times of movements)	Variable in full range, many alterations (>times of movements)
Isolated hand movements or hand and face movements	Cramped or abrupt	Poor repertoire or small in range (0–5 times of movement)	Variable in full range, many alternation (>5 times of movements)
Fingers movements	Unilateral or bilateral clenched fist, (neurological thumb)	Cramped invariable finger movements	Smooth and complex, variable finger movements
Gestalt perception of GM	Definitely abnormal	Borderline	Normal

(GA: gestational age; GM: general movements; HC: head circumference; SD: standard deviation)

in all aspects. Moreover, physiotherapy can improve in these patients their motoric system and even other parameters of the nervous system. Additionally, timely counseling from a psychologist could have long-term advantages for both the baby and its environment, regarding better parental mental health with less stress, improved parental-infant relationship and also children in preschool age present less internalizing behaviors. As there is little that could be done for the management of the infant with neurological retardation and because effectiveness of treatment is not optimal, the timely intervention is crucial for the better outcome.[4] Nevertheless, further research has to take place to define the ideal intervention which provides the optimal outcome.

REVIEW OF STUDIES: 10 YEARS EXPERIENCE OF KURJAK'S ANTENATAL NEURODEVELOPMENTAL TEST APPLICATION

Since the introduction of the KANET more than 10 years of clinical use have passed, many studies have been published and hundreds of

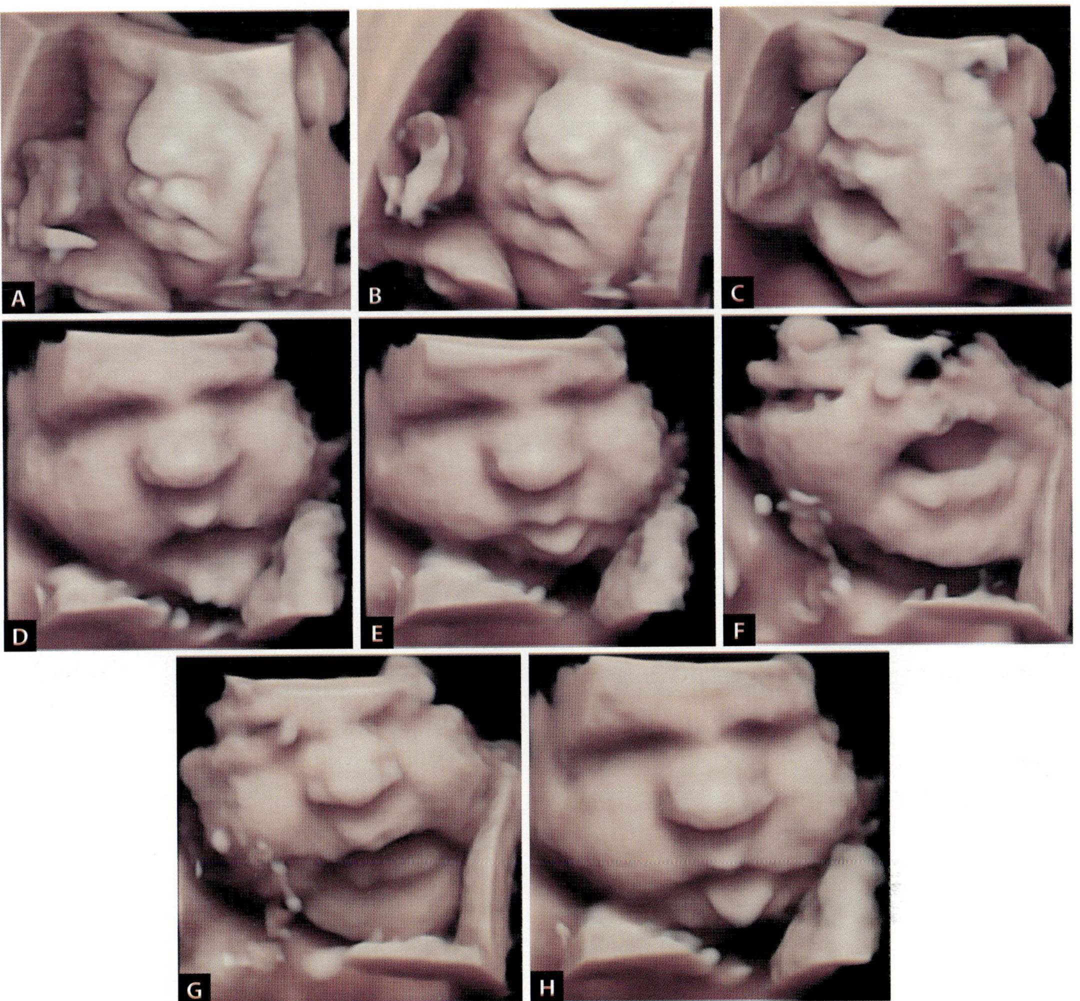

Figs. 2A to H: Facial alterations, grimacing, yawning, and tongue expulsion can be altered permanently or transiently by different maternal or environmental conditions.

test have been performed globally and the evidence they provide is really promising, as it seems that the KANET is able to detect severe neurological defects in utero and its results are in extreme accordance with the postnatal neurological outcome. Hence, the KANET has the potential to cover a great gap of fetal medicine regarding the diagnosis of neurological fetal conditions and detect pregnancies in high risk for neurodevelopmental impairment such as

CP, autism spectrum disorder (ASD), and others.[6]

Even before KANET introduction for fetal neurological assessment, Andonotopo et al., in 2006, studied prospectively with 4D imaging in utero behavior, in low-risk cases, and in fetuses complicated with growth restriction. Their goal was to assess whether these aspects of fetal behavior could predict the incidence of CP in growth restricted fetuses. The authors concluded that

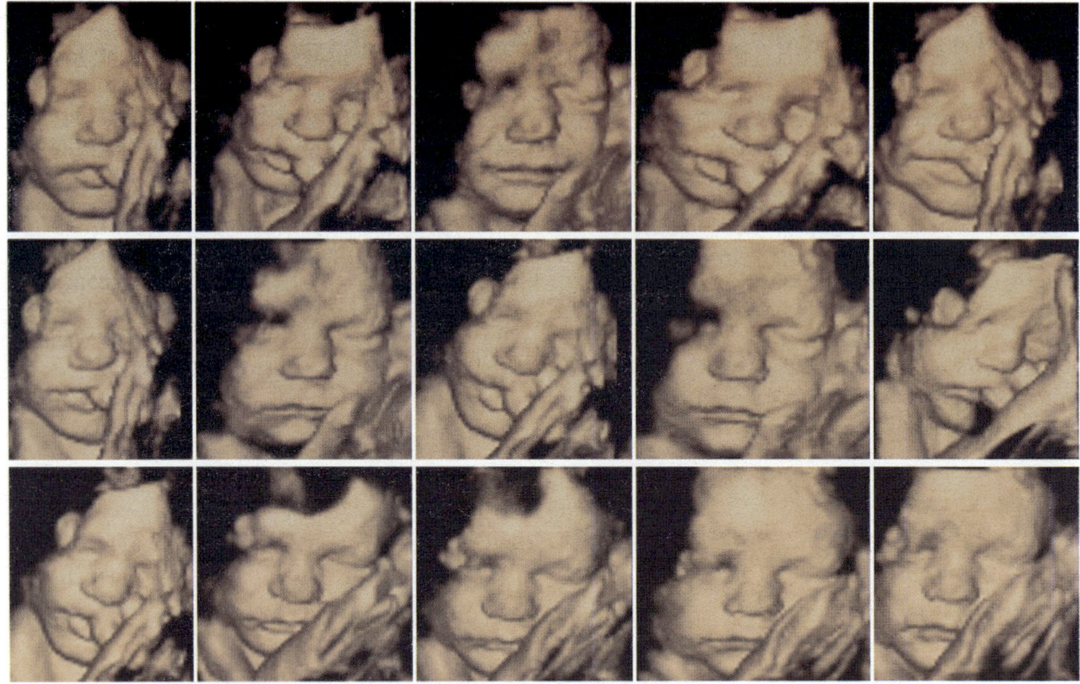

Fig. 3: Facial alteration is a landmark of fetal neurological assessment.

TABLE 4: Interpretation of KANET (Kurjak's antenatal neurodevelopmental test) scores.

Total score	Interpretation
0–5	Abnormal
6–9	Borderline
10–16	Normal

intrauterine growth restriction (IUGR) fetuses tended to be less active and they encouraged further investigation of the potential of 4D sonography to evaluate fetal behavior and therefore brain impairment.[48]

In the first multicenter study, four centers took part and were published in 2010 with almost 300 cases (Zagreb—Croatia, Istanbul—Turkey, Bucharest—Romania, and Doha—Qatar). Fetuses underwent KANET prenatally and ATNAT test at the first to third day of life. Concerning KANET test, 7 cases had abnormal score while 25 cases had borderline, identifying 32 fetuses in high risk for neurological defect. The seven neonates with the abnormal score were followed up postnatally since the 10th week of life and three of them (3/7) had also abnormal ATNAT test **(Fig. 4)**. These fetuses had arthrogryposis, vermis aplasia, and sibling with CP, respectively. The facial expressions of these fetuses were significantly decreased: the authors characterized them as masks due to the total absence of any expression at the time of examination. The other neonates showed no pathological findings. 22 cases that resulted not normal result (borderline score) showed also borderline ATNAT score. The underlying causes were variable including abnormal CNS anatomical findings or other fetal or maternal pathology. The remaining three (3/25) were cases with ventriculomegaly, intra-amniotic infection, and maternal thrombocytopenia had

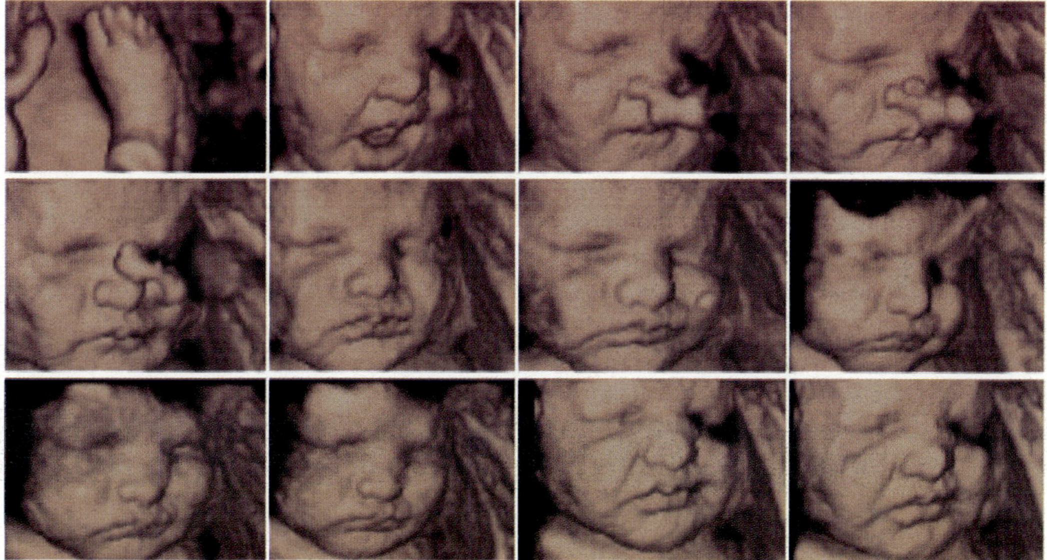

Fig. 4: Assessment of fetal neurobehavior. Four-dimensional (4D) ultrasound allows assessment of the fetus similarly to neonatal assessment.

normal ATNAT scores. In six cases there was a stillbirth and another five opted to stop their pregnancy. The authors drew the conclusion that the test can be helpful in prenatal detection of cases in high risk for neurodevelopmental impairment, especially in pregnancies with risk factors.[49]

Miskovic et al. published 10 years ago an article with really promising results. They studied 226 cases and three of them had a pathological score. These cases were chromosomally abnormal and also had postnatally abnormal ATNAT tests. The parameters of KANET test had also been assessed individually and there was a differentiation in eight of them between low- and high-risk pregnancies. When the two tests were compared (the antenatal KANET and the postnatal ATNAT), a moderate but statistically significant correlation between them was noticed, confirming that the postnatal ATNAT test agrees with the findings of the prenatal test.[50]

A large multicenter paper that included >600 cases confirmed the findings of previous studies regarding the differences in the KANET scores between normal and pathological cases, such as chromosomal abnormalities. Interestingly, the high-risk group with previous cases of CP had the higher percentage of pathological scores while in cases of maternal pyrexia antenatally the results of borderline scores were increased. When the parameters of the KANET test were evaluated one by one, the parameters that were statistically more frequently different from normal to pathological cases were identified. A new observation that derived from this study was the correlation of pathological score and the risk of stillbirth or even early postnatal-neonatal death. Out of 36 cases that had pathological score, the follow-up in 10 of them was found to have severe generalized spasticity, confirming the strength of predicting value of the KANET. Therefore, there were two conclusions concerning this study: an abnormal KANET score can predict not only neurological impairment but also intrauterine and neonatal mortality.[51]

The Dubai group study all cases up to three times between 28th and 38th gestational week. The fetuses were followed up postnatally just after birth and at 3 months of life including complete clinical assessment. The two scores of prenatal and postnatal assessment were assessed and the result was that normal prenatal tests were assertive of good postnatal outcome at both times, immediately after delivery and at 3 months of age.[52]

Talic et al. run an interesting trial, investigating movement behavior with the usage of KANET in normal fetuses (n = 100) and in fetuses with cerebral ventriculomegaly (n = 140), between 32nd and 36th gestational week. Only 6% of the fetuses in the normal brain structure resulted pathological scoring, while for the ventriculomegaly cases this percentage was 34.9%. When ventriculomegaly was related with other findings, especially anatomical abnormalities from CNS the risk of abnormal KANET score was higher. Interestingly, abnormal scores were not seen for fetuses with isolated—mild to moderate—ventriculomegaly. KANET results were in accordance with the postnatal neurological outcome. From this study, several important conclusions could be drawn: firstly, it is proved that the KANET can predict postnatal outcome of fetuses with ventriculomegaly, identifying also the degree that their behavior has been affected, so that not only an anatomical abnormality is detected but also at what level this affects the fetus. Secondly, it was clear that coexisting malformations besides ventriculomegaly affect KANET score and therefore neurological outcome. As ventriculomegaly is a finding whose clinical significance is not well-defined, KANET adds knowledge regarding the degree that this finding affects the fetus so that a more complete parental counseling and management can be achieved.[53,54]

Abo-Yaqoub also concluded to same results with the studies mentioned above: the KANET shows differences that are confirmed postnatally when studying pregnancies of different background and with different risk factors. Also, fetuses with abnormal KANET scores have higher odds to remain abnormal postnatally, while there was a tendency for fetuses with borderline KANET scores to normalize after birth. Moreover, they found which parameters could be more different in these populations.[53,54]

Additionally, the Romanian group applied KANET in almost 200 cases including high-risk cases. They came to the conclusion that KANET scores as long and fetal movements differed significantly between the two groups; 93.4% of fetuses on the low-risk group had normal scores, while almost 80% in the other group (high-risk) had a normal score. Accordingly, borderline scores resulted from fetuses in the high-risk group and more specifically from the subgroup of growth restriction and affected resistance index of middle cerebral artery (MCA-RI) or maternal hypertension. Concerning fetuses with abnormal KANET scores, the vast majority of them were complicated with preterm premature rupture of the membranes (PPROM). The predominant part of fetuses with Rh isoimmunization achieved a normal KANET score. Furthermore, when the subgroup of IUGR fetuses was assessed, it was noticed that the movements of the fetuses in this group were all different; number and duration of GM in addition with their organization were affected. Therefore, the authors ended up to the conclusion that the

KANET could be used for timely diagnosis of neurological defects.[32]

Honemeyer et al. in their second study applied a series of KANET evaluation in 56 singleton pregnancies—both low and risk—during 28 and 38 weeks of gestation, performing at total 117 tests. As one fetus underwent more than one test, they introduced the term "average KANET score". Although, they do not find any abnormal average scores, the vast majority [two-thirds (2/3)] in the middle group score (borderline) were presented in the cases with risk factors. Only one fetus with borderline score was found to be abnormal at postnatal neurological evaluation.[55]

In a study with >800 cases with main subject fetuses with IUGR and Doppler changes a significant difference was observed between these groups and completed the findings of previous studies that fetuses of high-risk groups have increased risk of borderline or pathological result in utero but also postnatally.[56]

Athanasiadis and his group examined about 150 cases of mixed high- and low-risk populations and compared the KANET scores and confirmed that the low-risk cases had higher scores. Additionally, when subgroups on the high-risk team were compared, fetuses whose pregnancies were complicated with diabetes mellitus (DM) achieved higher KANET scores than pregnancies complicated with IUGR or pre-eclampsia. Therefore, the authors stated that the KANET is a feasible technique for neurological assessment of pregnancies with high risk for adverse neurological outcome.[57]

Neto et al. in a pilot study confirmed that all pathological scores were from the group that contained the high-risk cases, while the low-risk cases had no pathological scores, concluding that neurobehavior depending on the risk factors of each pregnancy differ significantly.[58]

Hanaoka et al. performed a trial in 89 Japanese (Asian) and 78 Croatian (European) pregnant women in order to evaluate the effect on the test of different ethnical parameters and which parameters of the test could be affected. Differences between the two ethnic groups were noted and the specific parameters of the test that were affected were identified. This study drew a conclusion that ethnicity is a parameter that should be taken under consideration when fetal neurobehavior assessment is done and that this is more significant regarding some facial movements. However, these differences do not affect the overall and final KANET test score.[59]

Hata et al. from Kagawa, Japan published the study with the longest follow-up so far. They applied the KANET in 353 fetuses with uncomplicated pregnancies and they followed up them for 2 years. 95.4% (337/353) of fetuses achieved normal scores and the remaining 4.6% (16/353) resulted to a borderline score. Hence, there were not any abnormal scores. Five out of the 337 (1.48%) of fetuses with normal score were found to present postnatal developmental disability with mean age of diagnosis 3–24 months of age. Concerning fetuses with borderline scores, three out of 16 (18.75%) had also neurological defects: motor developmental delay (diagnosed at 6 months), Duchenne muscular dystrophy (diagnosed at 18 months) and ASD (diagnosed at 30 months). The authors noticed a difference in the postnatal assessment of neonates when there was a difference in the antenatal assessment as well and they reached to the conclusion that the KANET can be used as a diagnostic tool for the prediction of postnatal neurodevelopmental defects.[60]

Vladereanu et al. in their second trial performed KANET in 280 cases. 195 of them were categorized as low-risk cases while the remaining 85 were assigned in high-risk group for neurological impairment. Two cases had pathological KANET scores and nine were found to have borderline results. The remaining cases had been characterized as normal. From the pathological and borderline cases most of them were related to pathology fetal or maternal. In all cases, the assessment that was performed postnatally was uneventful.[45]

The Brazilian group after their pilot study performed a prospective cohort trial with 631 fetuses from singleton pregnancies which were divided into low- (n = 406) and high-risk (n = 225) group. They assessed KANET test to the fetuses between 28 and 38 weeks of gestation and they followed up the neonates in order to evaluate postnatal outcome. KANET scores between the two groups and the postnatal outcomes were compared. For the 19 fetuses with abnormal scores, five were related to pregnancy condition (pre-eclampsia, PPROM, and drug abuse) while the remaining 14 fetal condition were responsible (IUGR and trisomies 13, 18, 21). Follow-up was available for only 212 of the fetuses and according to the parents' knowledge, none of them has diagnosed with abnormal neurological findings or developmental problems so far.[45]

In Poland, a group of scientists examined the reaction in utero after acoustic stimulation, and especially the neurological effect of the acoustic stimulation and recorded that by applying KANET. The inspiration for this study came by data shown by previous studies that the vibroacoustic stimulation can cause changes in fetal heart rate patterns and that fetal motility can be altered particularly by an increase in fetal activity.[61] Indeed Bomba-Opon et al. showed that acoustic stimulation caused an increase in the pathological KANET scores and a decrease in the normal ones, without any improvement in the overall KANET score in any of the fetuses. They also managed to identify the parameters that are mainly affected by such interference which included: grimacing, eye blinking, and mouth opening, lower and upper extremity movements. The fact that fetal neurobehavior as shown by KANET is not affected by vibroacoustic stimulation shows that KANET is an objective way of assessing the fetus that is not altered by temporary external stimuli.

A more recent study that contained of almost 150 pregnancies confirmed the previous studies findings as from the low-risk group, there were no abnormal KANET results and from the high-risk cases derived all the nonnormal test results and most of the borderline cases and these were cases of severe IUGR and gestational diabetes.

Antsaklis et al. in Greece published a study including cases of pre-existing DM or gestational diabetes mellitus (GDM) that all required and were under treatment with insulin and applied antenatal neurological assessment with KANET. The authors compared these results with KANET scores from pregnancies that were uneventful and had normal oral glucose tolerance test (OGTT). Maternal characteristics concerning maternal and gestational age were not statistically significant different within the study sub-groups. For nondiabetic cases, the results of KANET appeared constantly and statistically significant higher. Hence, differences in neurobehavior were noted among the two groups. When further analysis of the parameters of KANET test was done, the three parameters that had the biggest differences were identified and these were blinking of the eyes, facial grimacing, and detailed movements of fingers. These were the movements that were noted to have with the biggest difference between the two groups.[62]

One of the most recent studies was that of the Indian group of KANET collaboration where they included only high-risk cases. Inclusion criteria were: DM (n = 13), diabetes diagnosed during pregnancy (GDM: n = 18), pregnancy-induced hypertension (PIH: n = 31), thyroid disease (n = 16), infection during pregnancy (n = 8), and cardiac disease (n = 1). They applied KANET after the 28th week of pregnancy until delivery and at least twice until then. Almost all fetuses that were assessed had normal KANET score, except for one case that showed a borderline result. A strong element of this particular study was that all fetuses that were examined antenatally also had a postnatal follow-up, which started immediately after delivery and lasted up to 2 years of life. Four postnatal assessments, from fetuses that derived from pregnancies that were complicated with GDM and PIH and during prenatal neurodevelopmental assessment had normal scores, recorded delay in the development of these neonates but not before 16 months after delivery. Another significant observation of this study was that even if KANET was normal during in utero life, if there was a significant drop from one score to the other (from the first to the second), then the risk of showing delay in some developmental milestones increased. But, even if the decrease was not significant there was a decrease from the first KANET to the second one was also considered to have worse prognosis compared to those that their KANET score increased during this 2–4 weeks antenatal period. When the KANET score was >14 the prognosis was better than when the KANET was 11–14, showing lower risk of postnatal neurological delay. The authors drew the conclusion that KANET is able to detect fetuses in increased risk for neurodevelopmental delay.[45]

Honemeyer et al. reported two really interesting cases of fetal akinesia deformation sequence. Examiners were surprised by the total immobility of the otherwise structural normal fetuses. When KANET was applied, both fetuses had extremely low scores (3 and 2 respectively).[45]

■ CONCLUSION

We may have reached a very good level regarding the assessment of fetal CNS anatomy but still there is a long way until we manage to assess the whole neurological system of the fetus. There is no doubt that fetal movement patterns reflect brain's maturation progress of every week of growth. Additionally, as sonography technology has made huge steps, introducing the 4D ultrasound in clinical routine, we are approaching the era when physicians could be able to have a clearer insight of the mysterious development of human brain.

Kurjak antenatal neurodevelopmental test can make the neurological evaluation for fetus and neonate just two tests in series. The primary goal of the KANET is the evaluation of fetal nervous system integrity and the timely diagnosis of functional and structural neurological impairment. So far, data from many multicenter studies are very promising, showing that the KANET is able to identify functional aspects of fetal behavior, enabling the detection of normal and abnormal fetal neurodevelopment. This information could be really valuable for timely intervention, better, and more accurate parental counseling. Nevertheless, further research is necessary for the establishment of the KANET in every day clinical practice. Worldwide, many studies have been started and very interesting results regarding the potential of KANET assessment on the timely diagnosis of fetuses in high risk for neurodevelopmental defects are yet to be published.

■ REFERENCES

1. Antsaklis P, Kurjak A, Izetbegovic S. Functional test for fetal brain: the role of KANET test. DSJUOG. 2013;7(4):385-99.
2. Kurjak A, Carrera JM, Stanojevic M, Andonotopo W, Azumendi G, Scazzocchio E, et al. The role of 4D sonography in the neurological assessment of early human development. Ultrasound Rev Obstet Gynecol. 2004;4(3):148-59.
3. Salihagic-Kadic A, Kurjak A, Medic M, Andonotopo W, Azumendi G. New data about embryonic and fetal neurodevelopment and behavior obtained by 3D and 4D sonography. J Perinat Med. 2005;33(6):478-90.
4. Stanojevic M, Zaputovic S, Bosnjak AP. Continuity between fetal and neonatal neurobehavior. Semin Fetal Neonatal Med. 2012;17(6):324-9.
5. Haak P, Lenski M, Hidecker MJC, Li M, Paneth N. Cerebral palsy and aging. Dev Med Child Neurol. 2009;51(Suppl 4):16-23.
6. Kurjak A, Antsaklis P, Stanojevic M, Porovic S. Fetal behavior assessed by four-dimensional sonography. Donald Sch J Ultrasound Obstet Gynecol. 2017;11(2):146-68.
7. Hadders-Algra M. General movements: A window for early identification of children at high risk for developmental disorders. J Pediatr. 2004;145(Suppl 2):S12-8.
8. Pomeroy SL, Voipe JJ. Development of the nervous system. In: Polin RA, Fox, WW (Eds). Fetal and Neonatal Physiology. Philadelphia-London-Toronto-Montreal-Sydney-Tokyo: WB Saunders Company; 1992. pp. 1491-509.
9. Kostovic I, Judas M, Petanjek Z, Simic G. Ontogenesis of goal-directed behavior: anatomo-functional considerations. Int J Psychophysiol. 1995;19(2):85-102.
10. Vasung L, Lepage C, Radoš M, Pletikos M, Goldman JS, Richiardi J, et al. Quantitative and qualitative analysis of transient fetal compartments during prenatal human brain development. Front Neuroanat. 2016;10:11.
11. Stanojevic M, Antsaklis P, Salihagic-Kadic A, Predojevic M, Vladareanu R, Vlădăreanu S, et al. Is Kurjak antenatal neurodevelopmental test ready for routine clinical application? Bucharest consensus statement. Donald Sch J Ultrasound Obstet Gynecol. 2015;9(3):260-5.
12. Schaher S. Determination and differentiation in the development of the nervous system. In: Kandel ER, Schwartz JH (Eds). Principles of Neural Science, 2nd edition. New York: Elsevier Science Publishing; 1985. pp. 730-2.
13. Kostovic I. Prenatal development of nucleus basalis complex and related fiber systems in man: a histochemical study. Neuroscience. 1986;17(4):1047-77.
14. Kurjak A, Antsaklis P, Stanojevic M. Fetal neurology: past, present and future. Donald Sch J Ultrasound Obstet Gynecol. 2015;9(1):6-29.
15. Andonotopo W, Medic M, Salihagic-Kadic A, Milenkovic D, Maiz N, Scazzocchio E. The assessment of fetal behavior in early pregnancy: comparison between 2D and 4D sonographic scanning. J Perinat Med. 2005;33(5):406-14.
16. Kurjak A, Stanojevic M, Andonotopo W, Salihagic-Kadic A, Carrera JM, Azumendi G. Behavioral pattern continuity from prenatal to postnatal life—a study by four-dimensional (4D) ultrasonography. J Perinat Med. 2004;32(4):346-53.
17. Kurjak A, Andonotopo W, Hafner T, Salihagic-Kadic A, Stanojevic M, Azumendi G, et al. Normal standards for fetal neurobehavioral developments—longitudinal quantification by four-dimensional sonography. J Perinat Med. 2006;34(1):56-65.
18. Kurjak A, Azumendi G, Vecek N, Kupesic S, Solak M, Varga D, et al. Fetal hand movements and facial expression in normal pregnancy studied by four-dimensional sonography. J Perinat Med. 2003;31(6):496-508.
19. Kurjak A, Vecek N, Kupesic S, Azumendi G, Solak M. Four dimensional ultrasound: how much does it improve perinatal practice? In: Carrera JM, Chervenak FA, Kurjak A (Eds). Eds). Controversies in Perinatal Medicine: Studies on the Fetus as a Patient. New York: A CRC press company, Parthenon Publishing; 2003. p. 222.
20. Nijhuis JG. Fetal behavior. Neurobiol Aging. 2003;24(Suppl 1):S41-6.

21. Arabin B, Bos R, Rijlaarsdam R, Mohnhaupt A, van Eyck J. The onset of inter-human contacts: longitudinal ultrasound observations in early twin pregnancies. Ultrasound Obstet Gynecol. 1996;8(3):166-73.

22. Prechtl HF. Ultrasound studies of human fetal behavior. Early Hum Dev. 1985;12(2):91-8.

23. Ianniruberto A, Tajani E. Ultrasonographic study of fetal movements. Semin Perinatol. 1981;5(2):175-81.

24. Joseph RG. Fetal brain behavior and cognitive development. Dev Rev. 2000;20(1):81-98.

25. Goto S, Kato TK. Early movements are useful for estimating the gestational weeks in the first trimester of pregnancy. In: Levski RA, Morley P (Eds). Ultrasound '82. Oxford: Pergamon Press; 1983. pp. 577-82.

26. Hata T, Kanenishi K, Sasaki M. Four-dimensional sonographic assessment of fetal movement in the late first trimester. Int J Gynaecol Obstet. 2010;109(3):190-3.

27. Kurjak A, Ahmed B, Abo-Yaquab S, Younis M, Saleh H, Shaddad AN, et al. An attempt to introduce neurological test for fetus based on 3D and 4D sonography. Donald Sch J Ultrasound Obstet Gynecol. 2008;2(4): 29-44.

28. D'Elia A, Pighetti M, Moccia G, Santangelo N. Spontaneous motor activity in normal fetuses. Early Hum Dev. 2001;65(2):139-47.

29. Patrick J, Campbell K, Carmichael L, Natale R, Richardson B. Patterns of gross fetal body movements over 24-hours observation intervals during the last 10 weeks of pregnancy. Am J Obstet Gynecol. 1982;142(4):363-71.

30. Kurjak A, Lausin I, Azumendi G. Assessment of fetal behavior by 3D and 4D sonography. In: Hata T, Kurjak A, Kozuma S (Eds). Current Topics on Fetal 3D/4D Ultrasound. UAE: Bentham Science Publishers; 2009. pp. 234-65.

31. Hadders-Algra M. The neuronal group selection theory: a framework to explain variation in normal motor development. Dev Med Child Neurol. 2000;42(8):566-72.

32. Vladareanu R, Lebit D, Constantinescu S. Ultrasound assessment of fetal neuro-behavior in high-risk pregnancies. Donald Sch J Ultrasound Obstet Gynecol. 2012;6(2):132-47.

33. Kurjak A, Barisic LS, Stanojevic M, Salihagic-Kadic A, Porovic S. Are we ready to investigate cognitive function of fetal brain? The Role of advanced four-dimensional sonography. Donald Sch J Ultrasound Obstet Gynecol. 2016;10(2):116-24.

34. Stanojevic M, Kurjak A. Continuity from fetal to neonatal behavior: lessons learned and future challenges. Donald Sch J Ultrasound Obstet Gynecol. 2011;5(2):107-18.

35. Stanojevic M, Talic A, Miskovic B, Vasilj O, Shaddad AN, Ahmed B, et al. An attempt to standardize Kurjak's Antenatal neuro-developmental test: Osaka consensus statement. DSJUOG. 2011;5(4):317-29.

36. Sekulić SR, Lukac DD, Naumović NM. The fetus cannot exercise like an astronaut: gravity loading is necessary for the physiological development during second half of pregnancy. Med Hypotheses. 2005;64(2):221-8.

37. Meigal AY. Synergistic action of gravity and temperature on the motor system within the lifespan: a "Baby Astronaut" hypothesis. Med Hypotheses. 2013;80(3):275-83.

38. Einspieler C, Prechtl HFR. Prechtl's assessment of general movements: a diagnostic tool for the functional assessment of the young nervous system. Ment Retard Dev Disabil Res Rev. 2005;11(1):61-7.

39. Moster D, Wilcox AJ, Vollset SE, Markestad T, Lie RT. Cerebral palsy among term and postterm births. JAMA. 2010;304(9):976-82.

40. de Vries JI, Visser GH, Prechtl HF. The emergence of fetal behaviour. I. Qualitative aspects. Early Hum Dev. 1982;7(4):301-22.

41. Nijhuis JG. Fetal Behaviour: Developmental and Perinatal Aspects. Oxford: Oxford University Press; 1992. p. 312.

42. Prechtl HF. State of the art of a new functional assessment of the young nervous system. An early predictor of cerebral palsy. Early Hum Dev. 1997;50(1):1-11.

43. Kurjak A, Luetic AT. Fetal neurobehavior assessed by three-dimensional/four-dimensional sonography. Zdrav Vestn. 2010; 79(11):790-9.

44. Seme-Ciglenečki P. Predictive value of assessment of general movements for neurological development of high-risk preterm infants: comparative study. Croat Med J. 2003;44(6):721-7.

45. Kurjak A, Barišić LS, Stanojević M, Antsaklis P, Panchal S, Honemeyer U, et al. Multicenter results on the clinical use of KANET. J Perinat Med. 2019;47(9):897-909.

46. Kurjak A, Stanojevic M, Andonotopo W, Scazzocchio-Duenas E, Azumendi G, Carrera JM. Fetal behavior assessed in all three trimesters of normal pregnancy by four-dimensional ultrasonography. Croat Med J. 2005;46(5):772-80.

47. Palmer FB. Strategies for the early diagnosis of cerebral palsy. J Pediatr. 2004;145(Suppl 2):S8-S11.

48. Andonotopo W, Kurjak A. The assessment of fetal behavior of growth restricted fetuses by 4D sonography. J Perinat Med. 2006;34(6):471-8.

49. Kurjak A, Abo-Yaqoub S, Stanojevic M, Yigiter AB, Vasilj O, Lebit D, et al. The potential of 4D sonography in the assessment of fetal neurobehavior—multicentric study in high-risk pregnancies. J Perinat Med. 2010;38(1):77-82.

50. Miskovic B, Vasilj O, Stanojevic M, Ivanković D, Kerner M, Tikvica A. The comparison of fetal behavior in high-risk and normal pregnancies assessed by four dimensional ultrasound. J Matern Fetal Neonatal Med. 2010;23(12):1461-7.

51. Talic A, Kurjak A, Ahmed B, Stanojevic M, Predojevic M, Salihagic-Kadic A, et al. The potential of 4D sonography in the assessment of fetal behavior in high-risk pregnancies. J Matern Fetal Neonatal Med. 2011;24(7):948-54.

52. Honemeyer U, Kurjak A. The use of KANET test to assess fetal CNS function. First 100 cases. 10th World Congress of Perinatal Med. 2011;8-11.

53. Talic A, Kurjak A, Stanojevic M, Honemeyer U, Badreldeen A, DiRenzo GC. The assessment of fetal brain function in fetuses with ventriculomegaly: the role of the KANET test. J Matern Fetal Neonatal Med. 2012;25(8):1267-72.

54. Abo-Yaqoub S, Kurjak A, Mohammed AB, Shadad A, Abdel-Maaboud M. The role of 4-D ultrasonography in prenatal assessment of fetal neurobehaviour and prediction of neurological outcome. J Matern Fetal Neonatal Med. 2012;25(3):231-6.

55. Honemeyer U, Talic A, Therwat A, Paulose L, Patidar R. The clinical value of KANET in studying fetal neurobehavior in normal and at-risk pregnancies. J Perinat Med. 2013;41(2):187-97.

56. Kurjak A, Talic A, Honemeyer U, Stanojevic M, Zalud I. Comparison between antenatal neurodevelopmental test and fetal Doppler in the assessment of fetal well being. J Perinat Med. 2013;41(1):107-14.

57. Athanasiadis AP, Mikos T, Tambakoudis GP, Theodoridis TD, Papastergiou M, Assimakopoulos E, et al. Neurodevelopmental fetal assessment using KANET scoring system in low and high risk pregnancies. J Matern Fetal Neonatal Med. 2013; 26(4):363-8.

58. Neto RM. KANET in Brazil: first experience. Donald Sch J Ultrasound Obstet Gynecol. 2015;9(1):1-5.

59. Hanaoka U, Hata T, Kananishi K, AboEllail MAM, Uematsu R, Konishi Y, et al. Does ethnicity have an effect on fetal behavior? A comparison of Asian and Caucasian populations. J Perinat Med. 2016;44(2):217-21.

60. Hata T, Kanenishi K, Mori N, AboEllail MAM, Hanaoka U, Koyano K, et al. Prediction of postnatal developmental disabilities using the antenatal fetal neurodevelopmental test: KANET assessment. J Perinat Med. 2018; 47(1):77-81.

61. Tan KH, Smyth RMD, Wei X. Fetal vibroacoustic stimulation for facilitation of tests of fetal wellbeing. Cochrane Database Syst Rev. 2013;(12):CD002963.

62. Antsaklis P, Porovic S, Daskalakis G, Kurjak A. 4D assessment of fetal brain function in diabetic patients. J Perinat Med. 2017;45(6): 711-5.

Brain Maturation and Development in Growth-restricted Fetuses: Functional Studies

Toshiyuki Hata, Riko Takayoshi, Aya Koyanagi, Yasunari Miyagi, Takahito Miyake

■ INTRODUCTION

Gould et al.[1] were the first to suggest that high-stress pregnancies accelerating the biochemical maturation of pulmonary surfactant may also accelerate fetal neurological maturation. In 51 infants from high-risk pregnancies (certain chronically stressed pregnancies), eight infants showed accelerated neurological maturation 3 or more weeks in excess of their gestational age.[2] Moreover, all 25 infants with documented acceleration of pulmonary surfactant showed accelerated neurological maturation. Amiel-Tison[3] suggested that unfavorable intrauterine conditions may induce an acceleration of neurologic development in infants with a number of forms of intrauterine stress. Moreover, neurological maturation in moderately to severely growth-restricted newborn infants might be accelerated by 3–4 weeks or more compared with appropriately grown infants of the same gestational age.[4] This phenomenon is particularly manifest in multiple pregnancies or hypertensive disorders of pregnancy (HDP). The authors suggested that the accelerated brain maturation and lung maturation in fetal growth restriction (FGR) may reflect an adaptation of the fetuses to early extrauterine life.

In 23 autopsies of preterm infants between 27 and 34 weeks of gestation born to women with HDP, 17 infants showed accelerated cerebral maturation 2 weeks or more in advance of their gestational age.[5] HDP and FGR were noted as significant risk factors in accelerated intrauterine cerebral maturation.

In this chapter, we present the current status of brain maturation and development in growth-restricted fetuses using four-dimensional (4D) ultrasound, and, on this basis, make recommendations for future research on fetal functional studies in FGR pregnancies.

■ TWO-DIMENSIONAL SONOGRAPHIC STUDIES

Fetal eye, body, and breathing movements were assessed in low-risk and growth-restricted fetuses using two-dimensional (2D) sonography in the third trimester of pregnancy, and the fetal heart rate was recorded simultaneously.[6] The mean frequency of fetal breathing movement was greater during active fetal periods (body and eye movements present, greater heart rate variability) than during quiescence (body and eye movements absent, reduced heart rate variability) in both groups. Moreover, the frequency of fetal breathing in growth-restricted fetuses was not different from that in low-risk fetuses.

Fetal mouthing, eye, and gross body movements were evaluated using 2D sonography in normal and uncomplicated growth-restricted fetuses.[7] The authors concluded that in mildly affected FGR fetuses with no evidence of hypoxia, there were no quantitative differences compared with normal fetuses regarding fetal activity. The only differences between fetuses were in the performance of such activities, suggesting a dysfunction of the central nervous system (CNS) resulting from a metabolic disturbance.

No clear effect of uncomplicated FGR was detected on the quality of general movements observed using 2D sonography.[8] However, general movements became slow and small in amplitude in cases with reduced amniotic fluid. With the onset of abnormal fetal heart rate patterns, the repertoire of general movements became restricted.

A qualitative and quantitative analysis of various fetal movement patterns was conducted using 2D sonography between appropriate-for-gestational age (AGA) and FGR fetuses.[9] A reduction of both the number and duration of general movements was noted in FGR fetuses. Markedly reduced frequencies of startle, twitch, and isolated limb movements were also evident in the FGR group. The qualitative analysis of general movements showed a reduction of the quicker components leading to slow and monotonous movement patterns. A marked reduction in variability of the speed and intensity of each movement was also identified in FGR fetuses. These reduced variabilities of motor patterns in FGR fetuses might be due to changes in the CNS function.

Fetal body and eye movements were observed using 2D sonography with continuous fetal heart rate monitoring in low-risk and uncomplicated FGR fetuses in the third trimester of pregnancy.[10] The appearance of states seemed to be delayed in FGR fetuses. Growth-restricted fetuses showed differences in the quality and quantity of somatic motility compared with low-risk fetuses. The authors suggest that some aspects of the CNS function

are disturbed in FGR fetuses, even in the absence of fetal distress.

Breathing and body movements were studied using 2D sonography before, during, and after heart rate decelerations in FGR fetuses.[11] These movements were significantly reduced during and after decelerations. The authors suggest that these changes might be mediated by a change in the brain activity state due to fetal hypoxemia.

Time intervals between two different behavioral states were studied using 2D sonography (fetal eye and body movements) and heart rate monitoring between healthy and FGR fetuses in near-term pregnancies.[12] In healthy fetuses, transitions usually lasted <3 minutes whereas FGR fetuses showed a longer duration when compared with healthy fetuses. Behavioral state transitions were different between healthy and FGR fetuses.

Sival et al.[13] studied the quantity of fetal general and breathing movements using 2D sonography in FGR fetuses. The quantity of general movements decreased from 25 weeks of gestation onward, whereas the quantity of fetal breathing movements increased. The quantity of general movements as well as that of breathing movements was low in FGR fetuses with abnormal fetal heart rate patterns, compared with uncomplicated FGR fetuses. In FGR fetuses with a reduced amount of amniotic fluid, only the quantity of breathing movements and not that of general movements was low.

FOUR-DIMENSIONAL ULTRASOUND STUDIES

With the introduction of and advances in 4D ultrasound, fetal facial expressions can now be easily and readily observed after 20 weeks of pregnancy.[14-21] The fetal facial expressions may mirror the fetal brain function and development in utero.[17,18] 4D ultrasound can differentiate several facial expressions (**Figs. 1 to 8**).

Andonotopo and Kurjak[22] evaluated the frequency of six fetal facial expressions (blinking, mouthing, yawning, tongue expulsion, grimacing, and swallowing) using 4D ultrasound between normal and FGR fetuses at 30–40 weeks of gestation. Frequencies of

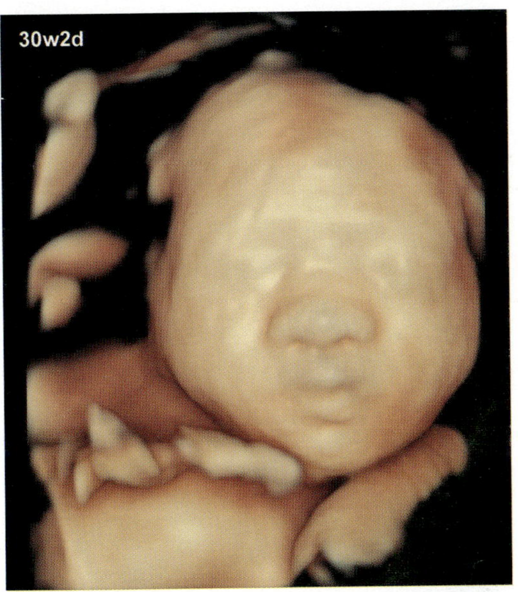

Fig. 1: Neutral fetal face.

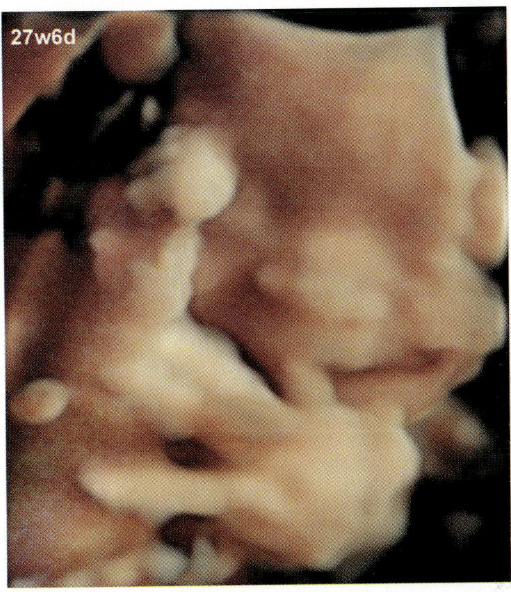

Fig. 3: Fetal sucking.

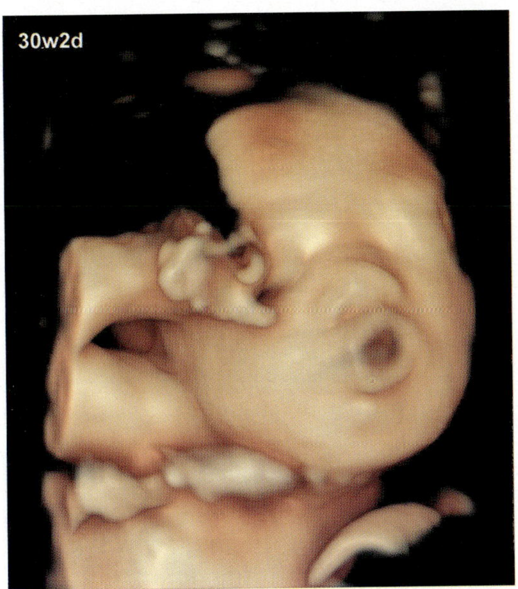

Fig. 2: Fetal mouthing.

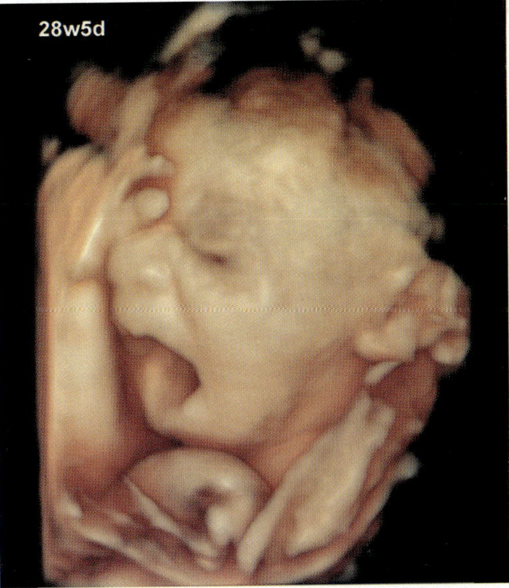

Fig. 4: Fetal yawning.

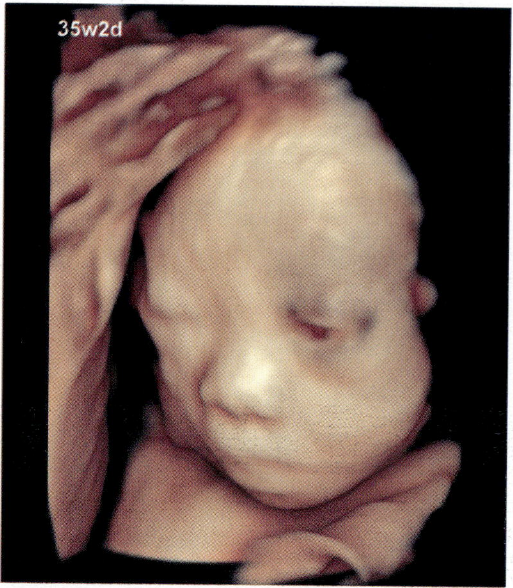

Fig. 5: Fetal blinking.

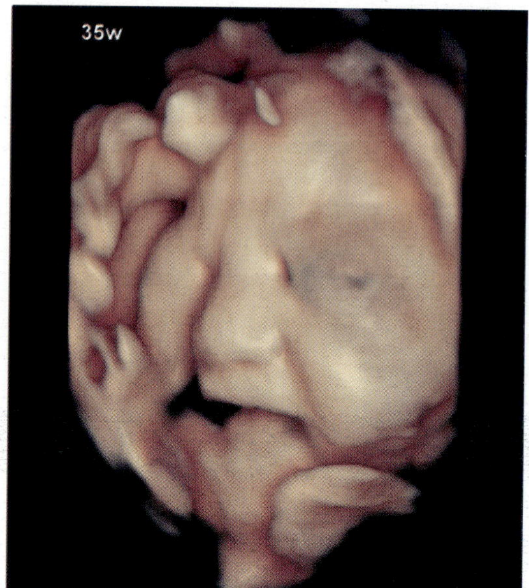

Fig. 7: Fetal scowling.

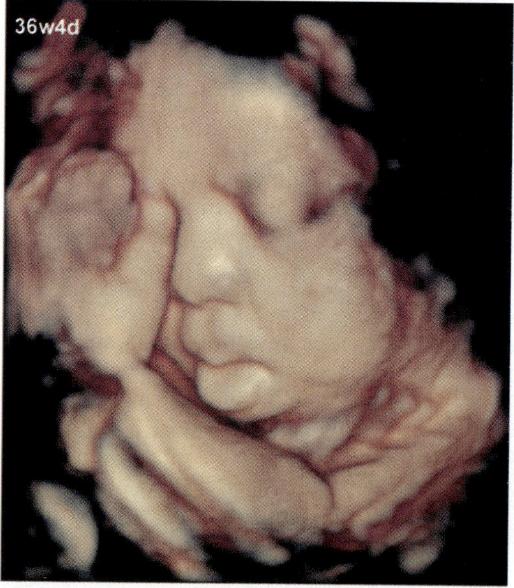

Fig. 6: Fetal tongue expulsion.

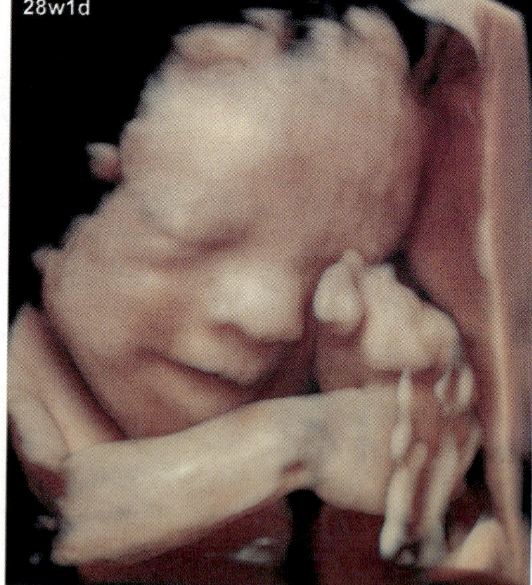

Fig. 8: Fetal smiling.

six facial expressions in FGR fetuses were significantly lower than those in normal fetuses. The neurological conditions in FGR fetuses could be assessed quantitatively and qualitatively using 4D ultrasound.

Chida et al.[23] assessed seven fetal facial expressions (blinking, mouthing, yawning, smiling, tongue expulsion, scowling, and sucking) using 4D ultrasound in normal and FGR fetuses between 26 and 39 weeks of gestation. There were no significant differences in frequencies of the seven facial expressions between two groups. The reason for no significant differences in fetal facial expressions between normal and FGR fetuses may be due to the small number of subjects studied (seven subjects in each group).

Mori et al.[24] examined seven facial expressions (blinking, mouthing, yawning, smiling, tongue expulsion, scowling, and sucking) of 50 AGA, 25 small-for-gestational age (SGA), and six FGR fetuses between 28 and 35 weeks of gestation. The frequencies of fetal facial expressions were not decreased in either SGA or FGR fetuses. The absence of a decrease in the frequency of each fetal expression in FGR fetuses might be due to increased brain blood flow because of the brain-sparing effect. Moreover, accelerated maturation and development of the brain function might be suspected in SGA and FGR fetuses.

Moreover, seven facial expressions (blinking, mouthing, yawning, smiling, tongue expulsion, scowling, and sucking) in 50 AGA and 34 FGR fetuses aged between 28 and 35 gestational weeks were assessed using 4D ultrasound.[25] The authors suggested that the number of significant correlations of fetal facial expressions in FGR fetuses increases more compared with that in AGA fetuses at 32–35 weeks of gestation. Due to the acceleration of neurological maturation and development in FGR fetuses, the control of facial expressions by the brain and CNS may be more evident compared with AGA fetuses during this period.

CONCLUSION

Four-dimensional ultrasound studies indicated that FGR fetuses show accelerations of neurological maturation and development in utero. Further studies involving a larger sample size are needed to fully understand the neurodevelopmental acceleration and development of the brain and CNS functions in FGR fetuses. 4D ultrasound assessment of the fetal response to vibroacoustic stimulation (VAS) has been reported to be a novel and simple technique for evaluation of the fetal brain function.[26] Its use may facilitate precise observation of fetal facial expressions and fetal movements, both spontaneous ones and those occurring in response to stimuli like VAS. Therefore, this technique might allow researchers to directly assess accelerated brain maturation and development in FGR fetuses in future studies.

Conflict of interest: The authors have no conflict of interest.

REFERENCES

1. Gould JB, Gluck L, Kulovich MV. The acceleration of neurologic maturation in high stress pregnancy and its relation to fetal lung maturity. Pediatr Res. 1972;6:335.
2. Gould JB, Gluck L, Kulovich MV. The relationship between accelerated pulmonary maturity and accelerated neurological maturity in certain chronically stressed pregnancies. Am J Obstet Gynecol. 1977;127(2):181-6.
3. Amiel-Tison C. Possible acceleration of neurological maturation following high-risk pregnancy. Am J Obstet Gynecol. 1980;138(3):303-6.
4. Amiel-Tison C, Pettigrew AG. Adaptive changes in the developing brain during intrauterine stress. Brain Dev. 1991;13(2):67-76.
5. Hadi HA. Fetal cerebral maturation in hypertensive disorders of pregnancy. Obstet Gynecol. 1984;63(2):214-9.
6. van Vliet MA, Martin CB Jr, Nijhuis JG, Prechtl HF. The relationship between fetal activity and behavioral states and fetal breathing movements in normal and growth-retarded fetuses. Am J Obstet Gynecol. 1985;153(5):582-8.
7. D'Elia A, Pighetti M, Moccia GF, Di Meo P. Computer-assisted analysis of fetal

movements in intrauterine growth retardation (IUGR). Early Hum Dev. 1998;51(2): 137-45.

8. Sival DA, Visser GH, Prechtl HF. The effect of intrauterine growth retardation on the quality of general movements in the human fetus. Early Hum Dev. 1992;28(2):119-32.

9. Bekedam DJ, Visser GH, de Vries JJ, Prechtl HF. Motor behavior in the growth retarded fetus. Early Hum Dev. 1985;12(2):155-65.

10. van Vliet MA, Martin CB Jr, Nijhuis JG, Prechtl HF. Behavioral states in growth-retarded human fetuses. Early Hum Dev. 1985;12(2):183-97.

11. Bekedam DJ, Visser GH. Effects of hypoxemic events on breathing, body movements, and heart rate variation: a study in growth-retarded human fetuses. Am J Obstet Gynecol. 1985;153(1):52-6.

12. Arduini D, Rizzo G, Caforio L, Boccolini MR, Romanini C, Mancuso S. Behavioral state transitions in healthy and growth retarded fetuses. Early Hum Dev. 1989;19(3):155-65.

13. Sival DA, Visser GH, Prechtl HF. The relationship between the quantity and quality of prenatal movements in pregnancies complicated by intra-uterine growth retardation and premature rupture of membranes. Early Hum Dev. 1992; 30(3):193-209.

14. Hata T, Dai SY, Marumo G. Ultrasound for evaluation of fetal neurobehavioral development: from 2-D to 4-D ultrasound. Inf Child Dev. 2010;19(1):99-118.

15. Hata T, Kanenishi K, Hanaoka U, Marumo G. HDlive and 4D ultrasound in the assessment of fetal facial expressions. Donald School J Ultrasound Obstet Gynecol. 2015;9(1):44-50.

16. Hata T. Current status of fetal neurodevelopmental assessment: four-dimensional ultrasound study. J Obstet Gynaecol Res. 2016;42(10):1211-21.

17. AboEllail MAM, Hata T. Fetal face and four-dimensional ultrasound. In: Kurjak A, Chervenak FA (Eds). Donald School Textbook of Ultrasound in Obstetrics & Gynecology, 4th Edition. New Delhi: Jaypee Brothers Medical Publishers (P) Ltd.; 2017. pp. 791-9.

18. AboEllail MAM, Hata T. Fetal face as important indicator of fetal brain function. J Perinat Med. 2017;45(6):729-36.

19. Hata T. Fetal face as predictor of fetal brain. Donald School J Ultrasound Obstet Gynecol. 2018;12(1):56-9.

20. AboEllail MAM, Kanenishi K, Mori N, Mohamed OAK, Hata T. 4D ultrasound study of fetal facial expressions in the third trimester of pregnancy. J Matern Fetal Neonatal Med. 2018;31(14):1856-64.

21. AboEllail MAM, Kanenishi K, Mori N, Hata T. Coordination of fetal facial expressions after 36 weeks of gestation. Donald School J Ultrasound Obstet Gynecol. 2018;12:156-61.

22. Andonotopo W, Kurjak A. The assessment of fetal behavior of growth restricted fetuses by 4D sonography. J Perinat Med. 2006;34(6):471-8.

23. Chida H, Kikuchi A, Kanasugi T, Isurugi C, Oyama R, Sugiyama T. Facial expressions of fetal growth restriction and appropriate-for-gestational age fetuses assessed by four-dimensional high-definition live ultrasound. Gynecol Obstet. 2017;7(10).

24. Mori N, AboEllail MAM, Tenkumo C, Kanenishi K, Nishimoto N, Hata T. Fetal facial expressions in small-for-gestational-age and growth-restricted fetuses. J Matern Fetal Neonatal Med. 2019;32(9):1426-32.

25. Mori N, Kanenishi K, AboEllail MAM, Nitta E, Hata T. Neurological development may be accelerated in growth-restricted fetuses: a 4D ultrasound study. J Perinat Med. 2019;47(4):429-33.

26. Ogo K, Kanenishi K, Mori N, AboEllail MAM, Hata T. Change in fetal behavior in response to vibroacoustic stimulation. J Perinat Med. 2019;47(5):558-63.

Is Fetus and Neonate the Same Individual in Terms of Behavior?

Milan Stanojević, Asim Kurjak

■ INTRODUCTION

For more than 20 years, the burden of mental and behavioral disorders in the world is becoming a main concern in terms of increased healthcare costs, decreased quality of life, without the possibility to intervene early enough to make a substantial change of this tendency.[1,2] Although biological, social, and psychological factors are considered to influence the mental and behavioral disorders, it should be pointed out that understanding of the brain development and function are of substantial significance to better understand etiology, pathophysiology, epidemiology, prevention, and therapy of those disorders.[1,2] It is well known that most of the disorders affecting human brain in perinatal period and infancy are prenatal in origin, making the perinatal period significant for the research of fetal and neonatal behavior.[3]

Neuroimaging methods like ultrasound (US) as the main screening and diagnostic method of brain structure and function, magnetic resonance imaging (MRI), electro-encephalography (EEG), magnetoencephalography (MEG), and near-infrared spectroscopy (NIRS) are used as a diagnostic tool for evaluation of structure and function of fetal brain.[3-8] As the dynamic of brain development is changing through gestation, the results obtained by those studies can be interpreted if one is aware of gestational age dependent brain developmental changes.[3-8] The early diagnosis of various structural and/or functional abnormalities of the brain as well as the distinction between normal and abnormal brain development could be better understood if fetal and infant behavior are studied in different gestations together with assessment of brain structure.[9-15]

Development of human brain is a long-lasting process in progress which is not completed in the time of delivery and even the decades afterward.[8-16] Nearly all injuries of the brain in perinatal period are prenatal in origin, while contrary to the common believe, infrequent are intrapartal and postnatal brain injuries.[3] That is why the diagnosis of brain damage is important during pregnancy which is difficult and tricky in terms of diagnostic methods and reproducibility, urging the development of fetal neurology.[3] Although the fetus and neonate are different, but from developmental point of view there is continuity between the two developmental periods of human life, which applies to fetal and neonatal movements as important indicator of developmental processes of the brain.[3]

The aim of the chapter is to present continuity of the behavior from fetus to neonate.

EPIDEMIOLOGY AND COURSE OF NEURODEVELOPMENTAL DISABILITY IN PERINATAL PERIOD

As stressed before, structural and functional abnormal brain development of fetuses can occur either pre- or postnatally.[4-8]

Fetal neurological assessment gives the opportunity to detect fetuses who are at neurological risk, which is the category from which most of neurologically disabled individuals will be recruited.[3] It has been learned from epidemiological studies that most of neurologically impaired fetuses and infants belong to low-risk group, whose development seemed to be normal in fetal, early neonatal life, and in infancy, meaning that screening and diagnostic methods used for the diagnosis of developmental disability from fetal life to infancy failed.[4-6] Higher the neurorisk higher the incidence of neurodevelopmental disorders. Exposure to only one or two risk factors poses a risk of developing neurodevelopmental disorder in 5% of those exposed, while increasing the number of risk factors from 5 to 7% increases the risk of neurodevelopmental disorder to 76% and 99%.[17,18] According to these data, more than half of infants and small children with neurodevelopmental disorders have five or more risk factors, among which the most common were child abuse, mental health disorders, minority status or low education of caregiver, a single parent, poverty, adolescent parent, domestic violence, four or more children in the household, addicted parents, and some others.[17,18] Risk factors can be prenatal, perinatal, and postnatal (neonatal), and are defined differently in different studies.[18,19]

According to the World Health Organization (WHO), the prevalence of neurodevelopmental disorders from the age of 2 years in developing countries is up to 10%, while in some regions and countries it ranges from 2.7 to 15.6% depending on the study.[1,19,20]

Recent research in developed countries revealed that the prevalence of cerebral palsy (CP) has not been changed in the last 60 years, ranging from 1.4 to 2.5/1,000 live births, despite a sixfold increase in the incidence of cesarean delivery in the same period.[21,22] According to data from Sweden, the prevalence of CP in all gestational ages was 1.96/1,000 live births, while for each gestational age group it was as follows: 59.0/1,000 live births for children born before 28 weeks of gestation, 45.7/1,000 live births for those between 28 and 31 weeks of gestation, 6.0/1,000 live births for those between 32 and 36 weeks, and after 36 weeks the prevalence was 1.2/1,000 live births of that gestational age.[23] One study found stagnant prevalence of CP in term infants, while it was increasing in preterm infants of all gestational ages, especially those extremely immature, probably due to their better survival.[24] It is thought that the slight increase in CP in the last 25 years is caused by higher prevalence of CP in preterm rather than term infants.[24] In the aforementioned Swedish study on the incidence of CP according to the clinical picture, hemiplegia was found in 44% of patients, diplegia in 34%, tetraplegia in 5%, the dyskinetic form of CP in 12%, and ataxia in 3%.[24] The following changes were found in the brains of children with CP by neuroimaging methods in the same study: congenital malformations of the brain in 12%, white matter lesions in 49%, cortical subcortical lesions in 15%, and basal ganglia damage in 11%.[24]

As for the time of onset of damage that caused CP, prenatal causes were found in 38%, perinatal causes in 38%, while there were 24% of unclassified cases.[24] According to data from another study, most of the brain damage (50–75% of them) in children with CP occurs between 24 weeks of postmenstrual age and term age.[25]

Cerebral palsy as a heterogeneous condition with various clinical manifestations in which sometimes hereditary elements could be found is one of the most often diagnosed developmental disability in infants.[22,26] If one child in the family is affected with CP, the next child has 4.8-fold risk, and if we are dealing with the twins than the risk is increasing to 29-fold.[22,26] It has been recently revealed that causative mutations could be found in 1–2% of (mostly) familial cases of CP.[3,27] It has been found by new generation exome-sequencing of sporadic cases of CP that 14% of them have likely causative single-gene mutations and almost 31% have clinically relevant copy number variations.[3,27] In the recently published genetic study of whole-genome sequencing in 250 children suffering from CP and their two parents it has been found that in 14% of cases excess of damaging de novo or recessive variants were revealed, with providing evidence for genetically-mediated dysregulation of early neuronal connectivity in CP.[27]

Severe childhood disability is most commonly caused by CP of largely undetected etiology.[22,28] The most important characteristic of this "umbrella" term is that CP as the disorder of development, movement, and posture is nonprogressive damage of developing brain.[28] Despite the intention for the early diagnosis of CP lasting for more than 2 centuries, CP is diagnosed late between 2 and 5 years retrospectively, exceptionally before the age of 6 months in only most severely affected infants.[28] Although the etiology of CP is poorly understood, it is well known that it does not result from a single event but in most of the times there is a sequence of interdependent adverse incidents providing to the condition.[28] Possibility of the diagnosis of CP in infancy should take into consideration this evolving adverse events timeframe, sometimes of crucial significance.[22] Only if the clinicians understand the profile of disability in child affected with CP as an ongoing sequence of adverse events in certain time window, they can plan appropriate personalized multidisciplinary treatment, which is sometimes not easy to achieve.[22] Early diagnosis (which often fails) of CP should be made whenever possible followed with factors related to pathogenesis, understanding of impairment, and functional limitations in every patient.[22,28]

ROLE OF NEUROLOGICAL CLINICAL ASSESSMENT IN NEONATAL PERIOD

Although we have very powerful imaging and other methods to find out the consequences of the brain damage, there is no doubt that clinical methods like the history and clinical assessment are of utmost importance. There are some recently published data concerning hereditary factors involved in the pathogenesis of CP.[22,28] For parents who had one affected child, the risk of recurrence of CP in another child was considerably increased.[22,28] In order to identify pathogenesis of the process, neuroimaging methods are used, among which the most frequently used in very low birthweight premature infants and in term infants with encephalopathy are cranial US, MRI, functional MRI, NIRS, magnetic resonance spectroscopy, and diffusion-weighted imaging.[22,28] Impairment of organs or systems by clinical assessment of muscle tone, strength, and control of voluntary movements for early detection of infants with the risk for CP has been frustrating for many decades, because 43% of 7-year-old children with CP had a normal newborn neurological examination.[29] Even recently, it is estimated that 25–50% of children with neonatal CP will not show signs of suspected CP and will not receive a recommendation for further monitoring of neurodevelopmental outcome.[30] According to a newly published systematic study, it is estimated that neurodevelopmental abnormalities after birth will be found in only one in 500 children who were later suspected of having CP.[31] It is questionable whether we can change this disappointing fact, which could enable timely diagnosis of CP in order to intervene. Before appearance of four-dimensional (4D) US the diagnosis of neurological impairment was mostly postnatal, but recently with technology improvements, it has been shifting toward prenatal period.[32] We are aware that in most of the CP cases (39.6%) no neurological risk factors could be identified, and for the solely intrapartum risk factors, contrary to the common believe, the percentages are even lower (24.7%).[33] Among all investigated risk factors, the only which reached statistical significance was birthweight below 2,500 g.[22] Are we approaching the era of the development of diagnostic tests to detect nonreassuring fetal status in its intrauterine life to intervene at appropriate time in order to decrease the CP rate?[28] This question is futuristic, because nothing has changed with the scarce possibility to diagnose neurological damage which will result in CP at the age of 6 months.[28] The question: Is there any possibility to improve timing of postnatal diagnosis of neurologically disabled infant remains unanswered? Postnatal assessment is probably easier to perform than prenatal, by using a simple and suitable for everyday work screening clinical test with good reliability, specificity, and sensitivity.[34,35] Such tests are still not widely used, while those complicated and time-consuming are used mostly for clinical research purposes. For many decades, clinicians are investigating the possibility to invent the simple and suitable clinical test for neurological assessment of term and preterm infants, with the possibility to find

possible causative link between pregnancy course and neurodevelopmental outcome.[34,35] Such tests are designed to detect impairment of movement and postural control which are the main characteristics of CP, and some of them can be helpful in detection of early neurological impairment.[34,35] Clinical neurological assessment proposed and practiced by Amiel-Tison could be very useful in the early detection of newborns at risk.[36] As stressed before, the development of central nervous system (CNS) is complex and extended process lasting from the time of conception to several decades after birth which is making assessment of its optimality complicated and challenging. Neurological Assessment at Term invented and published by Amiel-Tison (ATNAT) is one of the few tests taking into account ontogenesis of CNS assessing separately developmentally older so-called lower subcortical system consisting of reticular formation, vestibular nuclei and tectum, and developmentally younger upper cortical system developing from the corticospinal pathways.[36] The role of lower system is to maintain posture against gravity, while the upper system is responsible for the control of erect posture and for the movements of the extremities.[37] At the corrected age of 40 gestational weeks optimality assessment consists of head circumference measurement, assessment of cranial sutures, visual pursuit, social interaction, sucking reflex, raise-to-sit and reverse, passive tone in the axis, passive tone in the limbs, fingers and thumbs outside the fist, and autonomic control during assessment.[37] The ATNAT is used for neurological evaluation of term and preterm infants with acceptable assessment accuracy using simple scoring procedure, concentrating on the most important elements and finishing with so-called clinical synthesis at term by which all aspects of neurodevelopmental assessment are covered.[37] It was recognized that clinico-anatomic correlations using high resolution neuroimaging techniques could be helpful in the neurological assessment of newborns, while the neurological examination and the functional assessment of the developing CNS are bringing a new perspective of CNS status in neonatal period.[36] When assessing by ATNAT very low birthweight (VLBW) infants at corrected age of 40 weeks. ATNAT has low positive predictive value of 33% and high negative predictive value of 88%, respectively, with similar results at the corrected age of 3 months.[36] This means that we still need some other methods to be used in order to predict neurodevelopmental outcome of low- and high-risk infants.

IS NEUROIMAGING IMPORTANT FOR NEONATAL NEUROLOGICAL ASSESSMENT?

Typical patterns of brain injury, even in the early course of the disease, can be detected by conventional acquisition neuroimaging techniques together with modern diffusion tensor neuroimaging techniques which cannot be considered as pathognomonic despite their highly suggestive nature.[38-41] For example, different types of brain edema can be distinguished by diffusion tensor neuroimaging.[39,42]

Not all neuroimaging techniques could be used in neonatal intensive care units (NICUs) in critically sick newborns.[38-41] For many years, US has been considered as very important point of care diagnostic modality in NICUs.[38-41] It has fairly acceptable sensitivity and specificity in high- and low-risk neonatal population. The validity of the two-dimensional (2D) US scans was 85%, sensitivity 70%, specificity 90%, positive predictive value 72%, and negative predictive value 89%, respectively.[43]

The 2D US scans classified as low risk were followed by a normal neurological outcome in 74 (89%) of 83 infants; those classified as high risk for neurological impairment were followed by abnormal neurological outcome in 21 (72%) of 29 infants.[43] Other neuroimaging procedures like MRI or NIRS are also available and feasible in neonatal period with better sensitivity and specificity for the detection of hypoxic ischemic encephalopathy or focal cortical damage, but US remains as very important screening method for depiction of fetal and neonatal brain.[40] Neuroimaging is particularly useful to determine the timing of hypoxic-ischemic brain damage.[44] Cranial US has been used to determine the type and evolution of brain damage. MRI, functional MRI, and NIRS of the brain have also been used to detect antenatal, perinatal, and neonatal abnormalities and timing on the basis of standardized assessment of brain maturation.[40] In term and near-term neonates with CP, head MRI revealed focal arterial infarction in 22%, brain malformations in 14%, periventricular white matter abnormalities in 12%, generalized brain atrophy in 7%, hypoxic-ischemic brain injury in 5%, intracranial hemorrhage in 5%, delayed myelination in 2%, other abnormality in 6%, while in 37% of infants neuroimaging findings were normal.[45]

Due to a very limited availability of three-dimensional (3D) US equipment, benefits, and risks of 3D imaging should be taken under consideration when used in NICUs regardless of the fact that it is a low-risk procedure in neonates.[46,47] If there is a possibility to transport the 3D US equipment to critically sick newborn, then this method should be considered as method of choice for depiction of neonatal brain.[47] There is no difference between the indications for 2D and 3D US in neonatal period, but if 2D US is unreliable than 3D should be performed if available. 3D neurosonography is indicated for assessment of the following conditions developed either prenatally or postnatally:[46,47]

- Intracranial hemorrhage
- Hypoxic-ischemic brain damage
- Inflammatory disorders of the brain and its complications
- Ventriculomegaly and hydrocephaly (Doppler and volumetric studies included)
- Congenital brain defects, and
- Assessment of gestational age.

Perinatal and social risk factors are influencing development of neonatal brain particularly in very premature infants who are at greatest risk, especially if prenatal US findings have been abnormal while postnatally infant looked apparently well, which was the reason for thorough postnatal US evaluation.[48] A correlation was found between US findings in fetal and neonatal period and signs of neurological impairment in the neonatal period and later in childhood in some papers but not in the others.[49] Disabling and nondisabling CP at the age of 2 years in low birthweight infants who had severe motor impairment as 5-year-old children correlated well with cranial US in infancy.[49,50] Improving survival of very low birthweight infants in the last several decades contributed to the increased incidence of CP despite introduction of sophisticated brain sparing treatment methods of intensive care.[24] Disabling CP was mostly connected with the white-matter injury; however, neuroimaging methods of neonatal brain alone are not appropriate predictor of neurological outcome of high-risk neonates.[49] There is a need for more precise clinical and neuroimaging methods applicable in everyday practice in order to improve clinicians' ability to detect neurological handicap as early as possible and initiate treatment.[49]

WHY GENERAL MOVEMENTS COUNT?

It was ingenious idea of Heinz Prechtl who stated that spontaneous motility during human development might be used for assessment of fetuses and neonates bringing them into focus of many perinatologists prenatally and developmental neurologist postnatally.[30-51] Before Prechtl's research on spontaneous motility it was found that functional repertoire of developing neural structures must meet the requirements of human organism and its environment.[30,51] This concept is based on the theory of ontogenetic adaptation of human organism having the possibility to adapt to the internal and external requirements during each developmental stage.[51] Prechtl stated that spontaneous motility, as the expression of spontaneous neural activity, is a marker of brain proper or disturbed function.[30,51] The observation of unstimulated fetus or infant which is the result of spontaneous behavior without sensory stimulation is the best method to assess its CNS capacity.[51] All endogenously generated movement patterns from unstimulated CNS could be observed as early as from the 7 to 8 weeks of postmenstrual age, with developing a reach repertoire of movements within the next 2 or 3 weeks, continuing to be present for 5–6 months postnatally.[52] It can be concluded that there is a continuity of endogenously generated spontaneous activity from prenatal to postnatal life which is a great opportunity to detect fetuses at high neurological risk in whom development of neurological impairment is emerging. We have learned that most important movements are defined as general movements (GMs) which are involving the whole body in a variable sequence of movements from arm, leg, neck, and trunk with gradual onset and ending.[52] They wax and wane in intensity, force, and speed being fluent and elegant with the impression of complexity and variability.[52] GMs are called fetal or preterm from 28–36 to 38 weeks of postmenstrual age, while after that we have at least two types of movements: writhing present to 46–52 weeks of postmenstrual age and fidgety movements present till 54–58 weeks of postmenstrual age.[30,51,52] They can be considered as mildly abnormal if lacking the fluency and having considerable variation and complexity.[30] Definitely abnormal GMs miss complexity, variation, and fluency.[30] Quantity of movements is not that important as their quality which is complex perception of their speed, amplitude, and force.[30,51,52] Investigation of normal and neurologically impaired preterm infants showed that except for higher incidence of clone in the abnormal group, there was no marked difference in the quantity of different motor patterns studied.[30,51,52] However, video analysis of another group of sick preterm infants revealed a "reduction of elegance and fluency as well as variability, fluctuation in intensity, and speed rather than any change in incidence of distinct motor patterns".[53] Based on postnatal studies, it would be very important to seek for abnormal quantity and quality of prenatal movements in order to find fetuses neurologically at risk.[53]

The following facts may be very important in the assessment of GMs:[30,51]

- Evaluation of GMs either pre- or postnatally should be based on video-recorded movements.
- So called "gestalt perception" should be used as an overall impression of GMs recorded by standardized procedure.
- During perception of GMs their complexity, variability, and fluency should be assessed.

According to Hadders-Algra, GMs either pre- or postnatal could be classified as normal-optimal, normal-suboptimal, mildly abnormal, and definitely abnormal.[30] Assessment of the quantity of GMs is not that important as assessment of their quality which may be very important for the prognosis of neurodevelopmental outcome. They can better predict neurodevelopmental outcome than classical neurologic examination alone.[54]

Videotaped GMs by Prechtl's method enabled their reproducible assessment in the last 30 years which has been shown to be predictive of later CP.[51] The quality of GMs at 2–4 months post-term (so-called fidgety GMs age) has been found to have the highest predictive value in the detection of the infants at risk for CP development.[51,55] Early assessment of the quality of GMs seems to be a window of opportunity for early detection of children at high risk for developmental disorders.[55] Method is simple and it is based on so-called "gestalt perception", i.e., evaluation of GMs complexity, variation, and amplitude.[30,51,55] Assessment of GMs at 2–4 months post-term at so-called fidgety GM age has been found to have the highest predictive value for development of CP, if abnormal.[30,51,55] From that time on many studies on GMs have been done in high-risk infants among them meta-analysis of GMs in different age groups and risks, and comparison with other diagnostic methods.[56-59]

GENERAL MOVEMENTS AS A PREDICTOR OF NEUROLOGIC DISABILITY IN THE FUTURE: LESSON FOR PRENATAL ASSESSMENT

Neurological assessment of preterm infants has not been standardized and up to now, according to the research, at least

27 assessment measures were identified and among them eight fulfilled all clinimetric criteria for neuromotor assessment of preterm infants which were: suitable for use in preterm infants, discriminative, predictive, or evaluative, designed for serial/longitudinal use, and referenced as a norm.[35] Out of 27 analyzed clinimetric tests for premature infant neurological assessment, the following eight met the study inclusion criteria:[35]

Assessment of preterm infants' behavior (APIB), neonatal intensive care unit network neurobehavioral scale (NNNS), test of infant motor performance (TIMP), Prechtl's assessment of GMs, neurobehavioral assessment of the preterm infant (NAPI), Dubowitz neurological assessment of the preterm and full-term infant (Dubowitz), neuromotor behavioral assessment (NMBA), and the Brazelton neonatal behavioral assessment scale (NBAS).[35] In the absence of a criterion standard for neonatal neuromotor assessments, the NICU NNNS and APIB have strong psychometric qualities with better utility for research,[35] while the Prechtl's assessment of GMs, TIMP, and NAPI have strong psychometric qualities but better utility for clinical settings. In the Prechtl assessment of GMs have the best prediction of future outcome.[35]

Assessment of GMs has a positive predictive value of 89% and negative predictive value of 84% for prediction of motor outcome of VLBW infants; while neurodevelopmental assessment at corrected age of 40 weeks had positive predictive value of 33% and negative predictive value of 88%, respectively.[60] Similar results have been obtained at the corrected age of 3 months.[60] Assessment of GMs is a simple, repeatable, and nonintrusive technique, and may be a valuable method for the early detection of CNS impairment in VLBW infants.[60]

Recently published meta-analysis of 47 studies on Prechtl's GMs assessment in the writhing period (till 6 weeks post-term) revealed sensitivity of 93% [with 95% confidence interval (CI) 86–96] and specificity of 59% (95% CI: 45–71), respectively, while assessment of GMs in the fidgety period (from 10 to 20 weeks of corrected age) had the sensitivity of 97% (CI: 93–99) and specificity of 89% (CI: 83–93). Hadders-Algra GMs assessment had a pooled sensitivity 89% (CI: 66–97) and specificity 81% (CI: 64–91), respectively. Fidgety movements assessed by Prechtl's method reached the strongest predictive validity for later CP, but due to a false-positive results cannot be considered in isolation.[57] That is why earlier Hadders-Algra in her work proposed that the best prediction of CP can be achieved if complementary neuroimaging and functional techniques are used in longitudinal series.[30]

Assessment of GMs is time consuming, |and some investigators put the question whether this method could be used as a routine assessment of term and preterm infants, and can it replace physical neurological assessment which is considered not only the observation but also the relevant history taken, thorough examination and relevant plan for the other investigations together with two-way communication of clinician and caregivers.[61] In order to overcome time-consuming obstacle, artificial intelligence is being used for the assessment of GMs.[62,63] The investigation of artificial intelligence is based on the transfer the Prechtl's assessment of GMs from visual perception to computer-based analysis using innovative area of deep learning.[62]

Prechtl's method of GMs assessment used in prenatal and postnatal period enables better understanding of the function and development of CNS. Prechtl's new method and concept of GMs is using offline analysis and assessment after recording of examined infant, which is different than clinical examination in real time. That is the reason why Prechtl's method is time consuming, requiring some technology and expertise. Regardless of all obstacles and threats, this method has high prognostic value in everyday clinical practice giving opportunity to the clinicians to make more accurate and timely diagnosis of CP. Artificial intelligence use for the assessment of GMs is very promising new field of GMs assessment, which will probably solve the problem of time-consuming assessment for the individual clinician.[62] Classical postnatal assessment of GMs is well developed and established, while prenatal assessment needs sophisticated real-time 4D ultrasonographic or other technology to enable more precise evaluation of GM quality in fetuses. At the moment, to the best of our knowledge there is no artificial intelligence use for the assessment of fetal behavior yet.

POSSIBILITY OF LONGITUDINAL ASSESSMENT OF GENERAL MOVEMENTS FROM PRENATAL TO POSTNATAL LIFE

It could be learned from the postnatal studies of neonatal behavior that the assessment of behavior better predicts neurodevelopmental disorders than clinical neurological assessment alone.[54] Assessment of spontaneous infant motility introduced by Prechtl and associates was done "offline" after videotaping with quantitative and qualitative analysis of movements.[54] Such approach of assessment of GMs in high-risk infants has significantly better predictive value for neurological development than neurological examination.[54] 4D instead of 2D US has been used by Kurjak and associates for the assessment of fetal behavior, and

they revealed the continuity of behavior from prenatal/fetal to postnatal/neonatal life.[9-15] They have been speculating about the possibility that earlier diagnosis of neurological disability can improve the outcome. Even though many studies on the continuity of fetal to neonatal behavior have been conducted, it is still not clear whether it can improve our ability to earlier detect the brain pathology connected with neurodevelopmental disability. It is also speculative issue whether earlier diagnosis can possibly rise the opportunity for earlier intervention.[64] Early intervention programs for preterm infants have a positive influence on cognitive outcomes in the short to medium term.[64]

Our investigation of fetal to neonatal continuity revealed that there were no movements observed in the fetuses which were not present in neonates.[9,10] Hand-to-mouth and hand-to-face movements were the most frequent in fetuses and in neonates, while in fetuses hand-to-mouth and hand-to-face movements were more frequent than in neonates who less frequently expressed other hand movements as well.[9,10]

Systematic investigation of fetal behavior by 4D US showed different expressions and movements of fetal face, but the question was if they were indicating fetal awareness?[65] Is it the facial expression of the fetus that can help in understanding what fetus in utero would like to communicate? In concordance with our recent investigation, there is a behavioral continuity from fetal to neonatal life, which probably includes facial expression as well.[66] We can see on the fetal face whether it is satisfied or unhappy, smiling, or worried, self-confident or uncertain, but could the expression of fetal face be considered as the predictor of its normal neurological development?

PRENATAL USE OF POSTNATAL SIGNS OF NEUROLOGICAL ASSESSMENT

By no doubt ultrasonography is a powerful tool for the assessment of fetal behavior. It is 4D US which is making possible assessment by visual observation of two particularly important domains of fetal behavior: fetal finger movements and facial expressions.[4,66,67] 4D US as a new technology enables observation of the fetus in almost real time and evaluation of development of fetal CNS in normally developing fetuses and those at high neurodevelopmental risk.[68,69] A basic understanding of fetal neurology includes defining of motor pathways involved, chronology of their maturation, and direction of myelination.[70,71] Fetal sex is influencing behavior which means that it is different in male and female fetuses, but also maternal psychotropic drugs used in pregnancy influence fetal behavior in utero and postnatally, meaning that these facts should be taken under consideration not only for fetal behavioral assessment but for the neonate as well.[70,71] All these facts are helpful for the interpretation of fetal behavior and fetal movements.[34] The experience acquired with the ATNAT helps in interpretation of fetal movements.[72]

As pointed out before, activity limitation in CP is caused by disorders of movement and posture occurring at the time of fetal brain development.[22-25] Patients with CP besides motor disorders have associated disturbances of sensation, cognition, communication, perception, behavior, and/or with seizure disorder.[22-25] Expected pattern of brain maturation was impaired and not happening as expected for some reasons resulting in those "disturbances".[22-26] Sometimes brain can be morphologically changed, but morphology is not always

followed by neurological outcome.[22-26] The patients with CP are expecting and clinicians have a desire to make a long-term prognosis for each specific type of fetal brain damage, which then is followed by applicable plan for suitable treatment.[22-26]

According to the previously described prenatal neurological assessment of the neonate introduced by Amiel-Tison, fetal cranial sutures should be checked during 4D US assessment and if they are overlapping, then this is considered as an ominous sign of possible brain damage or improper brain growth.[34,72]

Four-dimensional ultrasound has many advantages for neurological assessment of the fetus, but it is commonly believed that early prediction of CP based on visual observation of the fetus by this valuable method is limited due to the "precompetent" stage of most of the motor behaviors observed in utero.[34] That is why another signs from prenatal neurological assessment should be searched for like high-arched palate which is a part of ATNAT postnatal assessment.[72] What was believed as prenatally undetectable became visible by 4D US. Recently, the 3D "reverse face technique" has been described in the assessment of high-arched palate and other fetal facial structures.[73,74] This technique overcomes shadowing of the fetal face by rotating the frontal facial image through 180° along the vertical axis, so that the palate, nasal cavity, and orbits become visualized.[74] New technique of image segmentation and computer analysis of 3D US volumes of the fetal face may provide an objective measure to quantify fetal facial features and identify abnormalities.[74] This technique is still not suitable for everyday clinical practice, because the volumes require additional manual segmentation, which is time consuming.[74]

Natural hand and finger positioning was assessed by Pooh and Ogura in their 3D/4D study of fetal hand and finger positioning.[75-77]

They found that between 9th and beginning of the 10th week of gestation fetal hands were located in front of the chest and no movements of wrists and fingers were visualized.[75-77] The first active arm movements occurred in the middle of the 10th week.[75] The significance of this study is showing that finger and thumb movements begun in the early stage of human life, long before the maturation of the upper system.[75] This study proved that motor activity of the hands and fingers are dependent on the development of the lower system, while upper system takes over not before 30–32 weeks.[34]

Four-dimensional ultrasound enables detection of so-called neurological thumb squeezed in a fist described by Amiel-Tison in her assessment of the neonate as well as overlapping cerebral sutures.[34,78]

Another important sign from postnatal neurological assessment used in neurological assessment of the fetus by 4D US is head retroflection which becomes visible between 10th and 11th gestational week.[34,79] It is known that the activity of flexor muscles is dependent on the upper system from 34 weeks of gestation, while before that it is mostly under lower system control.[34] The absence of active head flexion explored postnatally by the raise-to-sit maneuver is one of the major neurological signs at 40 weeks of gestation.[34]

IS GRAVITY AFFECTING PRENATAL AND POSTNATAL MOTOR DEVELOPMENT?

Very little is known about influence and significance of the gravity on fetal motor development. As pregnancy is advancing, gravity in utero is decreasing, which is the reason why the concept that the fetus floats in a state of weightlessness cannot be applied to the whole pregnancy.[80,81] After the birth, the fetus is exposed to the force of gravity, which is very stressful event for the neonate.[80,81] The fetus is exposed to quite different environment in utero then postnatally, which can be explained by the acronym GATO (gravity, age, thermoregulation, and oxygenation) meaning that there is gravity in utero during fetal period, the age of fetus is changing during gestation, and fetus is exposed to higher temperature and lower oxygen saturation than the neonate after birth.[81] This hypothesis is called a "Baby Astronaut" hypothesis which suggests to explain synergistic effect of these factors on development of the motor system.[81]

In utero fetus is exposed to the conditions of microgravity, but up to the end of pregnancy it is not in significant contact with the uterine walls and does not have the possibility to exert antigravity motor activity and sensory input arising from that activity.[80] It was revealed that fetus in utero until 21st week of gestation is in a condition similar to neutral buoyancy with apparent weight around 5%.[25] Exposure to the significant mechanical stress due to gravitation forces is apparent at around 26 weeks of gestation when the fetus has from 60 to 80% of apparent weight.[81] Antigravity control is developing in the first year of life when most of infants stand on their feet and begin walking. Exposure to 1 g force of gravity after birth and in the first months of life is frustrating for infants and for parents with many adjustments to the new hostile environment including the Moro reflex as the most important. Movement against gravity begins during the first month of life, and by 4 months of age increased flexion control balances the strong extensor muscle patterns.[80,81] These movements enable the child to develop weight shifting, which in turn stimulates righting and equilibrium responses.[80,81] The influence of the gravity on prenatal and postnatal development of motility could be considered as discontinuity from prenatal (low gravity) to postnatal life (high gravity); however, it proves that different environmental conditions significantly influence behavior and development. According to this theory, after birth neonate is exposed to the tyranny of gravity up to the age of 3–4 months, when antigravity forces of the neonate enable to overcome this developmental obstacle.[82]

SIGNIFICANCE OF EARLY INTERVENTION AND OTHER PROCEDURES TO IMPROVE NEURODEVELOPMENTAL OUTCOME IN CHILDREN WITH NEUROLOGICAL RISK

Neurodevelopmental disorders could be significant from a social, economic, medical, and individual point of view. Many interventions can have possibly positive impact on the course of disability depending on the time of onset of damage and its localization and severity. Accompanying comorbidity such as intellectual disabilities, behavioral, speech, and feeding disorders, epilepsy, sleep disorders, blindness, deafness, incontinence, hip dysplasia, and many others can influence the course and the outcome of the primary neurodevelopmental disability. In order to improve the neurodevelopmental outcome and reduce the consequences, it is necessary to include affected infant in early intervention programs (habilitation and rehabilitation) as early as possible.[83] It is important to start interventions in the perinatal period that act neuroprotectively and can possibly reduce the frequency of neurodevelopmental disorders postnatally.

Interventions in Pregnancy that Affect the Incidence of Neuro-developmental Disorders Postnatally

According to the results of systematic research, it has been proven that some interventions in pregnancy reduce the frequency of neurodevelopmental damage postnatally. According to the above meta-analysis (including 27 controlled randomized trials involving 32,490 children), it was found that the use of magnesium sulfate in pregnant women with threatened preterm birth for the purpose of fetal neuroprotection can postnatally reduce the incidence of CP. Prophylactic administration of antibiotics may increase the risk of developing CP in women who are in preterm labor with intact amniotic membranes and with fetus in a good condition during labor. Repeated doses of corticosteroids in pregnant women with threatened preterm birth have not shown a clear effect on reducing the risk of development of CP.[64] A recently published meta-analysis found that the use of magnesium sulfate prenatally in pregnant women with threatened preterm birth is very effective in reducing the incidence of CP in preterm infants postnatally.[84] In addition, an intervention that has a beneficial effect on the psychomotric development of infants and on the development of vision and speech is the use of omega-3 polyunsaturated fatty acids in pregnancy and postnatally.[85,86] It is believed that the use of other micronutrients such as vitamin B_{12}, folic acid in combination with omega-3 fatty acids may have a beneficial effect on reducing the incidence of preterm birth in pregnant women and behavioral disorders in infants.[87]

Neonatal Interventions Affecting the Incidence of Neurodevelopmental Disorders

In a systematic review of 96 studies in 15,885 children, the following neonatal interventions were found to be effective in reducing the incidence of CP: therapeutic hypothermia in proven intrapartum hypoxia and the development of hypoxic ischemic encephalopathy contributed to a reduction in the incidence of CP. Administration of methylxanthines (caffeine) in extremely immature infants either mechanically ventilated or not and methylxanthine administration prior to endotracheal extubation is neuroprotective.[31] In contrast, early postnatal administration of corticosteroids before the age of 8 days for chronic lung diseases contributed to an increase in the incidence of CP.[31] Postnatal procedures such as ethamsylate administration, volume expander administration, administration of collagen hydrolyzate instead of fresh frozen plasma, prophylactic administration of indomethacin, administration of synthetic surfactant, prophylactic phototherapy did not affect the incidence of CP in preterm infants.[31]

NEW PUBLISHED DATA ON THE CONTINUITY OF FETAL TO NEONATAL BEHAVIOR

In the recently published paper, postnatal follow-up of fetuses with borderline and abnormal KANET scores are presented in **Table 1**.[88] There were 153 fetuses with borderline scores and 52 fetuses with abnormal KANET scores, of whom 11 were terminated in utero or died postnatally, meaning that 41 could be evaluated postnatally.[88] In the group with borderline KANET scores, there were 145 with normal postnatal development, two had moderate and four had severe developmental delay, while two fetuses died in utero. In the group of 52 infants with abnormal KANET scores, 26 had normal development, one infant had slight developmental delay, one moderate, and 13 infants had severe developmental delay, while 11 died in utero.[88] Severe developmental delay was more frequent in the group with abnormal KANET scores, which was highly statistically significant **(Table 1)**. Out of 1,102 children

older than 2 years 36 had abnormal and 11 borderline KANET scores.[88] Of 47 children with borderline abnormal KANET scores in one >3-year-old child CP was diagnosed.[88] Out of 1,556 children with normal KANET scores 26 had developmental delay, of whom it appeared severe in 18.[88] One child from that group who had a normal KANET score developed severe developmental delay due to Kagami Ogata syndrome and is now 33 months old.[88]

CONCLUSION

It has been shown that neurological assessment of the fetus is not reliable using 2D US technology, but even with the sophisticated 4D US it is extremely difficult. Quantity of GMs is not that informative as assessment of their quality which is more predictive for detection of neurological impairment. "Gestalt perception" of premature GMs we are dealing with in utero and writhing GMs appearing several weeks postnatally are not as predictive for the detection of neurologically abnormal fetuses or newborns as fidgety GMs emerging from 54 to 58 weeks of postmenstrual age.[57] Therefore, some additional parameters should be added to the prenatal neurological examination to improve clinicians' ability to make the distinction between normal and abnormal fetuses or to assess optimality of CNS development.[34,37,71] Possibilities of 4D sonography are demonstrating the prenatal onset of a brain damage, based on morphological and functional signs. There is no doubt that this observation is helpful, even though that prenatally observed signs are not yet highly predictive due to the brain immaturity, their identification will be at least recognized as a retrospective marker for a prenatal insult.[88]

TABLE 1: Postnatal follow-up of infants who as fetuses had borderline and abnormal KANET[&] scores from low- and high-risk pregnancies including termination of pregnancy and postnatal death.[88]

Name of the investigator (N*)	KANET score (N*)	Postnatal developmental delay (N*)				Comment
		No	Slight	Moderate	Severe	
N = 482	Borderline N = 36	33	0	0	2	1 IUD[+]
	Abnormal N = 19	15	0	0	4	All severe congenital malformations
N = 520	Borderline N = 47	45	0	0	1	1 IUD[+]
	Abnormal N = 19	7	0	0	1[++]	5 died 6 terminated
N = 212	Borderline N = 39	39	0	0	0	-
	Abnormal N = 6	3	0	0	3	One case of trisomy 13, 18, and 21
N = 60	Borderline N =16	16	0	0	0	-
	Abnormal N = 2	1	1	0	0	IUGR** one with slight developmental delay
N = 145	Borderline N = 3	0	0	2	1	-
	Abnormal N = 0	0	0	0	0	-
N = 26	Borderline N = 2	2	0	0	0	-
	Abnormal N = 1	0	0	0	1	One with severe delay Kagami–Ogata syndrome
N = 35	Borderline N = 0	0	0	0	0	-
	Abnormal N = 1	0	0	1	0	IUGR**
N = 17	Borderline N = 3	3	0	0	0	-
	Abnormal N = 1	0	0	0	1	Trisomy 18, died in the first day of life
N = 76	Borderline N = 7	7	0	0	0	-
	Abnormal N = 3	3	0	0	3	Two severe congenital malformations and one IUGR**
Subtotal normal KANET	1,351 (86.8%)	1,348 (99.8%)	0	2 (0.1%)	1 (0.1%)	One with severe delay Kagami–Ogata syndrome
Subtotal borderline KANET	153 (9.8%)	145 (94.8%)	0	2 (1.3%)	4 (2.6%)	2 IUD (1.3%)
Subtotal abnormal KANET	52 (3.3%)	26 (50.0%)	1 (1.9%)	1 (1.9%)	13 (25.0%)	11 terminated or died (21.2%)
Total	1,556 (100.0%)	1,519 (97.6%)	1 (0.1%)	5 (0.3%)	18 (1.2%)	13 (0.8%)

$\chi^2 = 315.28$; d.f.[+++] = 6; p <0.01

[&]KANET: Kurjak's Antenatal Neurodevelopmental Test
*N: number of infants
[+]IUD: intrauterine death
[++]One infant with CP (with previous case of cerebral palsy in the family)
**IUGR: intrauterine growth restriction
[+++]d.f. = degrees of freedom

We have now applicable KANET screening neurological test for fetus and assessment of neonate is the continuation of that prenatal test, but standardized procedures for postnatal follow-up are still missing, because there are many neurological methods for postnatal evaluation and many of them are too complicated for everyday clinical use. The environment of prenatal and postnatal evaluation is quite different, which is the reason why issue of longitudinal GMs assessment from prenatal to postnatal life is questionable and should be further investigated as in utero we are dealing with quite different environment and less mature brain. Could neonatal assessment of neurologically impaired fetuses bring some new insights into their prenatal neurological status is still unclear and to be thoroughly and prospectively investigated. New KANET scoring system for prenatal neurological assessment of the fetus proposed by Kurjak et al. give some new possibilities to detect fetuses at high neurological risk, although it is obvious that dynamic and complicated process of functional CNS development is not easy to investigate. Although our journey of 15 years of investigating KANET test could probably be positively evaluated, we have still a long way to go.

■ REFERENCES

1. World Health Organization. (2001). World Health Report 2001. Chapter 2: Burden of mental and behavioral disorders. [online] Available from: https://www.who.int/whr/2001/en/whr01_en.pdf?ua=1 [Last accessed February, 2022).
2. Ismail FY, Shapiro BK. What are neuro-developmental disorders? Curr Opin Neurol. 2019;32(4):611-6.
3. MacLennan AH, Thompson SC, Gecz J. Cerebral palsy: causes, pathways, and the role of genetic variants. Am J Obstet Gynecol. 2015;213(6):779-88.
4. Kurjak A, Barisic LS, Stanojevic M, Salihagic-Kadic A, Porovic S. Are we ready to investigate cognitive function of fetal brain? The role of advanced four-dimensional sonography. Donald Sch JUltrasound Obstet Gynecol. 2016;10(2):116-24.
5. Kurjak A, Antsaklis P, Stanojevic M, Porovic S. Fetal behavior assessed by four-dimensional ultrasound. Donald Sch J Ultrasound Obstet Gynecol. 2017;11(2):169-73.
6. Neto RM, Kurjak A, Porovic S, Stanojevic M, Gaber G. Clinical study of fetal neurobehavior by the Kurjak antenatal neurodevelopmental test. Donald Sch J Ultrasound Obstet Gynecol. 2017;11(4):355-61.
7. Ouyang M, Dubois J, Yu Q, Mukherjee P, Huang H. Delineation of early brain development from fetuses to infants with diffusion MRI and beyond. Neuroimage. 2019;185:836-50.
8. Vasung L, Turk EA, Ferradal SL, Sutin J, Stout JN, Ahtam B, et al. Exploring early human brain development with structural and physiological neuroimaging. Neuroimage. 2019;187:226-54.
9. Kurjak A, Stanojevic M, Andonotopo W, Salihagic-Kadic A, Carrera JM, Azumendi G. Behavioral pattern continuity from prenatal to postnatal life—a study by four-dimensional (4D) ultrasonography. J Perinat Med. 2004;32(4):346-53.
10. Stanojevic M, Perlman JM, Andonotopo W, Kurjak A. From fetal to neonatal behavioral status. Ultrasound Rev Obstet Gynecol. 2004;4(1):59-71.
11. Stanojevic M, Kurjak A. Continuity between fetal and neonatal neurobehavior. Donald Sch J Ultrasound Obstetr Gynecol. 2008;2(3):64-75.
12. Stanojevic M, Kurjak A, Salihagić-Kadić A, Vasilj O, Miskovic B, Shaddad AN, et al. Neurobehavioral continuity from fetus to neonate. J Perinat Med. 2011;39(2):171-7.
13. Stanojevic M. Neonatal aspects: is there continuity? Donald Sch J ultrasound Obstet Gynecol. 2012;6(2):189-96.
14. Stanojevic M, Zaputovic S, Bosnjak AP. Continuity between fetal and neonatal neurobehavior. Semin Fetal Neonatal Med. 2012;17(6):324-9.

15. Stanojevic M. Antenatal and postnatal assessment of neurobehavior: which one should be used? Donald School J Obstet Gynecol. 2015;9(1):67-74.

16. Išasegi IZ, Radoš M, Krsnik Ž, Radoš M, Benjak V, Kostović I. Interactive histogenesis of axonal strata and proliferative zones in the human fetal cerebral wall. Brain Struct Funct. 2018;223(9):3919-43.

17. Barth RP, Scarborough A, Lloyd EC, Losby J, Casanueva C, Mann T. Developmental Status and Early Intervention Service Needs of Maltreated Children. Washington, DC: U.S. Department of Health and Human Services, Office of the Assistant Secretary for Planning and Evaluation; 2008. [online] Available from: http://aspe.hhs.gov/hsp/08/devneeds/report.pdf. [Last accessed February, 2018].

18. Jöud A, Sehlstedt A, Källén K, Westbom L, Rylander L. Associations between antenatal and perinatal risk factors and cerebral palsy: a Swedish cohort study. BMJ Open. 2020;10(8):e038453.

19. Tatishvili N, Gabunia M, Laliani N, Tatishvili S. Epidemiology of neurodevelopmental disorders in two-year-old Georgian children. Pilot study—population based prospective study in a randomly chosen sample. Eur J Paediatr Neurol. 2010;14(3):247-52.

20. Soleimani F, Vameghi R, Biglarian A, Rahgozar M. Prevalence of motor developmental disorders in children in alborz province, Iran in 2010. Iran Red Crescent Med J. 2014;16(12):e16711.

21. McIntyre S. The continually changing epidemiology of cerebral palsy. Acta Paediatr. 2018;107(3):374-5.

22. Patel DR, Neelakantan M, Pandher K, Merrick J. Cerebral palsy in children: a clinical overview. Transl Pediatr. 2020;9(Suppl 1):S125-S135.

23. Himmelmann K, Uvebrant P. The panorama of cerebral palsy in Sweden part XII shows that patterns changed in the birth years 2007-2010. Acta Paediatr. 2018;107(3):462-8.

24. Drummond PM, Colver AF. Analysis by gestational age of cerebral palsy in singleton births in north-east England 1970-94. Paediatr Perinat Epidemiol. 2002;16(2):172-80.

25. Reid SM, Dagia CD, Ditchfield MR, Carlin JB, Reddihough DS. Population-based studies of brain imaging patterns in cerebral palsy. Dev Med Child Neurol. 2014;56(3):222-32.

26. Hemminki K, Li X, Sundquist K, Sundquist J. High familial risks for cerebral palsy implicate partial heritable aetiology. Paediatr Perinat Epidemiol. 2007;21(3):235-41.

27. Jin SC, Lewis SA, Bakhtiari S, Zeng X, Sierant MC, Shetty S, et al. Mutations disrupting neuritogenesis genes confer risk for cerebral palsy. Nat Genet. 2020;52(10):1046-56.

28. te Velde A, Morgan C, Novak I, Tantsis E, Badawi N. Early Diagnosis and Classification of Cerebral Palsy: An Historical Perspective and Barriers to an Early Diagnosis. J Clin Med. 2019;8(10):1599.

29. Nelson KB, Ellenberg JH. Neonatal signs as predictors of cerebral palsy. Pediatrics. 1979;64(2):225-32.

30. Hadders-Algra M. Early diagnosis and early intervention in cerebral palsy. Front Neurol. 2014;5:185.

31. Shepherd E, Salam RA, Middleton P, Han S, Makrides M, McIntyre S, et al. Neonatal interventions for preventing cerebral palsy: an overview of Cochrane Systematic Reviews. Cochrane Database Syst Rev. 2018;6(6):CD012409.

32. Kurjak A, Miskovic B, Andonotopo W, Stanojevic M, Azumendi G, Vrcic H. How useful is 3D and 4D in perinatal medicine? J Perinat Med. 2007;35(1):10-27.

33. Gurbuz A, Karateke A, Yilmaz U, Kabaca C. The role of perinatal and intrapartum risk factors in the etiology of cerebral palsy in term deliveries in a Turkish population. J Matern Fetal Neonatal Med. 2006;19(3):147-55.

34. Amiel-Tison C, Gosselin J, Kurjak A. Neurosonography in the second half of fetal life: a neonatologist's point of view. J Perinat Med. 2006;34(6):437-46.

35. Noble Y, Boyd R. Neonatal assessments for the preterm infant up to 4 months corrected age: a systematic review. Dev Med Child Neurol. 2012;54(2):129-39.

36. Simard MN, Lambert J, Lachance C, Audibert F, Gosselin J. Interexaminer reliability of

Amiel-Tison neurological assessments. Pediatr Neurol. 2009;41(5):347-52.

37. Gosselin J, Gahagan S, Amiel-Tison C. The Amiel-Tison Neurological Assessment at Term: conceptual and methodological continuity in the course of follow-up. Ment Retard Dev Disabil Res Rev. 2005;11(1):34-51.

38. Groenendaal F, de Vries LS. Fifty years of brain imaging in neonatal encephalopathy following perinatal asphyxia. Pediatr Res. 2017;81(1-2):150-5.

39. Lemmon ME, Wagner MW, Bosemani T, Carson KA, Northington FJ, Huisman TAGM, et al. Diffusion Tensor Imaging Detects Occult Cerebellar Injury in Severe Neonatal Hypoxic-Ischemic Encephalopathy. Dev Neurosci. 2017;39(1-4):207-14.

40. Counsell SJ, Arichi T, Arulkumaran S, Rutherford MA. Fetal and neonatal neuro-imaging. Handb Clin Neurol. 2019;162:67-103.

41. Burkitt K, Kang O, Jyoti R, Mohamed AL, Chaudhari T. Comparison of cranial ultrasound and MRI for detecting BRAIN injury in extremely preterm infants and correlation with neurological outcomes at 1 and 3 years. Eur J Pediatr. 2019;178(7):1053-61.

42. Annink KV, de Vries LS, Groenendaal F, Vijlbrief DC, Weeke LC, Roehr CC, et al. The development and validation of a cerebral ultrasound scoring system for infants with hypoxic-ischaemic encephalopathy. Pediatr Res. 2020;87(Suppl 1):59-66.

43. Seme-Ciglenecki P. Predictive values of cranial ultrasound and assessment of general movements for neurological development of preterm infants in the Maribor region of Slovenia. Wien Klin Wochenschr. 2007;119(15-16):490-6.

44. Ophelders DRMG, Gussenhoven R, Klein L, Jellema RK, Westerlaken RJJ, Hütten MC, et al. Preterm Brain Injury, Antenatal Triggers, and Therapeutics: Timing Is Key. Cells. 2020;9(8):1871.

45. Millar LJ, Shi L, Hoerder-Suabedissen A, Molnár Z. Neonatal hypoxia ischaemia: mechanisms, models, and therapeutic challenges. Front Cell Neurosci. 2017;11:78.

46. Stanojevic M, Hafner T, Kurjak A. Three-dimensional (3D) ultrasound—a useful imaging technique in the assessment of neonatal brain. J Perinat Med. 2002;30(1):74-83.

47. Kurian J, Sotardi S, Liszewski MC, Gomes WA, Hoffman T, Taragin BH. Three-dimensional ultrasound of the neonatal brain: technical approach and spectrum of disease. Pediatr Radiol. 2017;47(5):613-27.

48. Wang Y, Chen X, Zhong S, Zhang R, Pan Y, An P, et al. Diagnostic Value of Two-Dimensional plus Four-Dimensional Ultrasonography in Fetal Craniocerebral Anomalies. Iran J Public Health. 2019;48(2):323-30.

49. Gotardo JW, Volkmer NFV, Stangler GP, Dornelles AD, Bohrer BBA, Carvalho CG. Impact of peri-intraventricular haemorrhage and periventricular leukomalacia in the neurodevelopment of preterms: a systematic review and meta-analysis. PLoS One. 2019;14(10):e0223427.

50. Brouwer MJ, van Kooij BJ, van Haastert IC, Koopman-Esseboom C, Groenendaal F, de Vries LS, et al. Sequential cranial ultrasound and cerebellar diffusion weighted imaging contribute to the early prognosis of neurodevelopmental outcome in preterm infants. PLoS One. 2014;9(10):e109556.

51. Einspieler C, Prechtl HFR, Bos AF, Ferrari F, Cioni G. Prechtl's method on the qualitative assessment of general movements in preterm, term and young infants. Cambridge: Mac Keith Press; 2004.

52. de Vries JI, Visser GH, Prechtl HF. The emergence of fetal behavior. I. Qualitative aspects. Early Hum Dev. 1982;7(4):301-22.

53. Seme-Ciglenečki P. Predictive value of assessment of general movements for neurological development of high-risk preterm infants: comparative study. Croat Med J. 2003;44(6):721-7.

54. Seesahai J, Luther M, Rhoden CC, Church PT, Asztalos E, Banihani R. The general movements assessment in term and late-preterm infants diagnosed with neonatal encephalopathy, as a predictive tool of cerebral palsy by 2 years of age: a scoping review protocol. Syst Rev. 2020;9(1):154.

55. Hadders-Algra M. General movements: a window for early identification of children

at high risk for developmental disorders. J Pediatr. 2004;145(Suppl 2):S12-8.

56. Darsaklis V, Snider LM, Majnemer A, Mazer B. Predictive validity of Prechtl's Method on the Qualitative Assessment of General Movements: a systematic review of the evidence. Dev Med Child Neurol. 2011;53(10):896-906.

57. Kwong AKL, Fitzgerald TL, Doyle LW, Cheong JLY, Spittle AJ. Predictive validity of spontaneous early infant movement for later cerebral palsy: a systematic review. Dev Med Child Neurol. 2018;60(5):480-9.

58. Hadders-Algra M, Philippi H. Predictive validity of the general movements assessment: type of population versus type of assessment. Dev Med Child Neurol. 2018; 60(11):1186.

59. Pires CS, Marba STM, Caldas JPS, Stopiglia MCS. Predictive value of the general movements assessment in preterm infants: a meta-analysis. Rev Paul Pediatr. 2020;38: e2018286.

60. Stahlmann N, Härtel C, Knopp A, Gehring B, Kiecksee H, Thyen U. Predictive value of neurodevelopmental assessment versus evaluation of general movements for motor outcome in preterm infants with birth weights <1500 g. Neuropediatrics. 2007;38(2):91-9.

61. Rosenbloom L. What is the role of the general movements assessment in clinical practice? Dev Med Child Neurol. 2018;60(1):6.

62. Irshad MT, Nisar MA, Gouverneur P, Rapp M, Grzegorzek M. AI approaches towards Prechtl's assessment of general movements: a systematic literature review. Sensors (Basel). 2020;20(18):5321.

63. Doroniewicz I, Ledwoń DJ, Affanasowicz A, Kieszczyńska K, Latos D, Matyja M, et al. Writhing movement detection in newborns on the second and third day of life using pose-based feature machine learning classification. Sensors (Basel). 2020; 20(21):5986.

64. Shepherd E, Salam RA, Middleton P, Makrides M, McIntyre S, Badawi N, et al. Antenatal and intrapartum interventions for preventing cerebral palsy: an overview of Cochrane systematic reviews. Cochrane Database Syst Rev. 2017;8(8):CD012077.

65. Kurjak A, Stanojevic M, Azumendi G, Carrera JM. The potential of four-dimensional (4D) ultrasonography in the assessment of fetal awareness. J Perinat Med. 2005;33(1):46-53.

66. AboEllail MAM, Hata T. Fetal face as important indicator of fetal brain function. J Perinat Med. 2017;45(6):729-36.

67. Kadic AS, Kurjak A. Cognitive functions of the fetus. Ultraschall Med. 2018;39(2):181-9.

68. Talic A, Kurjak A, Ahmed B, Stanojevic M, Predojevic M, Kadic AS, et al. The potential of 4D sonography in the assessment of fetal behavior in high-risk pregnancies. J Matern Fetal Neonatal Med. 2011;24(7):948-54.

69. Miskovic B, Vasilj O, Stanojevic M, Ivanković D, Kerner M, Tikvica A. The comparison of fetal behavior in high risk and normal pregnancies assessed by four dimensional ultrasound. J Matern Fetal Neonatal Med. 2010;23(12):1461-7.

70. Hata T, Hanaoka U, AboEllail MAM, Uematsu R, Noguchi J, Kusaka T, et al. Is there a sex difference in fetal behavior? A comparison of the KANET test between male and female fetuses. J Perinat Med. 2016;44(5):585-8.

71. Hata T, Kanenishi K, AboEllail MAM, Mori N, Koyano K, Kato I, et al. Effect of psychotropic drugs on fetal behavior in the third trimester of pregnancy. J Perinat Med. 2019;47(2):207-11.

72. Gosselin J, Amiel-Tison C. Neurological Assessment from Birth to 6 Years. Montreal: Editions du CHU Sainte-Justine; 2011. p. 181.

73. Hu JQ, Zhang YG, Feng W, Shi H. A pitfall in prenatal ultrasonic detection of submucous cleft palate. Ear Nose Throat J. 2020;145561320974867.

74. Clark AE, Biffi B, Sivera R, Dall'Asta A, Fessey L, Wong TL, et al. Developing and testing an algorithm for automatic segmentation of the fetal face from three-dimensional ultrasound images. R Soc Open Sci. 2020;7(11):201342.

75. Pooh RK, Ogura T. Normal and abnormal fetal hand positioning and movement in early pregnancy detected by three- and

four-dimensional ultrasound. Ultrasound Rev Obstet Gynecol. 2004;4(1):46-51.

76. Katz K, Mashiach R, Meizner I. Normal range of fetal finger movements. J Pediatr Orthop B. 2007;16(4):252-5.

77. Kubo S, Horinouchi T, Kinoshita M, Yoshizato T, Kozuma Y, Shinagawa T, et al. Visual diagnosis in utero: prenatal diagnosis of Treacher-Collins syndrome using a 3D/4D ultrasonography. Taiwan J Obstet Gynecol. 2019;58(4):566-9.

78. Ouyang YS, Zhang YX, Meng H, Wu XN, Qi QW. Adducted thumb as an isolated morphologic finding: an early sonographic sign of impaired neurodevelopment: A STROBE compliant study. Medicine (Baltimore). 2018;97(38):e12437.

79. AboEllail MAM, Kanenishi K, Mori N, Noguchi J, Marumo G, Hata T. Ultrasound study of fetal movements in singleton and twin pregnancies at 12-19 weeks. J Perinat Med. 2018;46(8):832-8.

80. Sekulic SR, Lukac DD, Naumovic NM. The fetus cannot exercise like an astronaut: gravity loading is necessary for the physiological development during second half of pregnancy. Med Hypotheses. 2005;64(2):221-8.

81. Meigal AY. Synergistic action of gravity and temperature on the motor system within the lifespan: a "Baby Astronaut" hypothesis. Med Hypotheses. 2013;80(3):275-83.

82. Mellor DJ. Preparing for life after birth: introducing the concepts of intrauterine and extrauterine sensory entrainment in mammalian young. Animals (Basel). 2019;9(10):826.

83. Spittle A, Orton J, Anderson PJ, Boyd R, Doyle LW. Early developmental intervention programmes provided post hospital discharge to prevent motor and cognitive impairment in preterm infants. Cochrane Database Syst Rev. 2015;2015(11):CD005495.

84. Wolf HT, Huusom LD, Henriksen TB, Hegaard HK, Brok J, Pinborg A. Magnesium sulphate for fetal neuroprotection at imminent risk for preterm delivery: a systematic review with meta-analysis and trial sequential analysis. BJOG. 2020; 127(10):1180-8.

85. Shulkin M, Pimpin L, Bellinger D, Kranz S, Fawzi W, Duggan C, et al. n-3 Fatty acid supplementation in mothers, preterm infants, and term infants and childhood psychomotor and visual development: a systematic review and meta-analysis. J Nutr. 2018;148(3):409-18.

86. Gawlik NR, Anderson AJ, Makrides M, Kettler L, Gould JF. The influence of DHA on language development: a review of randomized controlled trials of DHA supplementation in pregnancy, the neonatal period, and infancy. Nutrients. 2020;12(10):3106.

87. Dhobale M, Joshi S. Altered maternal micronutrients (folic acid, vitamin B12) and omega 3 fatty acids through oxidative stress may reduce neurotrophic factors in preterm pregnancy. J Matern Fetal Neonatal Med. 2012;25(4):317-23.

88. Stanojević M, Antsaklis P, Panchal S, Porovic S, Salihagić-Kadić A, Barišić LS, et al. A critical appraisal of Kurjak antenatal neurodevelopmental test: five years of wide clinical use. Donald Sch J Ultrasound Obstet Gynecol. 2021;14(4):304-10.

Twin Fetal Behavior and Facial Expression: Four-dimensional Ultrasound Study

Toshiyuki Hata, Riko Takayoshi, Aya Koyanagi, Takahito Miyake

■ INTRODUCTION

Two-dimensional (2D) sonography has been performed to assess twin fetal movements and behavioral patterns.[1-9] However, due to the characteristics of 2D sonographic scanning, fetal movements and behavioral patterns outside the scanning plane cannot be displayed on the monitor.[10] With the introduction of and advances in four-dimensional (4D) ultrasound, fetal movements, behavioral patterns, and facial expressions are now easily and readily observed in all three trimesters of pregnancy.[10-15] We herein discuss the current status of twin fetal behavioral and facial assessments using 4D ultrasound and provide our recommendations for further investigations on neurobehavioral development and brain function in twin pregnancies.

■ INTERTWIN CONTACT AND INTRAPAIR STIMULATION

Arabin et al.[5] previously examined the onset of interhuman contact using 2D sonography, and detected the first reaction to touch of a co-twin at 65 postmenstrual days. Contact of a longer duration between both twins, including the extremities, or complex contact was noted at 85 and 92 postmenstrual days, respectively. However, 4D ultrasound revealed intertwin contact and complex body movements earlier at 61 and 68 postmenstrual days, respectively.[16]

Hata et al.[17] were the first to demonstrate twin fetal intercontact using three-dimensional (3D) ultrasound, and 4D ultrasound now clearly shows various types of intertwin contacts in real time **(Figs. 1 to 4)**.

Sasaki et al.[18] used 4D ultrasound to investigate intertwin contact (10 different types of contact) at $11–13^{+6}$ weeks of gestation in monochorionic diamniotic (MD) and dichorionic diamniotic (DD) twins, and reported significant differences in the total number of contacts at $10–11^{+6}$ weeks of gestation between MD and DD twins. The total

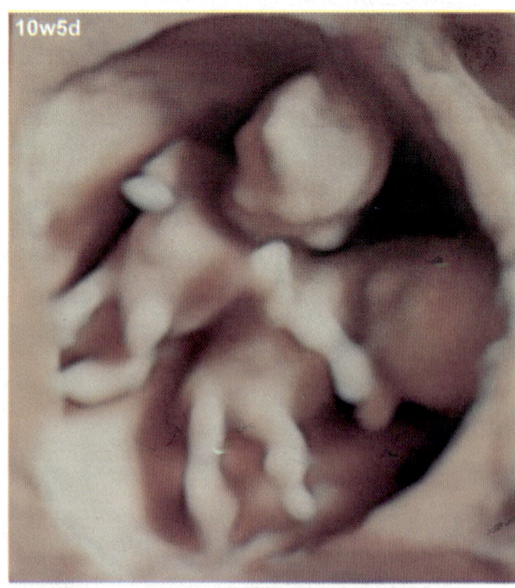

Fig. 1: Intertwin contact in monochorionic diamniotic twins at 10 weeks and 5 days of gestation.

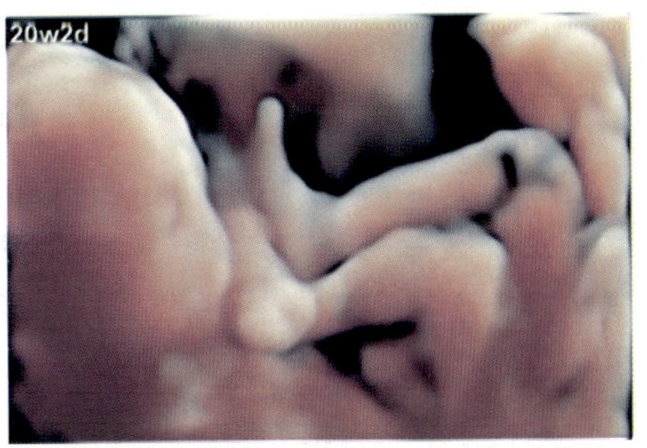

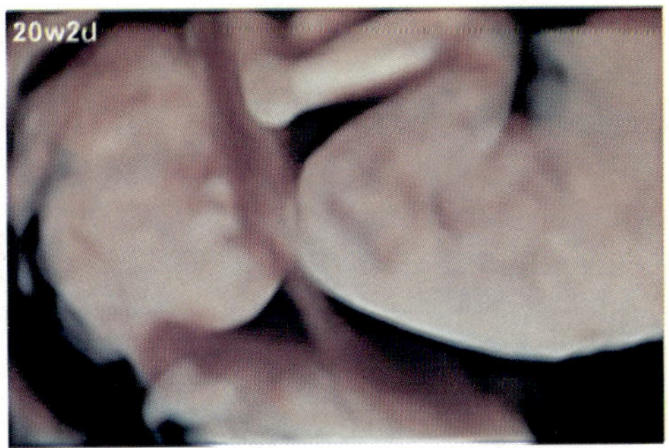

Fig. 2: Intertwin contact (kick in the face) in dichorionic diamniotic twins at 20 weeks and 2 days of gestation.

Fig. 3: Intertwin contact (simultaneous body-to-face and leg-to-face contacts) in dichorionic diamniotic twins at 20 weeks and 2 days of gestation.

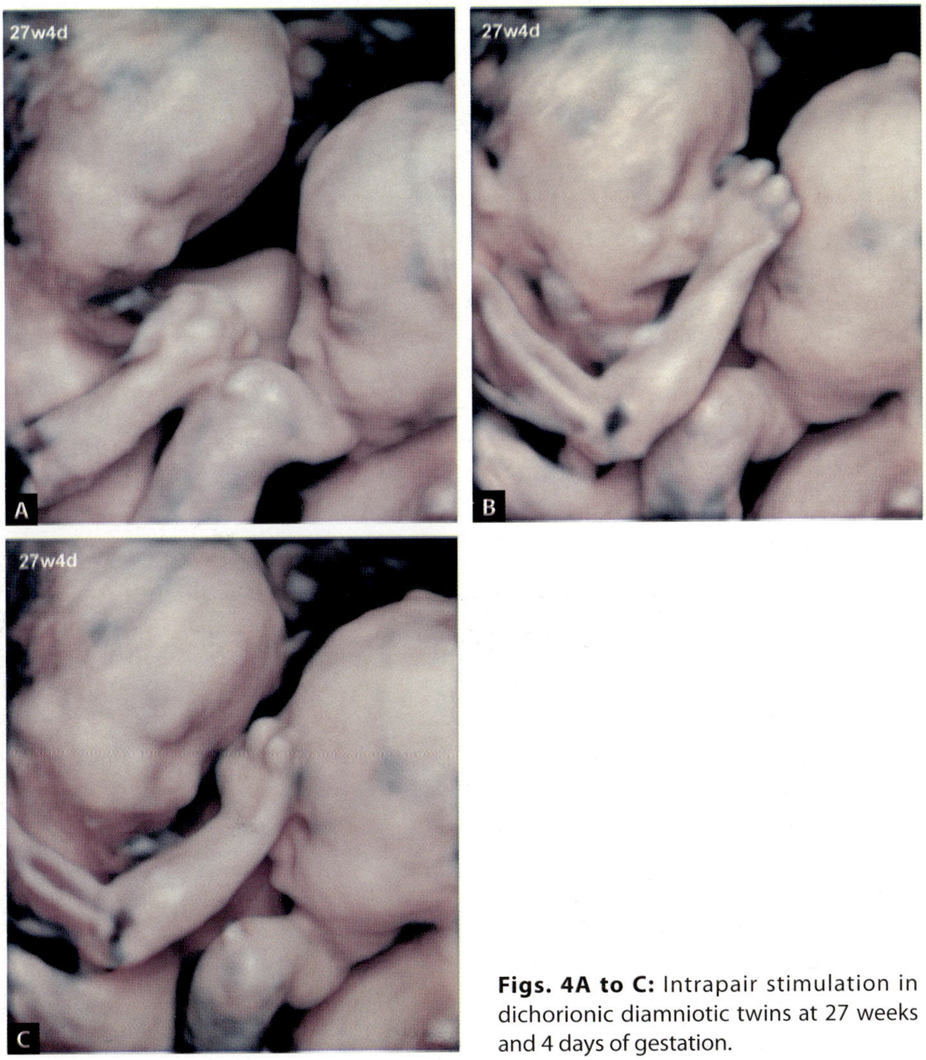

Figs. 4A to C: Intrapair stimulation in dichorionic diamniotic twins at 27 weeks and 4 days of gestation.

number of contacts also significantly differed between 10–11 and 12–13 weeks of gestation in DD twins. The higher number of and earlier intertwin contacts observed in MD twins were attributed to a smaller intertwin distance and thinner intertwin membranes. Furthermore, the position of one fetus relative to the other at 11–13[+6] weeks of gestation did not significantly differ between MD and DD twins.[19] However, the frequency of head-to-arm contact at 12–13[+6] weeks of gestation significantly differed between MD and DD twins. Moreover, significant differences were noted in head-to-arm, head-to-trunk, arm-to-arm, and arm-to-trunk contacts in MD twins between 10–11[+6] and 12–13[+6] weeks of gestation. Early fetal neuromuscular development and the differentiation of the neuromuscular system have been suggested to contribute to the differences observed in the frequencies of the various types of intertwin contacts in MD and DD twins.[19]

A previous study that used 2D sonography showed that the rate of evoked fetal movements simultaneously occurring in both twins at 10–21 weeks of gestation accounted for 4.96% of all fetal movements observed, whereas that of spontaneous fetal movements independently occurring in each fetus was 95.04%.[3] Hata et al.[20] employed 4D ultrasound to examine reactions to touch in utero between twin fetuses late in the first trimester of pregnancy; the frequencies of no reaction (although twins appear to touch, there is no clear reaction) and reaction (twins appear to touch and there is a clear reaction by the co-twin) movements were assessed. The median rate of reaction movements was 33.9% (range, 27–64.1%). These findings demonstrated that the incidence of a reflex movement by the co-twin to touch by the other twin late in the first trimester was higher using 4D than 2D sonography.

TWIN FETAL MOVEMENTS BEFORE 20 WEEKS

AboEllail et al.[21] used 4D ultrasound to compare differences in fetal behavioral patterns at 12–19[+6] weeks of gestation between singleton and twin fetuses. The frequencies of the following fetal movements: head anteflexion, head retroflexion, body rotation, hand-to-face movement, general movement, arm movement, leg movement, and mouthing, in 15-minute recordings were examined.[22] In comparison of fetal movements, a significant difference was only observed in arm movement at 12–13[+6] weeks between singleton and twin fetuses. Furthermore, the frequencies of all movements at 14–19[+6] weeks were significantly higher in singleton than in twin fetuses. Therefore, the limitation of available space and crowding of twin fetuses with advancing gestation appeared to have a more prominent effect on fetal movements in twin than in singleton fetuses, even in the first half of pregnancy.

Mori et al.[23] examined the effects of advancing gestation on the frequencies of singleton and twin fetal movements and used 4D ultrasound to compare the total number of fetal movements at 12–19[+6] weeks of gestation among singleton, active, and quiet twin fetuses. Significant increases in the frequencies of hand-to-face and leg movements were observed with advancing gestation, in contrast to significant decreases in the frequencies of general movements at 12–19[+6] weeks in singleton fetuses. Significant decreases were also noted in the frequencies of body rotation and general movements with advancing gestation, whereas a significant increase was observed in the frequency of mouthing movement at 12–19[+6] weeks in twin fetuses. The total number of fetal movements at 12–13[+6] weeks of gestation was significantly higher in singleton fetuses than in quiet twins, and significant differences were also noted in the total number of fetal movements at 14–19[+6] weeks between singleton and active or quiet twins. Therefore, the characteristics of fetal movements before 20 weeks of gestation appeared to differ between singleton and twin fetuses.

Castiello et al.[24] used 4D ultrasound to assess intrapair contact at 14 and 18 weeks of gestation in twin fetuses. A kinematic analysis showed a longer duration of movement and prolonged deceleration time for other-directed movements than for movements directed toward the uterine wall. Similar findings were obtained for movements directed toward the co-twin and self-directed movements toward the eye region (the most delicate region of the body). Therefore, movements directed toward the co-twin did not appear to be accidental, and movements specifically toward the co-twin had begun by 14 weeks of gestation.

Degani et al.[25] found significant differences in the total counts of fetal movements (general body, isolated head, isolated arm, and isolated leg movements) in active twins and their co-twins between 11 and 14 weeks of gestation using 4D ultrasound. Maternal reports on the temperament of twins as well as the more active twin in each pair after birth correlated with prenatal intertwin differences in activity. Therefore, differences in activity in early pregnancy, even before the emergence of fetal behavioral patterns, appear to be followed by postnatal differences in temperament.

TWIN FETAL FACIAL EXPRESSIONS

In order to provide further insights into twin fetal brain development and maturation, Nitta et al.[26] employed 4D ultrasound to examine the characteristics of twin fetal facial expressions at 30–33[+6] weeks of gestation. The frequencies of seven fetal facial expressions (mouthing, yawning, smiling, tongue expulsion, scowling, sucking, and blinking)[27] were assessed for 15 minutes. The most frequent facial expression in twin and singleton fetuses at 30–33[+6] weeks of gestation was mouthing, followed by blinking. Moreover, the frequencies of mouthing and blinking were significantly higher than those of other expressions. The findings obtained also revealed that the frequencies of mouthing and scowling were significantly lower in twin than in singleton fetuses, whereas no significant differences were observed in the frequencies of the five other facial expressions between these groups. These findings indicated that the frequencies of twin facial expressions early in the third trimester of pregnancy remained altered by restricted twin fetal behavioral patterns before 20 weeks of gestation.[21,23] Furthermore, the frequencies of facial expressions also differed between twin and singleton fetuses, which may reflect accelerated brain maturation and development in twin fetuses. Amiel-Tison et al.[28] also demonstrated that neurological and physical maturity was reached more rapidly in twins than in singletons after birth.

Kurjak et al.[16] evaluated Kurjak's antenatal neurodevelopmental test (KANET) scores obtained at 28–36 weeks of gestation using 4D ultrasound in singleton and twin fetuses. The findings obtained showed that abnormal, borderline, and normal KANET scores did not significantly differ between singletons and twins. However, significant differences were observed in the scores obtained for isolated eye blinking, mouthing, grimacing, hand-to-head movement, finger movements, Gestalt perception, and general movements between twins and singletons. Twins showed less activity than singletons as well as different behavioral patterns.

CONCLUSION

Four-dimensional ultrasound allows twin fetal movements and behavioral patterns as well as facial expressions to be clearly identified and assessed. Twin fetal behavior is restricted with advancing gestation between 12 and 19^{+6} weeks of gestational age. Since the restriction of fetal movements in twins early in pregnancy may affect fetal growth and development or personality development before and after birth, further studies are needed to assess this phenomenon. The limitation of available space in utero for twin fetuses early in the third trimester of pregnancy represents a stress condition, which may contribute to accelerated brain maturation, as indicated by less frequent mouthing and scowling movements than in singleton fetuses at the same gestational age. Observations of the actions of twin fetuses, their contact behaviors, and reactions represent an effective method for understanding the development of the brain and central nervous system. Twin research is expected to promote neurological studies involving fetuses and provide insights into the significance of interactions (consideration of and compassion for others) for humans. The impact of restricted space in utero on the functional development of the fetal brain and central nervous system in twins warrants further studies using a larger sample size or multicentric studies.

Conflict of interest: The authors have no conflict of interest.

REFERENCES

1. Sadovsky E, Ohel G, Simon A. Ultrasonographical evaluation of the incidence of simultaneous and independent movements in twin fetuses. Gynecol Obstet Invest. 1987;23(1):5-9.

2. Zimmer EZ, Goldstein I, Alglay S. Simultaneous recording of fetal breathing movements and body movements in twin pregnancy. J Perinat Med. 1988;16(2):109-12.

3. Samueloff A, Younis JS, Strauss N, Baras M, Sadovsky E. Incidence of spontaneous and evoked fetal movements in the first half of twin pregnancy. Gynecol Obstet Invest. 1991;31(4):200-3.

4. Arabin B, Gembruch U, von Eyck J. Registration of fetal behaviour in multiple pregnancy. J Perinat Med. 1993;21(4):285-94.

5. Arabin B, Bos R, Rijlaarsdam R, Mohnhaupt A, von Eyck J. The onset of inter-human contacts: longitudinal ultrasound observations in early twin pregnancies. Ultrasound Obstet Gynecol. 1996;8(3):166-73.

6. Piontelli A, Bocconi L, Kustermann A, Tassis B, Zoppini C, Nicolini U. Patterns of evoked behaviour in twin pregnancies during the first 22 weeks of gestation. Early Hum Dev. 1997;50(1):39-45.

7. Piontelli A, Bocconi L, Boschetto C, Kustermann A, Nicolini U. Differences and similarities in the intra-uterine behaviour of monozygotic and dizygotic twins. Twin Res. 1999;2(4):264-73.

8. Mulder EJH, Derks JB, de Laat MWM, Visser GHA. Fetal behavior in normal dichorionic twin pregnancy. Early Hum Dev. 2012;88(3): 129-34.

9. Tendais I, Figueiredo B, Mulder EJH, Lopes D, Montenegro N. Developmental trajectories of general and breathing movements in fetal twins. Dev Psychobiol. 2019;61(4):626-33.

10. Hata T, Dai SY, Marumo G. Ultrasound for evaluation of fetal neurobehavioural development: from 2-D to 4-D ultrasound. Inf Child Dev. 2010;19(1):99-118.

11. Hata T, Kanenishi K, Hanaoka U, Marumo G. HDlive and 4D ultrasound in the assessment of fetal facial expressions. Donald Sch J Ultrasound Obstet Gynecol. 2015;9(1):44-50.

12. Hata T. Current status of fetal neurodevelopmental assessment: four-dimensional ultrasound study. J Obstet Gynaecol Res. 2016;42(10):1211-21.

13. AboEllail MAM, Hata T. Fetal face and four-dimensional ultrasound. In: Kurjak A, Chervenak FA (Eds). Donald School Textbook of Ultrasound in Obstetrics and Gynecology, 4th Edition. New Delhi: Jaypee Brothers Medical Publishers (P) Ltd.; 2017. pp. 791-9.

14. AboEllail MAM, Hata T. Fetal face as important indicator of fetal brain function. J Perinat Med. 2017;45(6):729-36.

15. Hata T. Fetal face as predictor of fetal brain. Donald Sch J Ultrasound Obstet Gynecol. 2018;12(1):56-9.

16. Kurjak A, Talic A, Stanojevic M, Honemeyer U, Serra B, Prats P, et al. The study of fetal neurobehavioral in twins in all three trimesters of pregnancy. J Matern Fetal Neonatal Med. 2013;26(12):1186-95.

17. Hata T, Aoki S, Miyazaki K, Iwanari O, Sawada K, Tagashira T. Three-dimensional ultrasonographic visualization of multiple pregnancy. Gynecol Obstet Invest. 1998; 46(1):26-30.

18. Sasaki M, Yanagihara T, Naitoh N, Hata T. Four-dimensional sonographic assessment of inter-twin contact late in the first trimester. Int J Gynecol Obstet. 2010;108(2):104-7.

19. Hata T, Sasaki M, Yanagihara T. Difference in the frequency of types of inter-twin contact at 10–13 weeks' gestation: preliminary four-dimensional sonographic study. J Matern Fetal Neonatal Med. 2012;25(3):226-30.

20. Hata T, Kanenishi K, Sasaki M, Yanagihara T. Fetal reflex movement in twin pregnancies late in the first trimester: 4-D sonographic study. Ultrasound Med Biol. 2011;37(11): 1948-51.

21. AboEllail MAM, Kanenishi K, Mori N, Noguchi J, Marumo G, Hata T. Ultrasound study of fetal movements in singleton and twin pregnancies at 12-19 weeks. J Perinat Med. 2018;46(8):832-8.

22. Sajapala S, AboEllail MAM, Kanenishi K, Mori N, Marumo G, Hata T. 4D ultrasound study of fetal movement early in the second trimester of pregnancy. J Perinat Med. 2017;45(6):737-43.

23. Mori N, Kanenishi K, AboEllail MAM, Nitta E, Noguchi J, Marumo G, et al. Singleton and twin fetal movements before 20 weeks of gestation. Donald Sch J Ultrasound Obstet Gynecol. 2018;12(2):99-103.

24. Castiello U, Becchio C, Zoia S, Nelini C, Sartori L, Blason L, et al. Wired to be social: the ontogeny of human interaction. PLoS One. 2010;5(10):e13199.

25. Degani S, Leibovitz Z, Shapiro I, Ohel G. Twins' temperament: early prenatal sonographic assessment and postnatal correlation. J Perinatol. 2009;29(5):337-42.

26. Nitta E, Kanenishi K, Mori N, AboEllail MAM, Hata T. Twin fetal facial expressions at 30–33^{+6} weeks of gestation. J Perinat Med. 2019;47(9):963-8.

27. AboEllail MAM, Kanenishi K, Mori N, Mohamed OAK, Hata T. 4D ultrasound study of fetal facial expressions in third trimester of pregnancy. J Matern Fetal Neonatal Med. 2018;31(14):1856-64.

28. Amiel-Tison C, Maillard F, Lebrum F, Faucher P, Vitry F, Hottinger O, et al. Acceleration of neurologic and physical maturity in multiple pregnancies. Presented at European Congress of Perinatal Medicine, Helsinki, June, 1994.

Fetal Awareness

Milan Stanojević, Asim Kurjak, Aida Salihagić Kadić, Lara Spalldi Barišić, Miro Jakovljević

■ INTRODUCTION

Ultrasound (US) as a diagnostic modality has been introduced to the clinical practice as an important diagnostic tool in clinical medicine.[1,2] The intrauterine fetal life was mysterious and unknown until the advent of US as a diagnostic method introduced to obstetrics some 60 years ago.[3] In that way, intrauterine environment and fetal life became visible to the eyes of obstetricians and parents.[3] It took almost 40 years after introduction of US to the medicine to make two-dimensional (2D) image three-dimensional (3D), and adding motility to the image made it four-dimensional (4D).[4-6] The development of computer technology enabled that important advancement of the clinical use of US as an imaging technique which has made depiction of fetal anatomy more realistic with many details of normal and abnormal structures of many organs and organ systems.[4-6] Imaging X-ray methods were very important diagnostic modalities in the assessment of the brain and central nervous system (CNS) structure, entering firmly closed skull by introduction of computed tomography. 2D US enabled assessment of fetal CNS function by evaluation of Prechtl's fetal general movements (GMs).[7-9] Some 15 years ago, 4D US has been introduced in the field of fetal behavior with the development of Kurjak's antenatal neurodevelopmental test (KANET) aiming to detect fetuses at high neurodevelopmental risk by the assessment not only of fetal GMs and movements, but also some other signs from prenatal neurological assessment such as skull sutures, neurological thumb, and facial movements.[10-15] Introduction of 4D US in the assessment of fetal behavior enabled not only introduction of KANET but also depiction of spectacular fetal facial expressions which were resembling postnatal facial grimacing, which prompted us to speculate about fetal awareness and fetal cognitive function.[16,17] We were also trying to understand fetal emotional life and its readiness to separate from the intrauterine environment and begin independent life as a new individual.[16,17] This concept of looking at the fetus as a complete person is very important, because only by putting together all aspects of one's health even in utero is enabling better results of treatment. This means that at that time we have been thinking in the way of so-called personalized medicine, taking every fetus as a separate and unique individual.[18] Problem with fetus is that not all postnatal diagnostic tools are available prenatally, and the influence of intrauterine environment which is quite different from one postnatally is also disturbing and complicating our diagnostic means and approach.[19,20]

The aim of this chapter is to see whether by observing the fetus by 4D US we can enter fetal behavior, emotions, mental status, consciousness, awareness, and other states connected with fetal mind and ability of self-regulation.

HOW HUMAN AWARENESS CAN BE DEFINED?

Everything can be found on the "internet", even linguistic definition of awareness. According to the Webster Dictionary, awareness is the quality or state of being aware: knowledge and understanding that something is happening or exists.[21] MacMillan Dictionary is going further and more deeply into the definition of awareness distinguishing two aspects of awareness.[22]

1. Knowledge or understanding of a subject, issue, or situation
2. The ability to notice things.

Direct knowledge or identification, feeling something, or being aware of events, i.e., being conscious of something with informing environment about it is considered to be awareness.[23] It is not clear whether consciousness and awareness have synonymous meaning, although some investigators think about awareness in that way.[24] It is believed that consciousness consists of two components: awareness which is a content of consciousness, and arousal describing the level of consciousness.[25,26] Between awareness and arousal there is a positive correlation meaning that with decreased arousal awareness is decreasing and opposite.[25] At least two aspects could be recognized with the concept of awareness: the first focused on the intuitive feeling of something described as internal state, and the second directed toward the external events by means of sensory perception, when the brain is activated in certain ways enabling sensing something, which is process distinguished from observation and perceiving.[17] Depending on the subject to which awareness is directed, there can be at least two aspects of the state of awareness: if one is aware of one's own awareness state which is considered as self-awareness, and perception of external world which is other component called external awareness.[17,25] The organization of self-awareness denotes the inner experience of the subject which has a central role in the self-regulation.[27] One's awareness of internal and external world is defined as basic awareness and is dependent on the brainstem, while higher forms of awareness like self-awareness require cortical contribution.[27] Primary consciousness means ability to integrate sensations from the environment which are transposed to certain behavior.[27] This primary consciousness or basic awareness consists of the capacity to generate emotions and awareness of surrounding without ability to talk, label, or describe this experience. There are interconnected regions down the brainstem regulating the direction of the gaze and organize the decisions about one's next activity.[26,27]

HOW CONSCIOUSNESS AND AWARENESS ARE DEVELOPING?

As mentioned before, two main components of consciousness are arousal involving the activity of subcortical structures incorporating brainstem reticular formation, hypothalamus, and basal forebrain, and activity of frontoparietal associative areas which is related to the awareness.[25] While self-awareness networks include the posterior cingulate/precuneal cortices, medial frontal cortex, and bilateral temporoparietal junctions, the external awareness network encompasses lateral frontal and parietal cortices.[25,28]

At 7 weeks of gestation, brainstem is developed followed by development of cerebral hemispheres at 8 weeks of gestation.[29] From 7 weeks of gestation every minute is formed 250,000 neurons.[30] Differentiation and migration of neurons through newly formed cortical layers are happening early in gestation with the peak of migration around 12–20 weeks and it ends at around 26–29 weeks.[31-33] Cortical area differentiation begins approximately between 24 and 34 weeks and continues until the end of gestation.[34] The peak period of synaptogenesis begins at 34 weeks and continues well into early postnatal life.[35] Processing of sensory information and mental processes is becoming possible after formation of thalamocortical and cortico-cortical connections which are fundamental from developmental point of view.[36,37] The first such connections grow at 24–26 weeks of gestation.[36,37] The functional connection between periphery and cortex operates from 26 to 28 weeks onward enabling registration of evoked potentials from the cortex.[38,39]

ASSESSMENT OF BRAIN FUNCTION

Technical and ethical constrains are responsible for unavailability of diagnostic modalities for prenatal assessment of fetal brain function and morphology. To depict morphology of fetal CNS is much easier than to evaluate fetal brain function. Methods like functional magnetic resonance imaging (fMRI), diffuse correlation spectroscopy, and near-infrared spectroscopy, positron emission tomography (PET), magnetoencephalography, or electro-encephalography (EEG) can be used postnatally in premature infants and these data can be transposed to the fetuses of the same gestational age, but this comparison is not quite plausible at least because fetus and neonate are living in quite different environments, which may have substantial influence on the findings.[40-42] Most methods

rely on the idea to make assumptions about the timing or location of some activity pattern of the activated brain system.[25,43-47]

The EEG is more and more routinely recorded alongside fMRI to study spontaneous brain activity.[44,48] The EEG data provide access to very useful information regarding the timing of spontaneous brain activity. There are some differences between neonatal and adult brain activity shown by fMRI detecting the highest activity in the somatosensory, auditory, and visual cortex, whereas less activity is revealed in association area and the prefrontal cortex of the newborn brain as compared with adults.[49]

As we can see from the data of sophisticated neuroimaging and neurophysiological data used postnatally, neither of them has been routinely used in fetuses due to different technical and ethical constrains.[50,51] At the moment one of the available methods for functional assessment of fetal brain is 4D US for assessment of fetal behavior.

POSSIBILITIES OF FOUR-DIMENSIONAL ULTRASOUND IN ASSESSMENT OF FETAL BEHAVIOR

Fetal Sensory Perception

Tactile, vestibular, taste, olfactory, auditory, and visual sensations can be processed by the fetus.[52-55] Tactile experiences can be processed at a cortical level when thalamocortical connections are developed and functional.[51-55] It is estimated that fetus becomes aware of its body after 25 weeks of gestation, which is possibly associated with appearance of minimum level of consciousness.[56]

Wide spectrum of reactions can be observed in a fetus experiencing pain.[29,53,57-59] The first responses, motor reflexes appear at 7.5 weeks of gestation. Some of physiological reactions, such as activation of the hypothalamo-hypophysial axis and autonomic nervous system, do not reach the cerebral cortex. Development of nociceptors and sensory areas in cerebral cortex are prerequisites of sensing pain in fetal life with development of necessary connections occurring after 24–26 weeks of gestation.[57-59] Evidence of pain processing in the somatosensory cortex can be found by registration of somatosensory evoked potentials from the brain cortex from 29 weeks of gestation.[60] As shown by recent research, near-infrared spectroscopy can record cortical pain responses as early as from 25 weeks of gestation.[25,26] Facial expressions similar to those of adults sustaining pain have been observed in preterm infants after 25 weeks of gestation and these infants are probably conscious of pain. On the other hand, there is an opinion that the fetus may not be conscious of pain even after 25 weeks due to high endogenous sedatory and analgesic substances.[56] However, fetal facial expressions similar to those of children sustaining pain have been noticed by 4D sonography.[61]

Fetal Motoric Activity

According to the recent evidence, purpose of fetal motoric activity is development of some parts of CNS and muscles.[29] Based on our investigations by 4D US, general movements as the earliest, complex, and well-organized movement pattern including head, trunk, and limbs emerge at 8th gestational week.[62] They are the most frequent fetal movement pattern in the first trimester of pregnancy.[63] Right- or left-handed fetal behavior can be noticed at 10 weeks of gestation. Stimulation of the brain influences its organization and fetal motor activity induces the brain to develop "handedness" and subsequent lateralization of the function.[29] Goal-oriented hand movements and a target point can

be recognized for each hand movement from 13 weeks of gestation.[10] At 15 weeks of gestation, 16 different types of movement can be observed, including retroflection, anteflexion, and rotation of the head as well facial movements such as mouthing, yawning, hiccups, sucking, and swallowing.[29] Between 16 and 18 weeks of gestation the earliest eye movements can be observed.[62] Gradual organization of fetal movement patterns appears in the second half of pregnancy, with the periods of fetal quiescence increasing, together with recognizable rest-activity cycles. Based on our results, the most frequent facial movement patterns in the second trimester were isolated eye blinking pattern, grimacing, sucking, and swallowing.[62] The fetus can alter the frequency, patterning, and coordination of movement in response to sensory challenges, while retention of information from motor experience and motor learning may contribute to normal prenatal motor development.[64] Based on evaluation of fetal spontaneous motor activity by 4D US, a prenatal neurologic scoring test named KANET, was created.[12] This test has been used to assess almost 2,000 fetuses and our results have indicated that KANET has an ability to recognize normal, borderline, and abnormal behavior in fetuses from normal and pathological pregnancies.[65-76]

Fetus and Emotions

As mentioned before, fetal facial expressions are one of the important signs of fetal emotions. As early as in the 2nd and the 3rd trimesters of pregnancy, full range of fetal facial expressions similar to emotional expressions in adults can be recorded by 4D US including grimacing, smiling, and crying **(Figs. 1 to 5)**.[77-79] Appearance of more complex facial expressions like "cry-face gestalt" or "laughter-face gestalt" in the third trimester

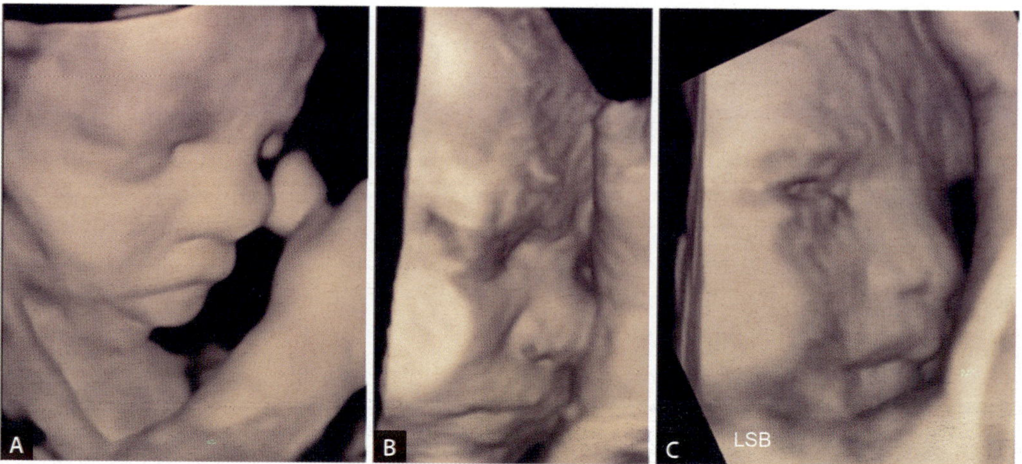

Figs. 1A to C: Three-dimensional (3D) surface rendering mode of the same fetal face, semi profile at 34 gestational weeks. (A) Fetus is relaxed at sleep; (B) Fetus is frowning with a sad expression on his face; (C) Fetus is awake with open eyes exploring the environment.
Courtesy: Lara Spalldi Barisic (LSB)

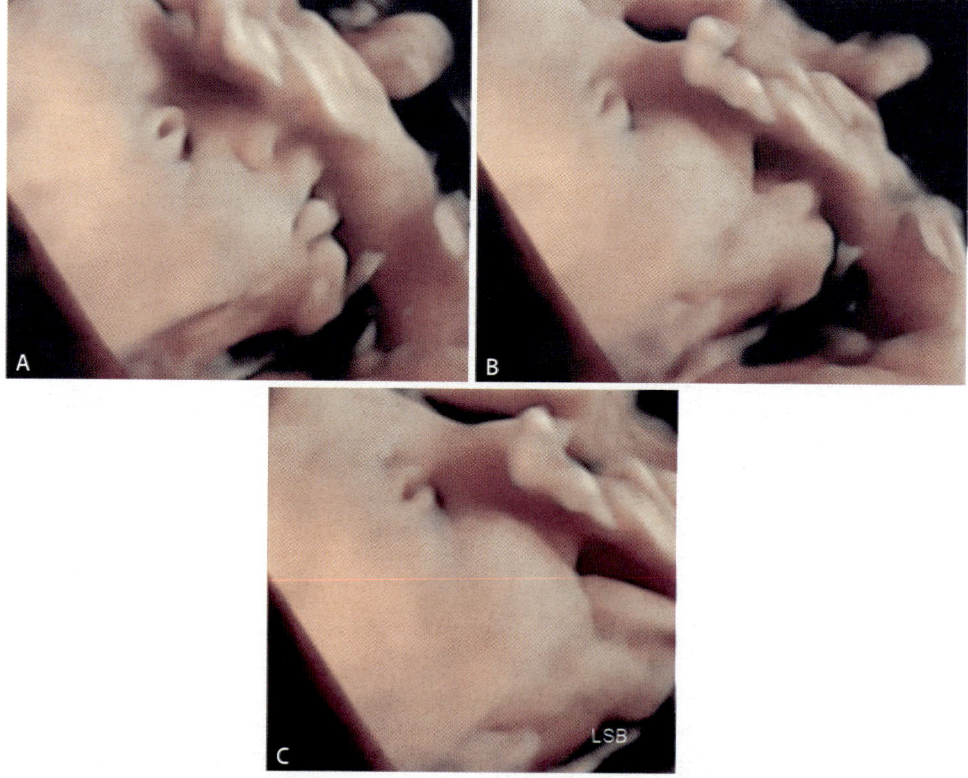

Figs. 2A to C: Three-dimensional (3D) HDlive surface rendering of the fetal face, profile. Fetus at 29 gestational weeks. Sequence of images where fetus is awake, with open eyes (A), opening the mouth (B), and licking his own hand (C).
Courtesy: Lara Spalldi Barisic (LSB)

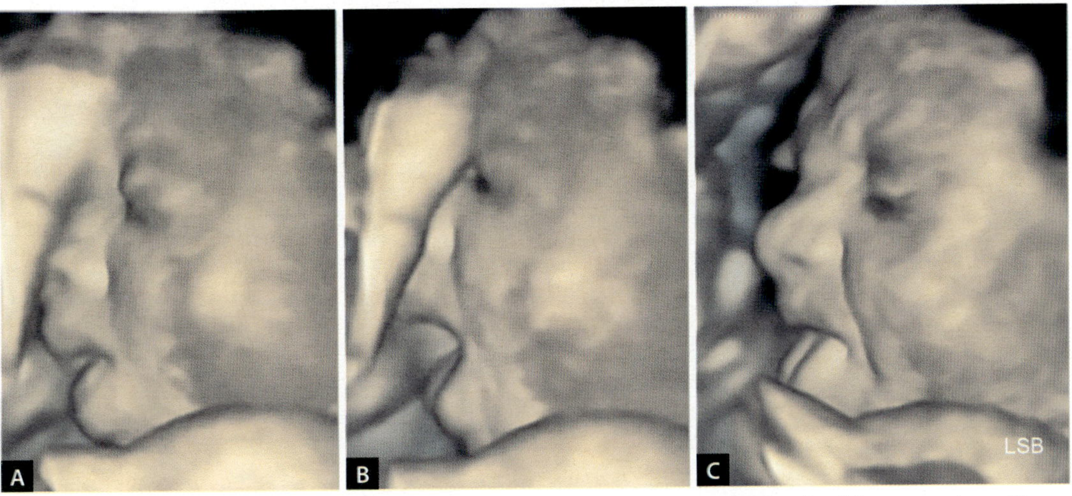

Figs. 3A to C: Three-dimensional (3D) surface rendering imaging of the fetal face, semi-profile at 32 gestational weeks. The fetus is swallowing amniotic fluid, tasting it (A), expelling the tongue (B), and making grimaces (C).
Courtesy: Lara Spalldi Barisic (LSB)

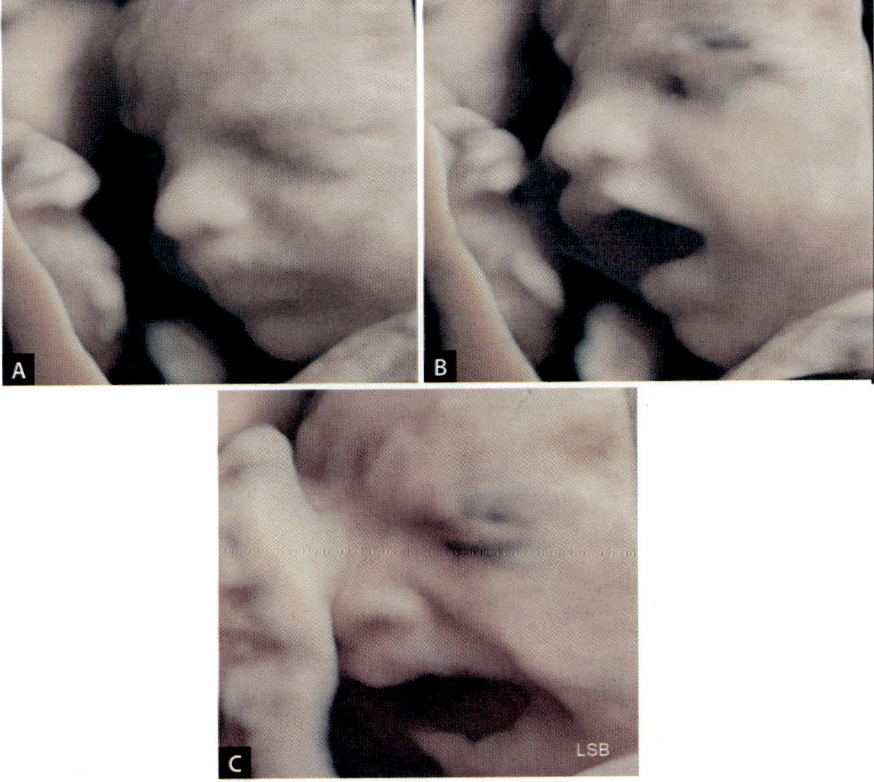

Figs. 4A to C: Three-dimensional (3D) HDlive surface rendering of the fetal semi-profile. A sequence of images showing the fetus and grimacing.
Courtesy: Lara Spalldi Barisic (LSB)

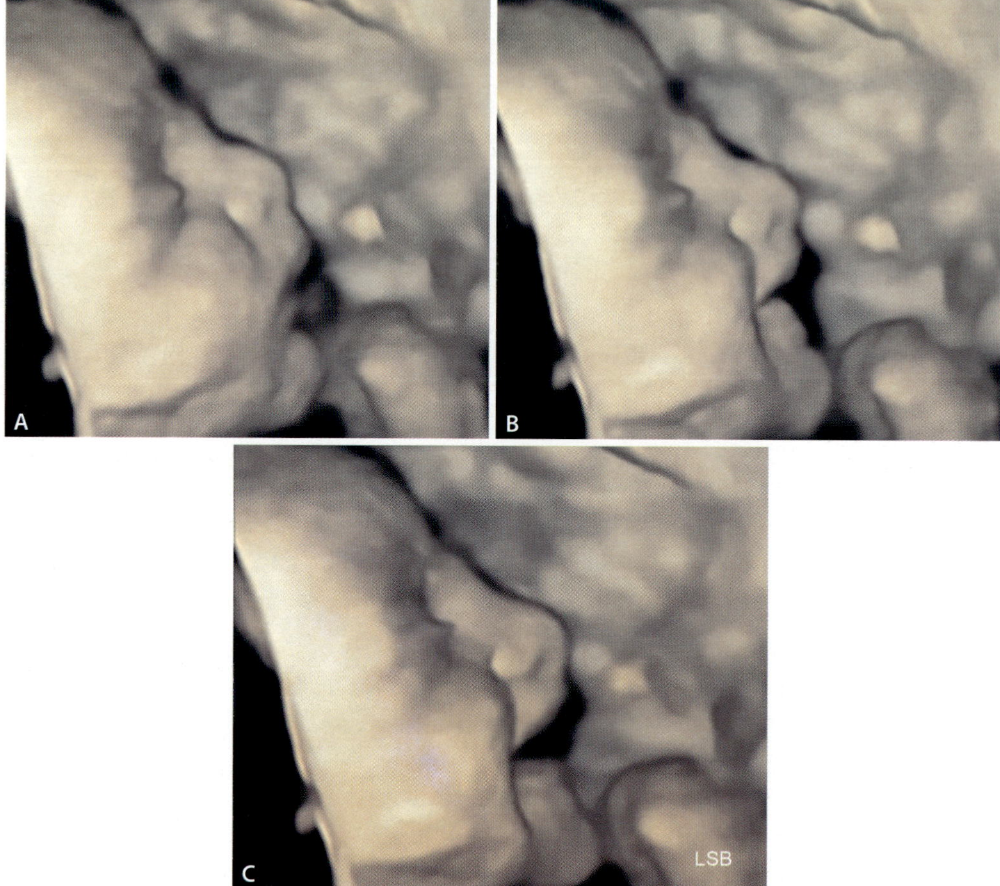

Figs. 5A to C: Three-dimensional (3D) surface rendering of the fetal profile at 32 gestational weeks. Fetus is awake with open eyes. Sequence of images captured fetal reaction on the mother's voice; notice the wide smile on the fetal face.
Courtesy: Lara Spalldi Barisic (LSB)

are signs of fetal neurological maturation.[57,79] Such facial expressions suggesting emotions may be beneficial for establishment of communication between mother and the fetus as the beginning of bonding continuing in postnatal life, as well as for the regulation of parental care.[80] Fetal facial expressions resembling stress or pain may be considered as an adaptive process which is useful to the fetus as training for postnatal life.[61,81] Do the facial expressions represent a part of reflexive behavior of the fetus? In fact, smiling as well as screaming and crying can be induced from the brainstem stimulation even with complete forebrain transection or destruction.[61,81] Based on 4D US research conducted till now, it can be speculated that fetal facial expressions and emotion-like behaviors may represent fetal emotions and awareness.[82] Moreover, recent data indicate that fetal movements serve not only to express different orientations, but also emotional states and manifestations of intentions.[83] The limbic forebrain is responsible for the expression and experience of emotions.[83] Amygdala, one of the important brain structures, is developed by the end of pregnancy and capable of mediating emotional memory, attention, arousal, and the experience of love, fear, pleasure, and joy.[77,78] It contains facial recognition neurons which discern the emotional significance of different facial expressions.[77,78] The evaluation of faces in social processing is an area of cognition specific to the amygdala.[83]

Is Fetus Capable of Learning and Memorizing?

Habituation methods, classical conditioning, and exposure learning have been used to investigate extensively fetal learning and memory.[84] From 22 weeks of gestation onward, it was observed that fetus is exerting decreased responsiveness on repeated presentation of the same stimulus which is defined as habituation.[85] Based on the research on fetal response to repeating vibroacoustic stimuli and habituation process, it was detected that number of stimuli needed to produce habituation was increased in younger gestational age, which means that habituation process is gestational age dependent.[86] The number of stimuli needed to produce habituation is decreasing with increasing gestational age.[86]

IMPORTANCE OF THE INVESTIGATION OF FETAL SELF-AWARENESS

The entire human life is marked with the process of the separation from the mother in order to begin the independent life and fulfill one's role during lifetime.[87,88] The crucial question is: when this process of separation begins and is it possible to investigate and detect this period of human life. This issue is very important from the philosophical and ethical point of view of the beginning of human life, which is fascinating many generations of investigators of different scientific disciplines. At the moment of conception, a new unique form of life is created and it is questionable when it begins to be called a life.[89,90] Development of human being is very complicated and with the onset of development probably the process of separation from the mother begins. The entire intrauterine development is marked with the preparation to be born, and being born means the physical moment of the separation. This separation can be successful and unsuccessful, and all components of this process should be orchestrated in the way to be successful, but very gradual and cautious. Some investigators claim that human product of conception is just a product of conception till the moment when it gains self-awareness, while the others consider embryo and the fetus as being a person from the conception.[91,92]

CONCLUSION

The fetus is living in protective intrauterine environment with plenty of stimulating matrix of motion as well as tactile, chemical, auditory, vestibular, and possibly other sensory information enabling all kinds of development, but provided in a manner to protect the fetus from overstimulation.[52] The fetus should be and is exposed to hundreds of specific and patterned stimuli each day, shaping the structure and function of the brain.[17,29] The fetus is capable of detecting, responding, and even memorizing for a long-time stimuli experienced during the prenatal and postnatal period, which may shape its behavior, development, and health postnatally.[93,94] It is proved that higher order sensory perception begins in fetal life, because functionally and structurally the fetus is ready to exert such behavior which is best studied by fetal awareness of noxious stimuli after development of functional thalamocortical connections.[53] Evidence for conscious sentience of pain during intrauterine life is indirect, but it is obvious that reaction on pain can be detected during fetal life and can impact reaction on pain postnatally, when analgesia is considered as a standard of care.[53,59] On the other hand, we have learned from the research that the fetus is capable of action planning and learning, meaning that probably the capability of being aware and conscious should proceed.[84] Fetal movements are reflecting the development of the brain, but at the same time they are stimulating the brain to develop, which can be applied to fetal senses and development of awareness as well. Emergence of spontaneous fetal movements culminating with presumed preferences for the sound of mother's voice are expression of behavioral complexity and progression which is reflection of maturational events taking place in the brainstem followed by forebrain structures.[81,82] More than 15 years of the investigation of fetal behavior by 4D US showed that fetal motor function undoubtedly reflects development of diverse cognitive, sensory, and motor systems.[17,26,29] The face is the mirror of the brain, many expressions can be depicted during fetal life which are proving that fetal life in utero is extremely dramatic and rich in different experiences.[17,29,57,58] Would it be possible without development of fetal awareness and consciousness?

■ REFERENCES

1. Newman PG, Rozycki GS. The history of ultrasound. Surg Clin North Am. 1998;78(2): 179-95.
2. Kurjak A, Stanojević M, Salihagić-Kadić A, Barišić LS, Jakovljević M. Is four-dimensional (4D) ultrasound entering a new field of fetal psychiatry? Psychiatr Danub. 2019;31(2):133-40.
3. McNay MB, Fleming JE. Forty years of obstetric ultrasound 1957-1997: from A-scope to three dimensions. Ultrasound Med Biol. 1999;25(1):3-56.
4. Baba K, Satoh K, Sakamoto S, Okai T, Ishii S. Development of an ultrasonic system for three-dimensional reconstruction of the fetus. J Perinat Med. 1989;17(1):19-24.
5. Merz E. Use of 3D ultrasound technique in prenatal diagnosis. Ultraschall Med. 1995; 16(4):154-61.
6. Kurjak A, Hafner T, Kos M, Kupesic S, Stanojevic M. Three-dimensional sonography in prenatal diagnosis: a luxury or necessity? J Perinat Med. 2000;28(3):194-209.
7. Prechtl HF. Qualitative changes of spontaneous movements in fetus and preterm infant are a marker of neurological dysfunction. Early Hum Dev. 1990;23(3):151-8.
8. Einspieler C, Prechtl HFR, Bos A, Cioni G, Ferrari F. Prechtl's method on the qualitative assessment of general movements in preterm, term and young infants. Cambridge: Mac Keith Press; 2004.
9. Hadders-Algra M. General movements: a window for early identification of children at high risk for developmental disorders. J Pediatr. 2004;145(Suppl 2):S12-8.
10. Kurjak A, Azumendi G, Vecek N, Kupesic S, Solak M, Varga D, et al. Fetal hand movements and facial expression in normal pregnancy studied by four-dimensional sonography. J Perinat Med. 2003;31(6):496-508.
11. Kurjak A, Stanojevic M, Andonotopo W, Salihagic-Kadic A, Carera JM, Azumendi G. Behavioral pattern continuity from prenatal to postnatal life—a study by four-dimensional (4D) ultrasonography. J Perinat Med. 2004;32(4):346-53.
12. Kurjak A, Miskovic B, Stanojevic M, Amiel-Tison C, Ahmed B, Azumendi G, et al. New scoring system for fetal neurobehavior assessed by three- and four-dimensional sonography. J Perinat Med. 2008;36(1):73-81.
13. Kurjak A, Abo-Yaqoub S, Stanojevic M, Yigiter AB, Vasilj O, Lebit D, et al. The potential of 4D sonography in the assessment

of fetal neurobehavior—multicentric study in high-risk pregnancies. J Perinat Med. 2010;38(1):77-82.

14. Amiel-Tison C, Gosselin J, Kurjak A. Neurosonography in the second half of fetal life: a neonatologist's point of view. J Perinat Med. 2006;34(6):437-46.

15. Amiel-Tison C, Gosselin J. From neonatal to fetal neurology: some clues for interpreting fetal findings. In: Pooh RK, Kurjak A (Eds). Fetal Neurology. New Delhi: Jaypee Brothers Medical Publishers (P) Ltd.; 2009. pp. 373-404.

16. Kurjak A, Stanojevic M, Azumendi G, Carrera JM. The potential of four-dimensional (4D) ultrasonography in the assessment of fetal awareness. J Perinat Med. 2005;33(1):46-53.

17. Kadic AS, Kurjak A. Cognitive functions of the fetus. Ultraschall Med. 2018;39(2):181-9.

18. Ingerslev HJ, Kesmodel US, Jacobsson B, Vogel I. Personalized medicine for the embryo and the fetus—options in modern genetics influence preconception and prenatal choices. Acta Obstet Gynecol Scand. 2020;99(6):689-91.

19. Sekulic SR, Lukac DD, Naumovic NM. The fetus cannot exercise like an astronaut: gravity loading is necessary for the physiological development during second half of pregnancy. Med Hypotheses. 2005;64(2): 221-8.

20. Meigal AY. Synergistic action of gravity and temperature on the motor system within the lifespan: a "Baby Astronaut" hypothesis. Med Hypotheses. 2013;80(3):275-83.

21. Merriam-Webster Dictionary. Awareness. [online] Available from: https://www.merriam-webster.com/dictionary/awareness [Last accessed February, 2022].

22. MacMillan Dictionary. Awareness. [online] Available from: https://www.macmillandictionary.com/dictionary/british/awareness [Last accessed February, 2022].

23. Wikipedia. Awareness. [online] Available from: https://en.wikipedia.org/wiki/Awareness [Last accessed February, 2022].

24. Hussain A, Aleksander I, Smith LS, Barros AK, Chrisley R, Cutsuridis V. Brain Inspired Cognitive Systems 2008. New York: Springer New York, 2010. p. 386.

25. Boly M, Phillips C, Tshibanda L, Vanhaudenhuyse A, Schabus M, Dang-Vu TT, et al. Intrinsic brain activity in altered states of consciousness: how conscious is the default mode of brain function? Ann N Y Acad Sci. 2008;1129:119-29.

26. Hata T, Kanenishi K, AboEllail MAM, Marumo G, Kurjak A. Fetal consciousness: four-dimensional ultrasound study. Donald Sch J Ultrasound Obstet Gynecol. 2015; 9(4):471-4.

27. Louis Sander, Amadei G, Bianchi I. Living Systems, Evolving Consciousness, and the Emerging Person: A Selection of Papers from the Life Work of Louis Sander. New York: Taylor & Francis; 2012. p. 296.

28. Droit-Volet S, Dambrun M. Awareness of the passage of time and self-consciousness: What do meditators report? Psych J. 2019; 8(1):51-65.

29. Kadić AS, Predojević M. Fetal neurophysiology according to gestational age. Semin Fetal Neonatal Med. 2012;17(5):256-60.

30. Budday S, Steinmann P, Kuhl E. Physical biology of human brain development. Front Cell Neurosci. 2015;9:257.

31. Anderson AL, Thomason ME. Functional plasticity before the cradle: a review of neural functional imaging in the human fetus. Neurosci Biobehav Rev. 2013;37(9 Pt B): 2220-32.

32. Faghiri A, Stephen JM, Wang YP, Wilson TW, Calhoun VD. Brain development includes linear and multiple nonlinear trajectories: a cross-sectional resting-state functional magnetic resonance imaging study. Brain Connect. 2019;9(10):777-88.

33. Jena A, Montoya CA, Mullaney JA, Dilger RN, Young W, McNabb WC, et al. Gut-Brain Axis in the Early Postnatal Years of Life: A Developmental Perspective. Front Integr Neurosci. 2020;14:44.

34. Kostović I, Judas M, Petanjek Z, Simić G. Ontogenesis of goal-directed behavior: anatomo-functional considerations. Int J Psychophysiol. 1995;19(2):85-102.

35. Tau GZ, Peterson BS. Normal development of brain circuits. Neuropsychopharmacology. 2010;35(1):147-68.

36. Kostović I, Judas M. The development of the subplate and thalamocortical connections in the human foetal brain. Acta Paediatr. 2010;99(8):1119-27.

37. Thomason ME. Development of brain networks in utero: relevance for common neural disorders. Biol Psychiatry. 2020;88(1): 40-50.

38. Klimach VJ, Cooke RW. Maturation of the neonatal somatosensory evoked response in preterm infants. Dev Med Child Neurol. 1988;30(2):208-14.

39. Nevalainen P, Lauronen L, Pihko E. Development of human somatosensory cortical functions—what have we learned from magnetoencephalography: a review. Front Hum Neurosci. 2014;8:158.

40. Laureys S, Goldman S, Phillips C, Van Bogaert P, Aerts J, Luxen A, et al. Impaired effective cortical connectivity in vegetative state: preliminary investigation using PET. Neuroimage. 1999;9(4):377-82.

41. Wintermark P, Hansen A, Warfield SK, Dukhovny D, Soul JS. Near-infrared spectroscopy versus magnetic resonance imaging to study brain perfusion in newborns with hypoxic-ischemic encephalopathy treated with hypothermia. Neuroimage. 2014;85[Pt 1(01)]:287-93.

42. Counsell SJ, Arichi T, Arulkumaran S, Rutherford MA. Fetal and neonatal neuroimaging. Handb Clin Neurol. 2019;162: 67-103.

43. Heiss WD. PET in coma and in vegetative state. Eur J Neurol. 2012;19(2):207-11.

44. Arichi T, Whitehead K, Barone G, Pressler R, Padormo F, Edwards AD, et al. Localization of spontaneous bursting neuronal activity in the preterm human brain with simultaneous EEG-fMRI. Elife. 2017;6.pii:e27814.

45. Andersen JB, Lindberg U, Olesen OV, Benoit D, Ladefoged CN, Larsson HB, et al. Hybrid PET/MRI imaging in healthy unsedated newborn infants with quantitative rCBF measurements using ^{15}O-water PET. J Cereb Blood Flow Metab. 2019;39(5):782-93.

46. Giovannella M, Contini D, Pagliazzi M, Pifferi A, Spinelli L, Erdmann R, et al. BabyLux device: a diffuse optical system integrating diffuse correlation spectroscopy and time-resolved near-infrared spectroscopy for the neuromonitoring of the premature newborn brain. Neurophotonics. 2019;6(2):025007.

47. O'Sullivan M, Temko A, Bocchino A, O'Mahony C, Boylan G, Popovici E. Analysis of a Low-cost EEG monitoring system and dry electrodes toward clinical use in the neonatal ICU. Sensors (Basel). 2019;19(11). pii:E2637.

48. Salek-Haddadi A, Friston KJ, Lemieux L, Fish DR. Studying spontaneous EEG activity with fMRI. Brain Res Brain Res Rev. 2003;43(1):110-33.

49. Lagercrantz H. The emergence of consciousness: science and ethics. Semin Fetal Neonatal Med. 2014;19(5):300-5.

50. Di Mascio D, Sileo FG, Khalil A, Rizzo G, Persico N, Brunelli R, et al. Role of magnetic resonance imaging in fetuses with mild or moderate ventriculomegaly in the era of fetal neurosonography: systematic review and meta-analysis. Ultrasound Obstet Gynecol. 2019;54(2):164-71.

51. Hart AR, Embleton ND, Bradburn M, Connolly DJA, Mandefield L, Mooney C, et al. Accuracy of in-utero MRI to detect fetal brain abnormalities and prognosticate developmental outcome: postnatal follow-up of the MERIDIAN cohort. Lancet Child Adolesc Health. 2020;4(2):131-40.

52. Clark-Gambelunghe MB, Clark DA. Sensory development. Pediatr Clin North Am. 2015;62(2):367-84.

53. Bellieni CV. New insights into fetal pain. Semin Fetal Neonatal Med. 2019;24(4): 101001.

54. Podzimek Š, Dušková M, Broukal Z, Rácz B, Stárka L, Dušková J. The evolution of taste and perinatal programming of taste preferences. Physiol Res. 2018;67(Suppl 3):S421-S429.

55. Donovan T, Dunn K, Penman A, Young RJ, Reid VM. Fetal eye movements in response to a visual stimulus. Brain Behav. 2020;10(8):e01676.

56. Lagercrantz H. The emergence of the mind: a borderline of human viability? Acta Paediatr. 2007;96(3):327-8.

57. Kurjak A, Azumendi G, Andonotopo W, Salihagic-Kadic A. Three- and four-dimensional ultrasonography for the structural and

functional evaluation of the fetal face. Am J Obstet Gynecol. 2007;196(1):16-28.

58. Reissland N, Francis B, Mason J. Can healthy fetuses show facial expressions of "pain" or "distress"? PLoS One. 2013;8(6):e65530.

59. Pierucci R. Fetal pain: the science behind why it is the medical standard of care. Linacre Q. 2020;87(3):311-6.

60. Bellieni CV, Vannuccini S, Petraglia F. Is fetal analgesia necessary during prenatal surgery? J Matern Fetal Neonatal Med. 2018;31(9):1241-5.

61. Bernardes LS, Ottolia JF, Cecchini M, Filho AGA, Teixeira MJ, Francisco RPV, et al; Fetal Pain Study Group. On the feasibility of accessing acute pain-related facial expressions in the human fetus and its potential implications: a case report. Pain Rep. 2018;3(5):e673.

62. Kurjak A, Andonotopo W, Hafner T, Kadic AS, Stanojevic M, Azumendi G, et al. Normal standards for fetal neurobehavioral developments—longitudinal quantification by four-dimensional sonography. J Perinat Med. 2006;34(1):56-65.

63. Andonotopo W, Medic M, Salihagic-Kadic A, Milenković D, Maiz N, Scazzocchio E. The assessment of fetal behavior in early pregnancy: comparison between 2D and 4D sonographic scanning. J Perinat Med. 2005;33(5):406-14.

64. Robinson SR. Spinal mediation of motor learning and memory in the rat fetus. Dev Psychobiol. 2015;57(4):421-34.

65. Kurjak A, Stanojević M, Predojević M, Laušin I, Salihagić-Kadić A. Neurobehavior in fetal life. Semin Fetal Neonatal Med. 2012;17(6):319-23.

66. Salihagić Kadić A, Stanojević M, Predojević M, Poljak B, Grubišić-Cabo B, Kurjak A. Assessment of the fetal neuromotor development with the new KANET test. In: Reissland N, Barbara S, Kisilevsky BS (Eds). Fetal Development Research on Brain and Behavior, Environmental Influences, and Emerging Technologies. Heidelberg, New York, Dordrecht, London: Springer International Publishing Switzerland; 2016. pp.177-89.

67. Kurjak A, Antsaklis P, Stanojevic M, Vladareanu R, Vladareanu S, Neto RM, et al. Multicentric studies of the fetal neurobehavior by KANET test. J Perinat Med. 2017;45(6):717-27.

68. Kurjak A, Antsaklis P, Stanojevic M, Porovic S. Fetal behavior assessed by four-dimensional ultrasound. Donald Sch J Ultrasound Obstet Gynecol. 2017;11(2):169-73.

69. Neto RM, Kurjak A, Porovic S, Stanojevic M, Gaber G. Clinical study of fetal neurobehavior by the Kurjak Antenatal Neurodvelopmental Test. Donald Sch J Ultrasound Obstet Gynecol. 2017;11(4):355-61.

70. Stanojević M, Antsaklis P, Panchal S, Porovic S, Salihagic-Kadic A, Barišić LS, et al. A Critical Appraisal of Kurjak Antenatal Neurodevelopmental Test: Five Years of Wide Clinical Use. Donald Sch J Ultrasound Obstet Gynecol. 2021;14(4):304-10.

71. Stanojevic M, Perlman JM, Andonotopo W, Kurjak A. From fetal to neonatal behavioral status. Ultrasound Rev Obstet Gynecol. 2004;4(1):459-71.

72. Stanojevic M, Kurjak A. Continuity between fetal and neonatal neurobehavior. Donald Sch J Ultrasound Obstet Gynecol. 2008;2(3):64-75.

73. Stanojevic M, Kurjak A, Salihagić-Kadić A, Vasilj O, Miskovic B, Shaddad AN, et al. Neurobehavioral continuity from fetus to neonate. J Perinat Med. 2011;39(2):171-7.

74. Stanojevic M. Neonatal aspects: Is there continuity? Donald Sch J Ultrasound Obstet Gynecol. 2012;6(2):189-96.

75. Stanojevic M, Zaputovic S, Bosnjak AP. Continuity between fetal and neonatal neurobehavior. Semin Fetal Neonatal Med. 2012;17(6):324-9.

76. Stanojevic M. Antenatal and postnatal assessment of neurobehavior: which one should be used? Donald Sch J Obstet Gynecol. 2015;9(1):67-74.

77. AboEllail MAM, Hata T. Fetal face as important indicator of fetal brain function. J Perinat Med. 2017;45(6):729-36.

78. Nitta E, Kanenishi K, Mori N, AboEllail MAM, Hata T. Twin fetal facial expressions

at 30-33^{+6} weeks of gestation. J Perinat Med. 2019;47(9):963-8.

79. Mori N, AboEllail MAM, Tenkumo C, Kanenishi K, Nishimoto N, Hata T. Fetal facial expressions in small-for-gestational-age and growth-restricted fetuses. J Matern Fetal Neonatal Med. 2019;32(9):1426-32.

80. de Jong-Pleij EAP, Ribbert LSM, Pistorius LR, Tromp E, Mulder EJH, Bilardo CM. Three-dimensional ultrasound and maternal bonding, a third trimester study and a review. Prenat Diagn. 2013;33(1):81-8.

81. Cunen NB, Jomeen J, Xuereb RB, Poat A. A narrative review of interventions addressing the parental-fetal relationship. Women Birth. 2017;30(4):e141-e151.

82. van Manen MA. towards the womb of neonatal intensive care. J Med Humanit. 2019;40(2):225-37.

83. Rolls ET. The cingulate cortex and limbic systems for action, emotion, and memory. Handb Clin Neurol. 2019;166:23-37.

84. Borsani E, Vedova AMD, Rezzani R, Rodella LF, Cristini C. Correlation between human nervous system development and acquisition of fetal skills: an overview. Brain Dev. 2019;41(3):225-33.

85. Dirix CEH, Nijhuis JG, Jongsma HW, Hornstra G. Aspects of fetal learning and memory. Child Dev. 2009;80(4):1251-8.

86. Hepper PG, Dornan JC, Lynch C. Sex differences in fetal habituation. Dev Sci. 2012;15(3):373-83.

87. Kossowsky J, Wilhelm FH, Roth WT, Schneider S. Separation anxiety disorder in children: disorder-specific responses to experimental separation from the mother. J Child Psychol Psychiatry. 2012;53(2):178-87.

88. Bergman NJ. Birth practices: Maternal-neonate separation as a source of toxic stress. Birth Defects Res. 2019;111(15):1087-109.

89. Kurjak A. Controversies on the beginning of human life-science and religions closer and closer. Psychiatr Danub. 2017;29(Suppl 1):89-91.

90. Kurjak A, Carrera JM, McCullough LB, Chervenak FA. Scientific and religious controversies about the beginning of human life: the relevance of the ethical concept of the fetus as a patient. J Perinat Med. 2007;35(5):376-83.

91. Watt H, McCarthy A. Targeting the fetal body and/or mother-child connection: vital conflicts and abortion. Linacre Q. 2020;87(2):147-60.

92. Peterfy A. Fetal viability as a threshold to personhood. A legal analysis. J Leg Med. 1995;16(4):607-36.

93. Marx V, Nagy E. Fetal behavioral responses to the touch of the mother's abdomen: a frame-by-frame analysis. Infant Behav Dev. 2017;47:83-91.

94. Miranda-Morales RS, D'Aloisio G, Anunziata F, Abate P, Molina JC. Fetal alcohol programming of subsequent alcohol affinity: a review based on preclinical, clinical and epidemiological studies. Front Behav Neurosci. 2020;14:33.

Neurosonogenetics

Ritsuko K Pooh

▪ INTRODUCTION

Neuronal embryology shows the rapid development of central nervous system (CNS) during pregnancy. Various disorders due to genetic mutation, trauma, viral infection, and other factors, and unexpected events during developmental stages can result in multiple phenotypes of congenital CNS abnormalities. It is essential to know the congenital CNS diseases related to each developmental stage of the CNS, such as neurulation, prosencephalic development, cell proliferation, neuronal migration, organization, and myelination.

Most fetal abnormalities can be diagnosed in early pregnancy or during the first trimester due to recent advanced fetal ultrasound.[1-3] However, it is challenging to detect brain malformations because the CNS structure is not accomplished in the early stage. The proliferation of neuronal cells, neuronal migration from the ganglionic eminence, and ventricular zone (VZ) start from 3 months of gestation. The recent advance of three-dimensional (3D) ultrasound technology has enabled us to conduct precise prenatal neuroimaging as if it were postnatal magnetic resonance imaging (MRI). The transfontanelle neuroimaging procedure combined with the 3D ultrasound **(Figs. 1A and B)** has been introduced. Systematic and accurate neuroimaging contributes to the detection of various congenital brain abnormalities, including the malformations of cortical development (MCD).

▌ CRANIAL DYSRAPHISM (NEURULATION DISORDER)

The neural tube is a single tubular structure from the head to the tail during development and is the primordium of the brain and spinal cord that constitutes the CNS. The neural tube is derived from the neural plate, which has a simple squamous epithelial structure. The formation of a vascular structure is initiated by forming a neural ridge near the boundary between the neural plate and the epidermal ectoderm and a neural grove in the middle of the neural plate. The actin cytoskeleton is abundant on the apical side of the neural epithelial cells that make up the neural plate, contracts, causing distortion in the neural plate, and bending the neural plate. After that, the left and right ridges of the neural plate are fused, and the neural plate finally breaks from the epidermal ectoderm and changes to a tubular structure. Such a mode of development is called primary neurulation. On the other hand, in the tail of mammalian and avian embryos, neural tube formation is observed due to epithelialization of mesoderm mesenchymal cells. This mode is called secondary neurulation.

It is known that over 200 genes cause neural tube defects (NTDs) in mice. In humans, the occurrence pattern is a multifactorial polygenic or oligogenic etiology.[4,5] In acranial and anencephalic embryos, the complete or incomplete defect of the

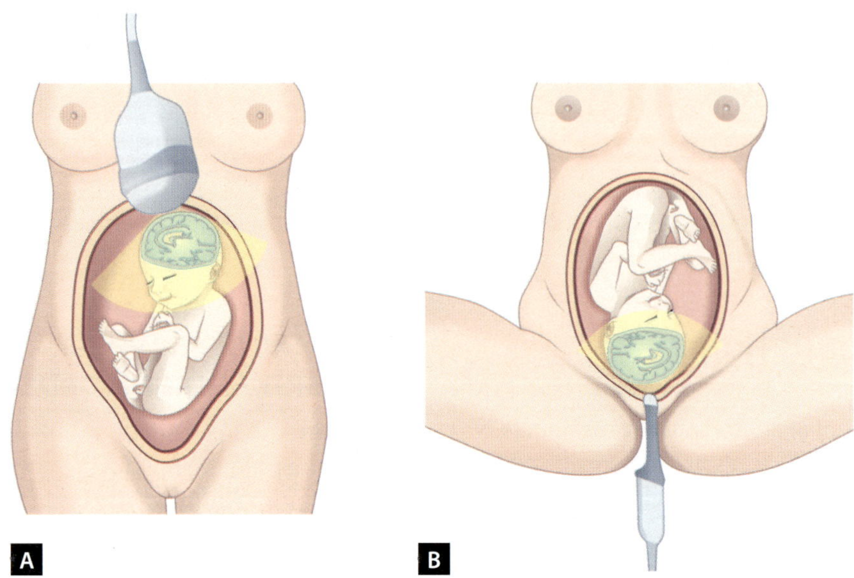

Figs. 1A and B: Fetal transfontanelle neuroimaging. (A) Transabdominal neuroimaging; (B) Transvaginal neuroimaging.

brain tissue and calvaria. The feature of craniorachischisis is anencephaly associated with a contiguous spinal defect and neural tissue exposure. The pathogenesis of encephalocele has not been well established. Encephalocele was classified as one of the NTDs. It has been, however, controversial whether encephalocele is NTD or a postneurulation defect. Rolo and colleagues used the mice model experiment and described that the encephalocele is not the consequence of the failure of neural tube closure but rather due to a later disruption of the surface ectoderm which covers the already closed neural tube.[6] However, the true pathogenesis remains unknown. The other considerable etiologies include single gene mutation, multifactorial inheritance, specific drugs such as valproic acid, and environmental factors. For a long time, it was thought that maternal serum alfa-fetoprotein level increases in NTDs. However, in skin-covered encephalocele or NTD

fetuses, maternal serum alfa-fetoprotein level is normal. Therefore, neurosonography is a powerful tool for detecting NTDs during pregnancy.

HOLOPROSENCEPHALY (PROSENCEPHALIC DISORDER)

The incidence of holoprosencephalic infants is one out of 15,000–20,000 live births. However, it has been described that the initial incidence in aborted human embryos might be more than 60 times higher than the incidence of live births.[7,8] Holoprosencephalies are mainly classified into three varieties; alobar, semilobar, and lobar types. Seventy-five percent of holoprosencephalic individuals have no genetic cause identified; the rest are due to genetic factors. The most common chromosomal aberration is trisomy 13. There are several gene mutations that were identified as genetic causes of holoprosencephaly, such as *Sonic Hedgehog (SHH)* located on 7q36, *SIX3* on 2p21, *ZIC2* on

13q32, and *TGIF* on 18p11.3.[9-12] In individuals with normal karyotypes, point mutations or pathogenic copy number variation, including those genes, are identified in approximately 22%.[10] Approximately 80% are accompanied by facial abnormalities due to hypoplasia of the midline of the face, such as hypotelorism, cyclopia, nasal septum defect, proboscis, rhinoplasty, cleft lip, and cleft palate,[13] as shown in **Figures 2A to D**. In mild familial cases, there are cases with only a single central incisor.

AGENESIS OF THE CORPUS CALLOSUM

The corpus callosum (CC) is the most extensive fiber-tract structure in the cerebrum, connecting the right and left cerebral hemispheres, integrating the motor and sensory information, and influencing higher cognition.[14] An essential gene is *FGF8* for early forebrain patterning, commissural plate development. *ZIC2*, *EMX1*, *NFIA*, and *SIX3* are responsible genes for developing the CC, the hippocampus, and anterior commissure. By 20 postconceptional weeks, the CC's final form is accomplished, although axonal growth continues still after birth. The CC is not formed in the early stage of CNS development, but early cerebral events, such as combining morphogenetic gradients that, together with developing thalamocortical circuits,[15,16] are essential to forming the CC.

Agenesis of the corpus callosum (AOCC) is brain malformation that occurs isolated or associated with syndromic diseases. AOCC includes complete AOCC (total absence of CC, **Figs. 3A and B**), partial AOCC, and hypoplastic CC (thin CC) with a normal anterior to a posterior extent).[14] The causal factors of AOCC are related to the events in each step of neuronal, glial proliferation, midline patterning,

callosal neuronal migration, specification, axon guidance, and postguidance.[14] Various copy number variations are related to AOCC, such as 1q42-q44 deletion,[17,18] 4p16.3 deletion (Wolf-Hirschhorn syndrome),[19] 8p rearrangements,[20-22] 17p13, 3 deletion (Miller–Dieker lissencephaly syndrome),[23,24] and others.

The *ARX* gene mutation[25-28] is responsible for X-linked lissencephaly with an absent CC and ambiguous genitalia (XLAG). *L1CAM* mutations cause L1 syndrome.[29,30] As an *L1CAM* (L1 cell adhesion molecule) gene is located on Xq28, the primarily male baby is affected. L1 is an essential gene for neuronal adhesion. *L1CAM*-affected patients have severe disorders with mental retardation, lower limb spasticity, and paraplegia.

Causative genes have not been identified in some of the syndromes with AOCC. Aicardi syndrome,[30] featured by AOCC, infantile spasms, and chorioretinal lacunae including microphthalmia, coloboma, is X-linked dominant inherited and has a paired X chromosome. Therefore, the affected individuals are mostly females, but males with XXY karyotypes (Klinefelter syndrome) can be affected. An age-adjusted prevalence is 0.63 per 100,000 females.[31] Intrahemispheric cysts (**Figs. 3C and D**) or pericallosal lipoma can be associated with AOCC.

MALFORMATIONS OF CORTICAL DEVELOPMENT

The cortex of the brain is formed as a consequence of the complicated dynamic process. There are three stages of the process of cortical development.[32] The first stage is the cell proliferation phase, in which stem cells increase in number and differentiate into neurons or glial cells in the VZ and

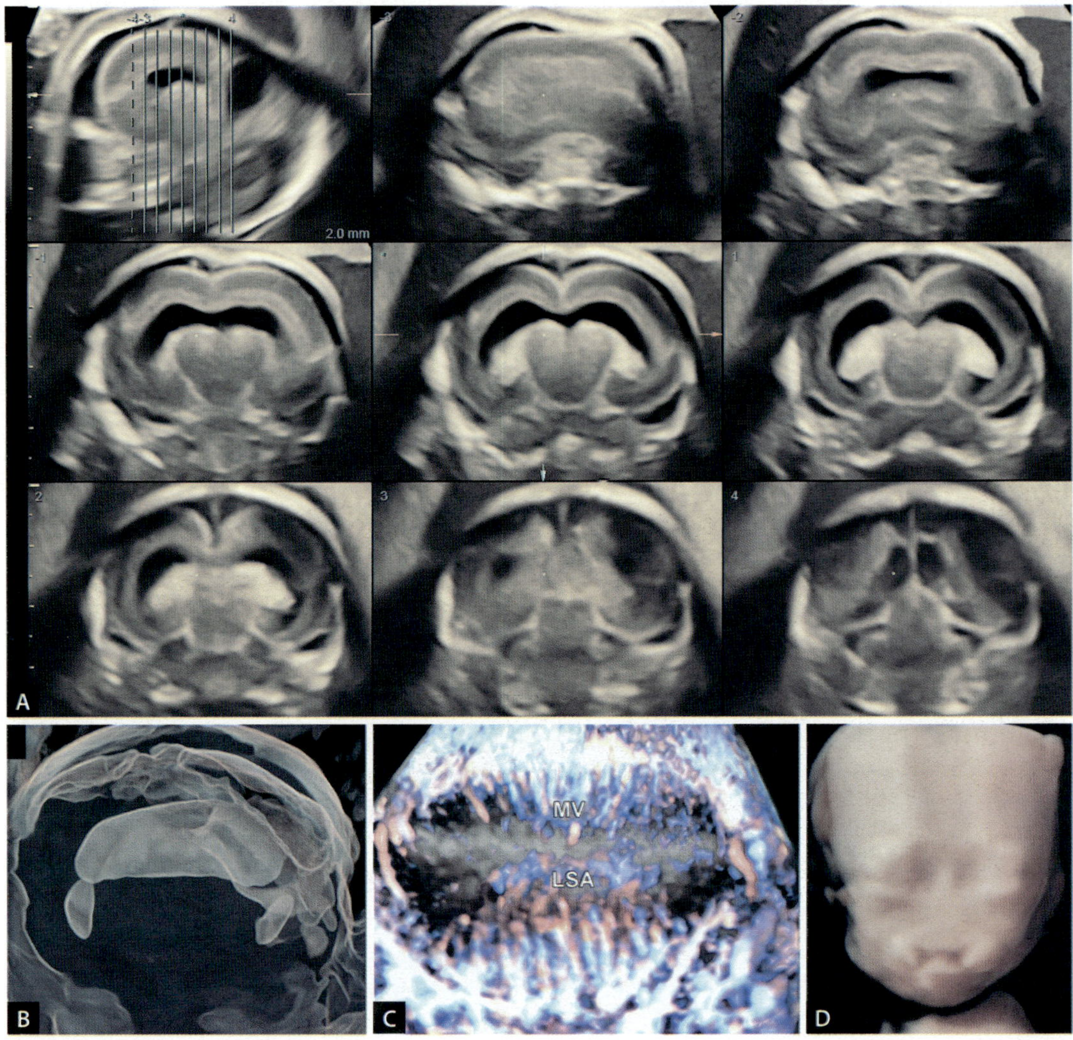

Figs. 2A to D: Neurosonographic images of fetal holoprosencephaly. (A) The coronal tomographic ultrasound images. Note a fused ventricle between the left and right ventricles; (B) HD live silhouette image of the fused ventricle; (C) HD flow image in the coronal section; (D) 3D surface image of the fetal face. Arrhinia and cleft lip are clearly demonstrated. (MV: medullary veins; LSA: lenticulostriate arteries)

subventricular zone (SVZ). The second stage is the neuronal cell migration phase. The neurons are tangentially migrating toward the cerebral surface from the ventricular surface with inside-out mode. This third stage is the organization phase, in which the six layers of the cortex are formed.[33]

As described above, it is obvious that the cerebral cortex is formed during the fetal period, and MCD, dysplasia of the cerebral cortex, is a disease that is completed during the fetal period. However, MCD is rarely noticed during the fetal period, and it is mostly discovered after birth by

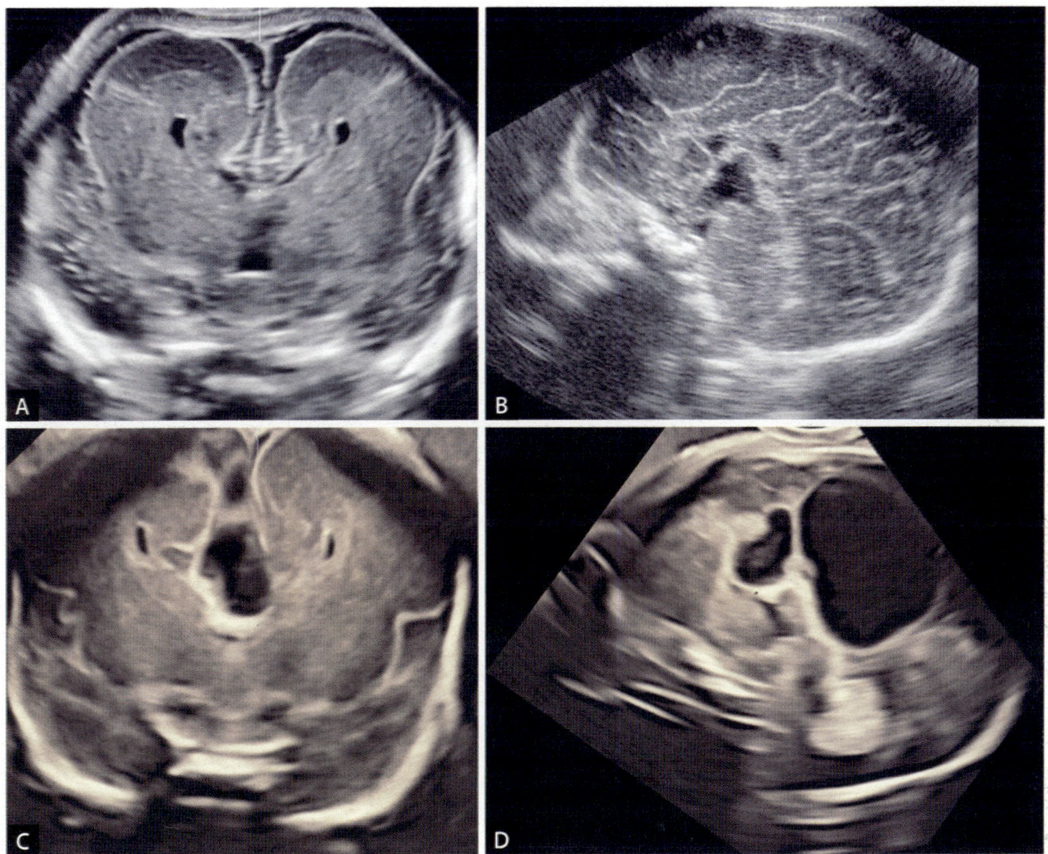

Figs. 3A to D: Neuroimages of agenesis of the corpus callosum (AOCC) and AOCC-related interhemispheric cysts. (A) Neuroimage in the coronal section. Note the defect of the corpus callosum; (B) Neuroimage in the mid-sagittal section; (C) Interhemispheric cysts in the coronal section, in the case of AOCC; (D) Interhemispheric cysts in the mid-sagittal section.

detailed examinations such as MRI due to developmental delay or epilepsy, and then the causal factors are investigated by genetic examinations.[34] MCD is classified into three groups according to the three developmental stages described above. More than 100 genes were identified, being responsible for MCD. However, because MCD-related genes are involved in multiple developmental stages, it has been assumed that the tissues of proliferation, migration, and postmigration are genetically and functionally interdependent, it has turned out that it is difficult to classify MCDs into these three groups.[35,36]

PROLIFERATION AND APOPTOSIS DISORDERS

Microcephaly is a proliferation disorder secondary to degeneration of normal growth and subsequent loss of neuronal cells.[37] Microcephaly vera, actual microcephaly, or primary microcephaly, results in intellectual disability after birth. Infants with microcephaly vera have no apparent brain malformations despite small brains. The phenotypes are not always uniform. There is a continuum between microcephaly with regular gyral formation and microcephaly associated with other malformation,[38-40] such as microlissencephaly. The causal factors of microcephaly include fetal infections by rubella virus, cytomegalovirus (CMV), ZIKA virus and toxoplasmosis, and single-gene mutations. There are several responsible genes for microcephalies, such as Microcephalin (*MCPH1*[39,41,42]), *ASPM*,[43] *CDK5RAP2*,[44] *CENPJ*,[34,44,45] *STIL*,[40,45] *WDR62*,[38,40,46] and *CEP152*[47] and others. In the case of microcephaly, neurosonographic observation of the intracranial structure through the cranial fontanelle is often very difficult because the cranial fontanelle and sutures are very narrow due to microcephaly. For a detailed evaluation of intracranial structure in cases with microcephaly, MRI is recommended.

Neuronal Migration Disorders

On the brain surface, the gyri and sulci are detectable by neurosonogram after the late 7 months' gestation. The further gyral elaboration continues during the rest of fetal life and shortly after birth. Neuronal cell migration is controlled by a complex series of chemical guidance and signals. If these signals are incorrect or absent, neuronal cells will not be able to reach where they should belong. This can result in structurally abnormal or missing areas in any part of the intracranial structure, such as the cerebral hemispheres, cerebellum, hippocampus, and brainstem. Neuronal migration disorders include agyria, pachygyria, lissencephaly, microgyria, polymicrogyria, neuronal heterotopias such as periventricular nodular heterotopia and band heterotopia. The gyral development aberration often cause seizures and neurological dysfunction from early in life. Migration disorders are prominent in the cerebral cortex in late pregnancy. Therefore, it seems impossible to detect migration disorder at midgestation when the gyri and sulci are not formed. Toi and his colleagues[48] showed a regular gyrus pattern detected by transabdominal sonography. The cortex develops macroscopically at the end of the second trimester, and the most obvious morphological difference is the changing appearance of Sylvian fissure.[49-51] The Sylvian fissure is one of the markers of cortical development due to normal migration. According to the development of the brain, the change in the appearance of Sylvian fissure is remarkable. Poon et al.[52] proposed the Sylvian fissure angle explaining a significant angle decrease as the gestational age progressed. Furthermore, Pooh et al.[53] showed 22 MCD cases between 18 and 30 weeks of gestation, with the delayed development of the Sylvian fissure with a wider Sylvian angle than before gyrus formation.

Lissencephaly is characterized as a cortical malformation associated with abnormal neuronal migration and gyrus formation. The spectrum of lissencephaly includes agyria, pachygyria, and subcortical band heterotopia. Lissencephaly was traditionally divided into two types. Lissencephaly type I was with a smooth brain and type II with a cobblestone appearance. However, many responsible genes for migration disorders were clarified, and classification was changed depending on the pathogenesis. *LIS1* on 17p13.3, *PAFAH1B1* gene mutation, which subdivides into Miller–Dieker syndrome, *DCX* causes lissencephaly due to doublecortin mutation. Cobblestone lissencephaly includes muscle-eye-brain (MEB) disease, Walker–Warburg syndrome due to *POMGnT1*,[54,55] Fukuyama syndrome due to *Fukutin*.[56-59] *ARX* gene on Xq22.13[60-63] mutation causes X-linked lissencephaly. *Reelin* gene on 7q22.1[64-66] causes Norman–Roberts syndrome, and microlissencephaly.[34,67-72]

However, with recent rapid advances in molecular genetics, a conventional classification system became inadequate to distinguish various patterns of lissencephaly to predict the most likely causative gene mutations; a new classification based on imaging was proposed in 2017.[73] Several reports on the prenatal diagnosis of lissencephaly have been published.[48,51,74-78]

Postmigrational Disorders

Polymicrogyria is the most common MCD relate postmigrational causes. Copy number variations of 1p36.3 deletion, 22q11.2 deletion, and mechanistic target of rapamycin (*mTOR*)-related genes are often associated with polymicrogyria and macrocephaly. Germline mutations that affect the *PI3K/AKT/mTOR* pathway are involved in certain hereditary diseases. The loss of the tumor suppressor phosphatase and tensin homolog (*PTEN*) causes congenital diseases, such as Cowden syndrome, Bannayan–Riley–Ruvalcaba syndrome, *PTEN*-related Proteus syndrome, and Proteus-like syndrome. The author and colleagues recently reported a rare case with megalencephaly with cortical maldevelopment due to *PTEN* mutation, as shown in **Figures 4A to C**.[77]

Perisylvian bilateral polymicrogyria[78,79] is often associated with schizencephaly. Schizencephaly is characterized by congenital cerebral clefts, lined by pial-ependyma, with communication between the subarachnoid space laterally and the lateral ventricles medially. Schizencephaly occurs unilaterally in 63% and 37% bilaterally. A considerable cause is a vascular disruption during cortical development, genetic factors such as *WDR62* mutation,[45,80] which causes schizencephaly as well as microcephaly,[46] indicating relations between processes of proliferation and schizencephaly pathogenesis, and *COL4A1* mutation.[81-83]

■ VENTRICULOMEGALY

Ventriculomegaly is defined when a diameter of an atrial width is measured 10 mm or higher. Ventriculomegaly during fetal life is categorized into mild (10–12 mm), moderate (13–15 mm), or severe (>15 mm) types. The incidence of mild to moderate type is approximately 1%. Mild ventriculomegaly seems to be a normal variant if other associated abnormalities do not exist, and genetic examination is normal.[84]

Hydrocephalus and ventriculomegaly are the terms that indicate the pathological condition with enlarged lateral ventricles. Hydrocephalus is mainly associated with increased intracranial pressure (ICP) by occlusion or stenosis of cerebrospinal fluid (CSF) flow pathway, and neuroimaging reveals dangling choroid plexus inside the enlarged ventricles. In contrast, normal-pressure hydrocephalus (NPH) is associated with enlarged ventricles without increased ICP, with the normal appearance of choroid plexus. Hydrocephalus commonly occurs due to congenital stenosis of the cerebral aqueduct stenosis. However, secondary ventriculomegaly can occur due to vascular disease, cortical maldevelopment, intra-cranial tumor, or cysts, intracerebral or intraventricular hemorrhage (IVH), Chiari malformation due to myelomeningocele, encephalopathy, meningitis, and other CNS abnormalities. The causal factors of hydro-cephalus and ventriculomegaly vary widely: neuronal adhesion, vesicle trafficking, dystroglycanopathies, ciliopathies, RAS-opathies, planar cell polarity, and NTDs, lysosomal storage disorders, growth factors, Wnt signaling pathway, and *PI3K/AKT/mTOR* pathway to transcription factors.

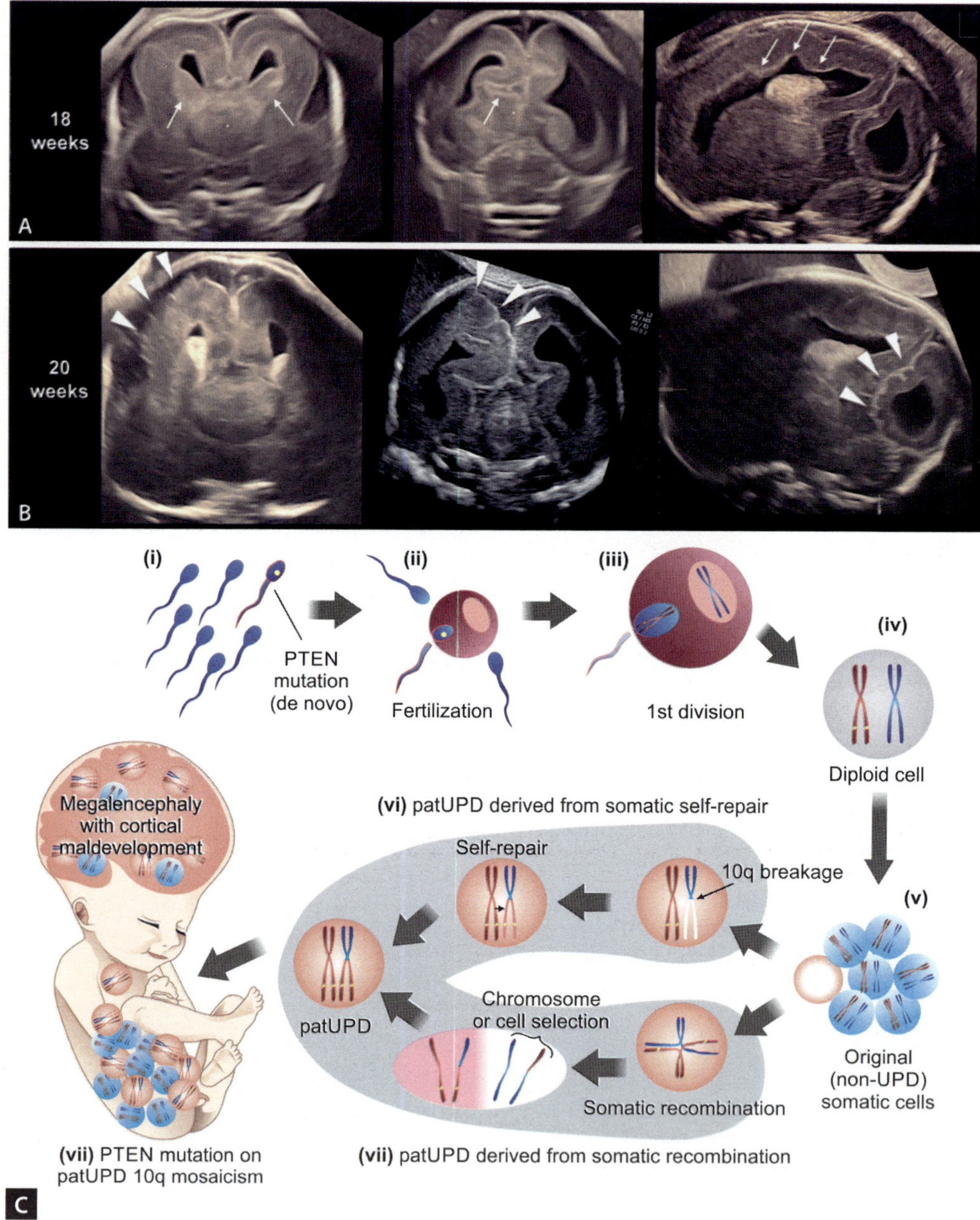

Figs. 4A to C: Neurosonographic images and the schematic illustration of the fetus's genetic events with phosphatase and tensin homolog (*PTEN*) mutation on paternal UPD (patUPD) 10q mosaicism.[77] (A) Neuroimaging at 18th gestational week. Macrocephaly with asymmetrical megalencephaly due to PTEN mutation. Arrows indicate the persistence of ganglionic eminence, abnormal sulcation, and the irregular ventricular wall; (B) Neuroimaging at 20th week. From left, anterior coronal, posterior coronal, and parasagittal views. Sonogram depicted the remarkable polygyria that were not seen in the 18th week; (C) Schematic illustration of genetic events.

Owing to recent advances in sequencing technologies, four genes have been well known to cause congenital hydrocephalus:[85] *L1CAM*, *AP1S2* (X-linked), *CCDC88C*,[86] and *MPDZ*[87] (autosomal recessive). Further, over 100 genes have been identified as the causal factors of genetic hydrocephalus or ventriculomegaly.[88]

L1CAM[30,89-91] located at Xq28, mediates cell–cell adhesion, the guidance of neurite outgrowth, bundling, myelination, pathfinding, long-term potentiation, neuronal cell survival, migration, and synaptogenesis.[92] Mutated *L1CAM* results in invariable neurological phenotypes, such as hydrocephalus, AOCC or hypoplasia, and adducted thumbs **(Figs. 5A to G)**. Because of X-linked recessive inheritance, the carrier mother's male fetus has a 50% chance of being affected.

The CSF flow pathway is also affected by abnormal beating or asynchronism of the ependymal cilia lining the ventricular system. Therefore, ciliopathies such as Bardet–Biedl syndrome (*CEP290*[93]), Meckel syndrome (*MKS1, TMEM67*[94-96]), and Joubert syndrome (*TMEM216*,[97,98] *CC2D2A*[99]) are often associated with ventriculomegaly.

Muscular dystrophies are associated with the aberrant glycosylation of α-dystroglycan and collectively termed dystroglycanopathies.[88,100] Dystroglycanopathies are often associated with brain and ocular pathology. In cases of dystroglycanopathy, a disorder of neuronal cell migration results in cortical maldevelopment and subsequent ventricular enlargement. Walker–Warburg syndrome (*POMT1, PONT2,* and *B3GALNT2*), MEB disease (*POMGnT1*), and Fukuyama congenital muscular dystrophy (*FKTN*) are representative dystroglycanopathies.

PI3K/AKT/mTOR pathway-related genes are identified in several other over growth syndromes. The megalencephaly polymicrogyria-polydactyly-hydrocephalus syndrome (MPPH) and megalencephaly-capillary malformation-polymicrogyria syndrome (MCAP) are spectrums of megalencephaly-associated syndromes[88,101] characterized by megalencephaly, polymicrogyria, ventriculomegaly, and Chiari malformation. In megalencephaly-associated syndromes, the mechanism of ventriculomegaly is that megalencephaly induces polymicrogyria and cerebellar overgrowth, leading to oppression of the posterior fossa cerebellar tonsillar herniation, which eventually obstructs CSF flow. However, as Chiari malformation does not always exist, CSF flow obstruction may occur within the overgrown brain.

Mutations of growth factors related to genes such as *FGFR3* can lead to skeletal dysplasia (thanatophoric dysplasia) with enlarged ventricles associated with overgrown and hyperconvoluted temporal lobe,[102] as shown in **Figures 6A to D**.

The term "Isolated" ventriculomegaly is often used when no other structural abnormalities are notified prenatally. However, in many "antenatally isolated" ventriculomegaly cases, extra-CNS abnormalities or single-gene mutations are often found after birth. Detailed observation of ventricular shapes, intracerebral, and extra-CNS morphology may lead to identifying causal factors and prognostic evaluation far more than atrial width (AW) measurement. To find out causal factors, chromosomal microarray, exome sequencing, or genome sequencing, as well as viral antibody analysis, may be recommendable. Furthermore, longitudinal study during the fetal period by neurosonography is essential because spontaneous resolution of enlargement during pregnancy is seen in some isolated ventriculomegaly cases.

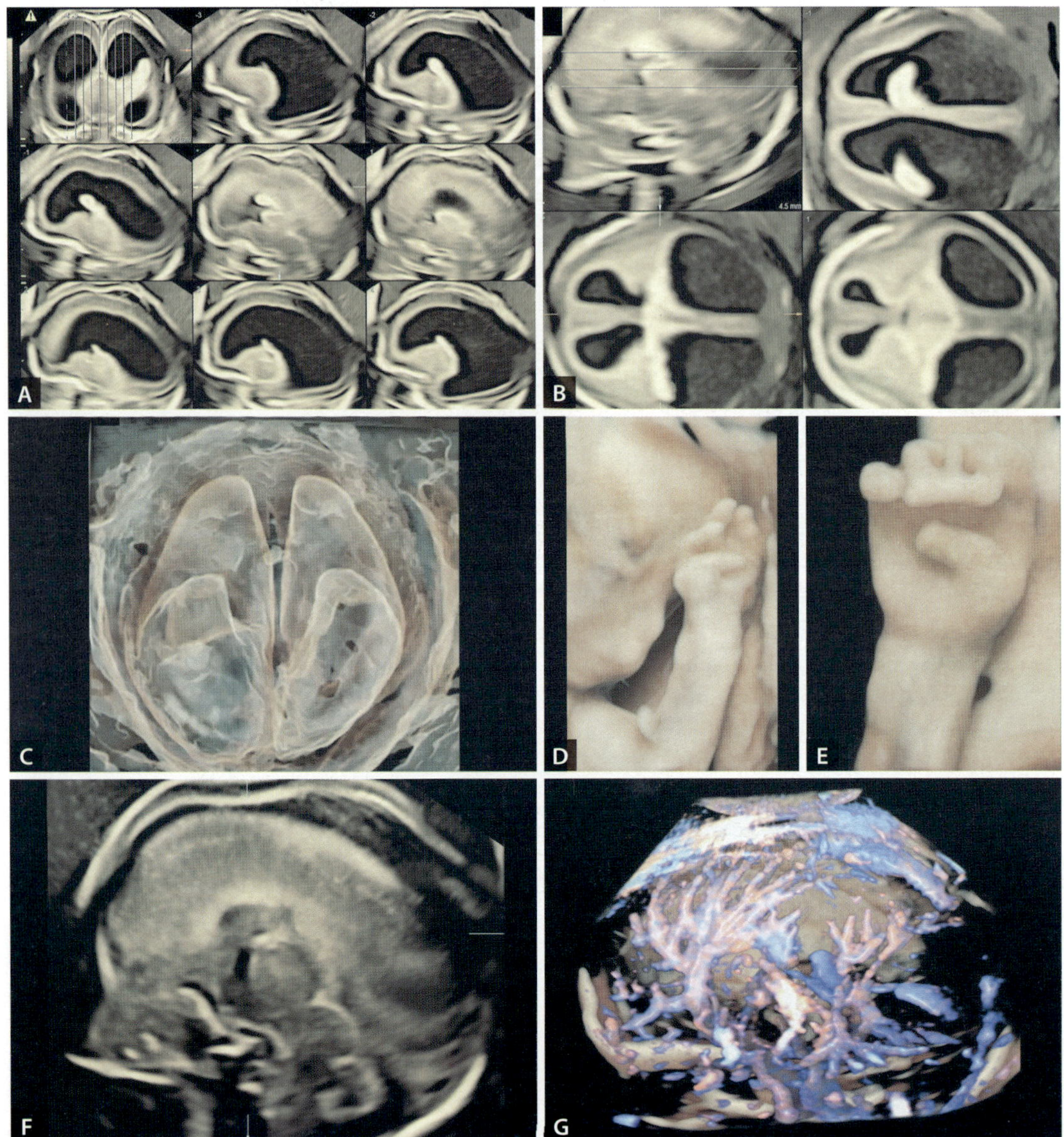

Figs. 5A to G: X-linked (L1) hydrocephalus at 20th gestational week. (A) 3D sagittal tomographic images; (B) 3D axial tomographic images; (C) HD live silhouette image of enlarged ventricles; (D) The adducted thumb of the left hand by 3D ultrasound; (E) The adducted thumb of the right hand by 3D ultrasound; (F) The midsagittal plane of the fetal brain. Note the hypoplastic corpus callosum; (G) HD flow image of the midsagittal brain.

IN UTERO BRAIN INJURY AND DAMAGE

In the cases of neonatal encephalopathy and cerebral palsy, *"When is the timing of causal events, antepartum, intrapartum or postpartum?"* is a point of interest to discuss because it involves medico-socio-legal-ethical issues. Brain insults may be

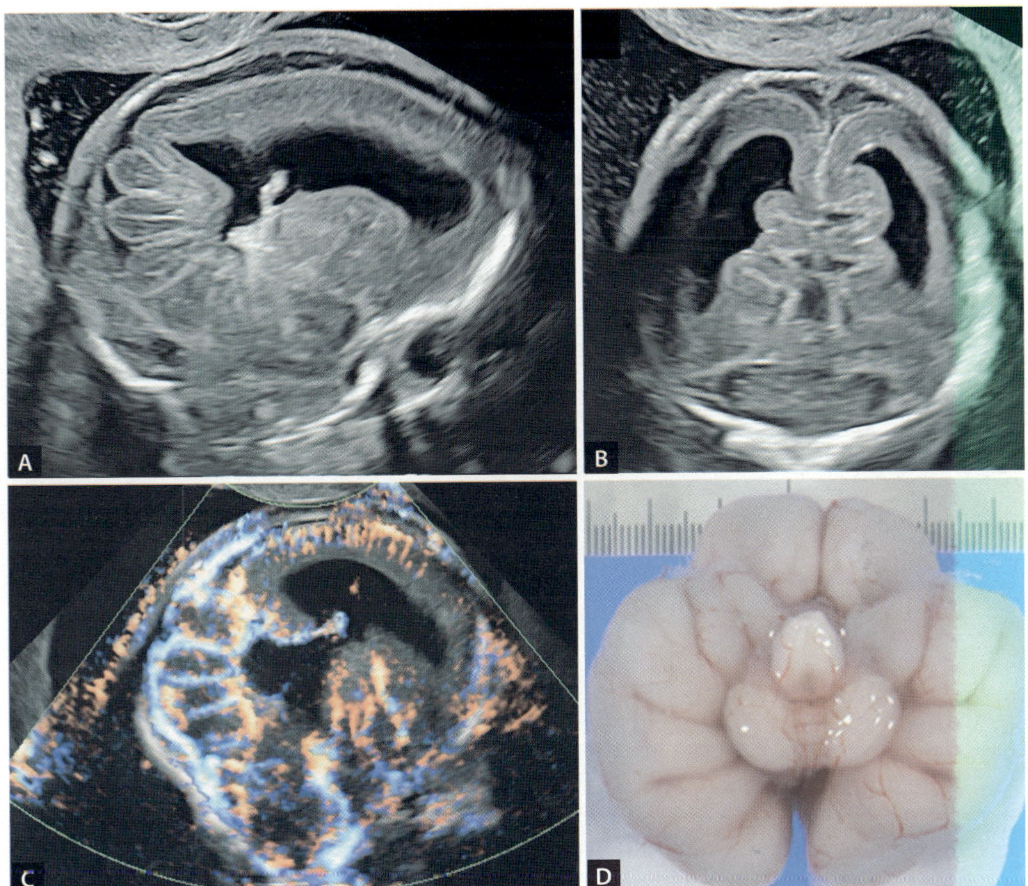

Figs. 6A to D: *FGFR3*-related thanatophoric dysplasia with ventriculomegaly associated with overgrown and hyperconvoluted temporal lobe. (A) Neurosonographic image in the parasagittal fetal brain at 16 weeks. Note the serpentine appearance of the overgrown brain parenchyma; (B) Neurosonographic image in the posterior coronal fetal brain at 16 weeks; (C) Power Doppler image in the parasagittal section. The superficial cerebral vessels run along the serpentine-shaped cerebrum; (D) The autopsy findings at 21 weeks. The view from the basilar. Note the abnormal sulci of the cerebri.

related to antenatal events such as cerebral hemorrhage, encephalopathy, migration disorder, as shown in **Figures 7A to D**. It is not always possible to specify when the event occurred. Occasionally the causative event for encephalopathy may be speculated, for example, single intrauterine fetal death (sIUFD) or fetal intervention for twin-to-twin transfusion syndrome in cases of monochorionic twins. However, it is challenging to grasp prenatal evidence of in utero brain injury, which causes postnatal neurological deficits. Neurosonography and neuro-MRI are reliable modalities for detecting silent encephalopathy.

In many cases with cerebral palsy with in utero brain insults. Especially term-delivered infants with reassuring fetal heart rate monitoring at delivery are not suspected of having brain damage or injury. Therefore, it is hard to identify the exact incidence.

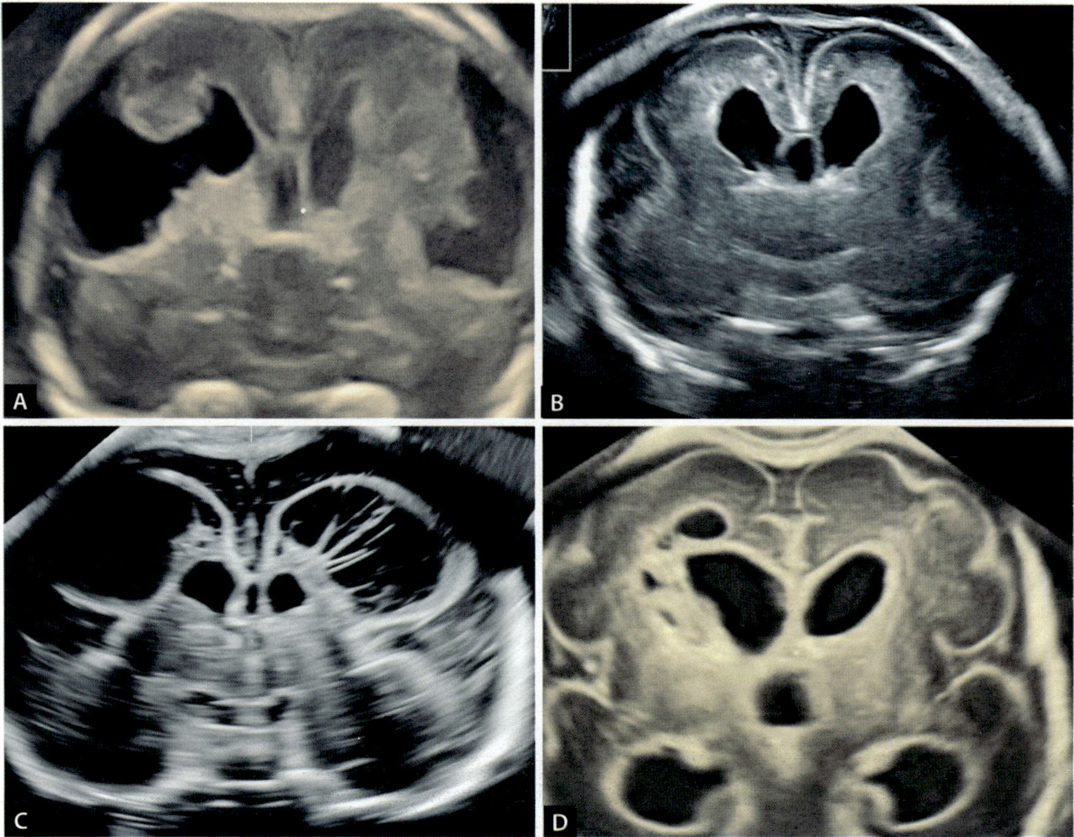

Figs. 7A to D: In utero brain injury due to various causal factors. (A) Intracranial bleeding with porencephalic change due to *COL4A1* gene mutation; (B) Bilateral multiple intracranial hemorrhages is seen in a hydropic fetus. The cause might be the increased cardiac output due to congenital heart disease; (C) Destructive encephalopathy after single intrauterine fetal death (sIUFD) of monochorionic twin; (D) Cerebral hemorrhage with ventriculomegaly. The causal factor was uncertain.

Fetal intracranial bleeding is a rare condition and has been called a fetal stroke after 2004[103-106] and other various descriptions were used in published reports, such as fetal cerebrovascular disorder or perinatal brain injury.[107] It was reported that fetal stroke is an event between the 14th week and labor onset and cited an incidence of about 17–35 of 100,000 live births,[103] or 0.5–1.0 per 1,000 pregnancies.[108] In a report in 1985, a series of stillbirth autopsies showed 6% with the evidence of fetal intracranial hemorrhage.[109]

Various etiologies of fetal intracranial bleeding or hemorrhage are considered, including idiopathic, alterations of fetal blood pressure, fetomaternal hemorrhage, umbilical abnormalities, placental abnormalities, fetal infection, single-gene mutations, trauma, alloimmune and idiopathic thrombocytopenia, von Willebrand disease, illicit drug (cocaine) abuse or specific medications (warfarin), congenital factor X and factor V deficiencies, twin-to-twin transfusion, vascular diseases, intracranial tumor, and the sIUFD of monochorionic twin. Several reports described *COL4A1* and *COL42A* gene mutations strongly related to perinatal cerebral bleeding and porencephaly.[110-116] Fetal neuroimaging demonstrates hyperechoic lined ventricular wall, avascular intracranial mass, parenchymal echogenicity, porencephalic cysts, hyperechoic acute clot adherent to choroid plexus, and hyperechoic nodular ependyma, and increased periventricular white matter echogenicity is demonstrated in cases with cerebral bleeding. Secondary ventriculomegaly is often observed because of the Monro stenosis or obstruction by blood clots.

Primary IVH is defined, when intraventricular events such as choroid plexus tumor or bleeding are apparent. The incidence of primary IVH is approximately 30%, and the rest 70% is secondary IVH. The most common cause of secondary IVH is intraparenchymal bleeding, which is expanding into the ventricular system. The IVH grading system in the infant was first reported by Papile et al.[117] Grade I is isolated to the periventricular (subependymal) germinal matrix; Grade II implies IVH (10–50%) without ventricular dilatation; Grade III is IVH (>50% or with ventriculomegaly); and Grade IV is with parenchymal hemorrhage or periventricular hemorrhagic infarction.[118]

FUTURE PERSPECTIVE

As shown in this article, the recent advances in 3D neurosonography have enabled us the systematic evaluation of fetal brain morphology. Owing to the rapid progress of molecular genetics, it has been clarified that more than a hundred genes are responsible for congenital cortical abnormalities. Most congenital CNS disorders are deeply associated with developmental stages, genetic causes, environmental factors, and intrauterine insults and events. Prenatal counseling for parents was conducted according to a morphology-based diagnosis. Nowadays, however, as CNS diagnoses can be made, detailed neuroimaging, genetic examination of chromosomal microarray, exome sequencing, and genome sequencing add causal genetic factors. Prenatal genetic counseling in cases with fetal brain abnormalities is done according to all those results. Detailed neurosonography combined with molecular genetics has established "Neurosonogenetics", a new field in multidisciplinary fetal neurology, for precise perinatal management and care, and treatment and prevention in the future.[119,120]

REFERENCES

1. Pooh RK, Kurjak A. 3D/4D Sonography moved prenatal diagnosis of fetal anomalies from the second to the first trimester of pregnancy. J Matern Fetal Neonatal Med. 2012;25(5):433-55.
2. Pooh RK, Shiota K, Kurjak A. Imaging of the human embryo with magnetic resonance imaging microscopy and high-resolution transvaginal 3-dimensional sonography: Human embryology in the 21st century. Am J Obstet Gynecol. 2011;204(1):77.e1-16.
3. Pooh RK. Sonoembryology by 3D HDlive silhouette ultrasound - what is added by the "see-through fashion"? J Perinat Med. 2016; 44(2):139-48.
4. Copp AJ, Greene NDE. Genetics and development of neural tube defects. J Pathol. 2010;220(2):217-30.
5. Greene NDE, Copp AJ. Development of the vertebrate central nervous system: formation of the neural tube. Prenat Diagn. 2009;29(4):303-11.
6. Rolo A, Galea GL, Savery D, Greene NDE, Andrew J. Novel mouse model of encephalocele: post-neurulation origin and relationship to open neural tube defects. Dis Model Mech. 2019;12(11):dmm040683.

7. Cohen Jr MM. Perspectives on holoprosencephaly: Part I. Epidemiology, genetics, and syndromology. Teratology. 1989;40(3):211-35.

8. Matsunaga E, Shiota K. Holoprosencephaly in human embryos: epidemiologic studies of 150 cases. Teratology. 1977;16(3):261-72.

9. Cohen Jr MM. Holoprosencephaly: clinical, anatomic, and molecular dimensions. Birth Defects Res A Clin Mol Teratol. 2006;76(9):658-73.

10. Roessler E, Muenke M. The molecular genetics of holoprosencephaly. Am J Med Genet C Semin Med Genet. 2010;154C(1):52-61.

11. Robbins DJ, Nybakken KE, Kobayashi R, Sisson JC, Bishop JM, Thérond PP. Hedgehog elicits signal transduction by means of a large complex containing the kinesin-related protein costal2. Cell. 1997;90(2):225-34.

12. Robbins DJ, Fei DL, Riobo NA. The Hedgehog signal transduction network. Sci Signal. 2012;5(246):re6.

13. Blaas HGK. Holoprosencephaly. In: Odibo AO, Tutschek B, Gratacos E, Feltovich H, Copel J, Platt L, et al. (Eds). Obstetric Imaging: Fetal Diagnosis and Care, 2nd edition. Philadelphia: Elsevier Health Sciences; 2017. p. 190.

14. Edwards TJ, Sherr EH, Barkovich AJ, Richards LJ. Clinical, genetic and imaging findings identify new causes for corpus callosum development syndromes. Brain. 2014;137(Pt 6):1579-613.

15. O'Leary DDM, Chou SJ, Sahara S. Area patterning of the mammalian cortex. Neuron. 2007;56(2):252-69.

16. Hoerder-Suabedissen A, Hayashi S, Upton L, Nolan Z, Casas-Torremocha D, Grant E, et al. Subset of cortical layer 6b neurons selectively innervates higher order thalamic nuclei in mice. Cereb Cortex. 2018;28(5):1882-97.

17. Puthuran MJ, Rowland-Hill CA, Simpson J, Pairaudeau PW, Mabbott JL, Morris SM, et al. Chromosome 1q42 deletion and agenesis of the corpus callosum. Am J Med Genet A. 2005;138(1):68-9.

18. Filges I, Röthlisberger B, Boesch N, Weber P, Wenzel F, Huber AR, et al. Interstitial deletion 1q42 in a patient with agenesis of corpus callosum: phenotype-genotype comparison to the 1q41q42 microdeletion suggests a contiguous 1q4 syndrome. Am J Med Genet A. 2010;152A(4):987-93.

19. Righini A, Ciosci R, Selicorni A, Bianchini E, Parazzini C, Zollino M, et al. Brain magnetic resonance imaging in Wolf-Hirschhorn syndrome. Neuropediatrics. 2007;38(1):25-8.

20. O'Driscoll MC, Black GCM, Clayton-Smith J, Sherr EH, Dobyns WB. Identification of genomic loci contributing to agenesis of the corpus callosum. Am J Med Genet A. 2010;152A(9):2145-59.

21. Heide S, Keren B, de Villemeur TB, Chantot-Bastaraud S, Depienne C, Nava C, et al. Copy number variations found in patients with a corpus callosum abnormality and intellectual disability. J Pediatr. 2017;185:160-6.

22. Schell-Apacik CC, Wagner K, Bihler M, Ertl-Wagner B, Heinrich U, Klopocki E, et al. Agenesis and dysgenesis of the corpus callosum: clinical, genetic and neuroimaging findings in a series of 41 patients. Am J Med Genet A. 2008;146A(19):2501-11.

23. Chen CP, Chang TY, Guo WY, Wu PC, Wang LK, Chern SR, et al. Chromosome 17p13.3 deletion syndrome: aCGH characterization, prenatal findings and diagnosis, and literature review. Gene. 2013;532(1):152-9.

24. Chen CP, Chien SC. Prenatal sonographic features of Miller-Dieker syndrome. J Med Ultrasound. 2010;18(4):147-52.

25. Kitamura K, Yanazawa M, Sugiyama N, Miura H, Iizuka-Kogo A, Kusaka M, et al. Mutation of ARX causes abnormal development of forebrain and testes in mice and X-linked lissencephaly with abnormal genitalia in humans. Nat Genet. 2002;32(3):359-69.

26. Kato M, Das S, Petras K, Kitamura K, Morohashi KI, Abuelo DN, et al. Mutations of ARX are associated with striking pleiotropy and consistent genotype-phenotype correlation. Hum Mutat. 2004;23(2):147-59.

27. Dobyns WB, Berry-Kravis E, Havernick NJ, Holden KR, Viskochil D. X-linked lissencephaly with absent corpus callosum and

ambiguous genitalia. Am J Med Genet. 1999;86(4):331-7.

28. Bonneau D, Toutain A, Laquerrière A, Marret S, Saugier-Veber P, Barthez MA, et al. X-linked lissencephaly with absent corpus callosum and ambiguous genitalia (XLAG): clinical, magnetic resonance imaging, and neuropathological findings. Ann Neurol. 2002;51(3):340-9.

29. Fransen E, Vits L, Van Camp G, Willems PJ. The clinical spectrum of mutations in L1, a neuronal cell adhesion molecule. Am J Med Genet. 1996;64(1):73-7.

30. Aicardi J. Aicardi syndrome. Brain Dev. 2005;27(3):164-71.

31. Lund C, Bjørnvold M, Tuft M, Kostov H, Røsby O, Selmer KK. Aicardi syndrome: an epidemiologic and clinical study in Norway. Pediatr Neurol. 2015;52(2):182-6.e3.

32. Parrini E, Conti V, Dobyns WB, Guerrini R. Genetic basis of brain malformations. Mol Syndromol. 2016;7(4):220-33.

33. Guerrini R, Dobyns WB. Malformations of cortical development: clinical features and genetic causes. Lancet Neurol. 2014;13(7):710-26.

34. Desikan RS, Barkovich AJ. Malformations of cortical development. Ann Neurol. 2016; 80(6):797-810.

35. Barkovich J. Complication begets clarification in classification. Brain. 2013;136(Pt 2):368-73.

36. Severino M, Geraldo AF, Utz N, Tortora D, Pogledic I, Klonowski W, et al. Definitions and classification of malformations of cortical development: practical guidelines. Brain. 2020;143(10):2874-94.

37. Gilmore EC, Walsh CA. Genetic causes of microcephaly and lessons for neuronal development. Wiley Interdiscip Rev Dev Biol. 2013;2(4):461-78.

38. Yu TW, Mochida GH, Tischfield DJ, Sgaier SK, Flores-Sarnat L, Sergi CM, et al. Mutations in WDR62, encoding a centrosome-associated protein, cause microcephaly with simplified gyri and abnormal cortical architecture. Nat Genet. 2010;42(11):1015-20.

39. Jackson AP, Eastwood H, Bell SM, Adu J, Toomes C, Carr IM, et al. Identification of microcephalin, a protein implicated in determining the size of the human brain. Am J Hum Genet. 2002;71(1):136-42.

40. Nicholas AK, Khurshid M, Désir J, Carvalho OP, Cox JJ, Thornton G, et al. WDR62 is associated with the spindle pole and is mutated in human microcephaly. Nat Genet. 2010;42(11):1010-4.

41. Trimborn M, Bell SM, Felix C, Rashid Y, Jafri H, Griffiths PD, et al. Mutations in microcephalin cause aberrant regulation of chromosome condensation. Am J Hum Genet. 2004;75(2):261-6.

42. Brunk K, Vernay B, Griffith E, Reynolds NL, Strutt D, Ingham PW, et al. Microcephalin coordinates mitosis in the syncytial Drosophila embryo. J Cell Sci. 2007;120(Pt 20):3578-88.

43. Bond J, Roberts E, Mochida GH, Hampshire DJ, Scott S, Askham JM, et al. ASPM is a major determinant of cerebral cortical size. Nat Genet. 2002;32(2):316-20.

44. Bond J, Roberts E, Springell K, Lizarraga SB, Scott S, Higgins J, et al. A centrosomal mechanism involving CDK5RAP2 and CENPJ controls brain size. Nat Genet. 2005;37(4):353-5.

45. Kumar A, Girimaji SC, Duvvari MR, Blanton SH. Mutations in STIL, encoding a pericentriolar and centrosomal protein, cause primary microcephaly. Am J Hum Genet. 2009;84(2):286-90.

46. Bilgüvar K, Öztürk AK, Louvi A, Kwan KY, Choi M, Tatli B, et al. Whole-exome sequencing identifies recessive WDR62 mutations in severe brain malformations. Nature. 2010;467(7312):207-10.

47. Guernsey DL, Jiang H, Hussin J, Arnold M, Bouyakdan K, Perry S, et al. Mutations in centrosomal protein CEP152 in primary microcephaly families linked to MCPH4. Am J Hum Genet. 2010;87(1):40-51.

48. Toi A, Lister WS, Fong KW. How early are fetal cerebral sulci visible at prenatal ultrasound and what is the normal pattern of early fetal sulcal development? Ultrasound Obstet Gynecol. 2004;24(7):706-15.

49. Pooh RK. The role of imaging detection of congenital defects in the era of PGT-A and NIPT. J Perinat Med. 2019;47(eA):92.

50. Pooh RK. Fetal brain imaging. Ultrasound Med Biol. 2017;43(1):S132.

51. Pooh RK. Fetal Neuroimaging of neural migration disorder. Ultrasound Clin. 2008; 3(4):541-52.

52. Poon LC, Sahota DS, Chaemsaithong P, Nakamura T, Machida M, Naruse K, et al. Transvaginal three-dimensional ultrasound assessment of Sylvian fissures at 18-30 weeks' gestation. Ultrasound Obstet Gynecol. 2019;54(2):190-8.

53. Pooh RK, Machida M, Nakamura T, Uenishi K, Chiyo H, Itoh K, et al. Increased Sylvian fissure angle as early sonographic sign of malformation of cortical development. Ultrasound Obstet Gynecol. 2019; 54(2):199-206.

54. Yoshida A, Kobayashi K, Manya H, Taniguchi K, Kano H, Mizuno M, et al. Muscular dystrophy and neuronal migration disorder caused by mutations in a glycosyltransferase, POMGnT1. Dev Cell. 2001;1(5):717-24.

55. Hehr U, Uyanik G, Gross C, Walter MC, Bohring A, Cohen M, et al. Novel POMGnT1 mutations define broader phenotypic spectrum of muscle-eye-brain disease. Neurogenetics. 2007;8(4):279-88.

56. Godfrey C, Clement E, Mein R, Brockington M, Smith J, Talim B, et al. Refining genotype phenotype correlations in muscular dystrophies with defective glycosylation of dystroglycan. Brain. 2007;130(Pt 10):2725-35.

57. Kobayashi K, Nakahori Y, Miyake M, Matsumura K, Kondo-Iida E, Nomura Y, et al. An ancient retrotransposal insertion causes Fukuyama-type congenital muscular dystrophy. Nature. 1998;394(6691):388-92.

58. Toda T, Kobayashi K, Kondo-Iida E, Sasaki J, Nakamura Y. The Fukuyama congenital muscular dystrophy story. Neuromuscul Disord. 2000;10(3):153-9.

59. Takeda S, Kondo M, Sasaki J, Kurahashi H, Kano H, Arai K, et al. Fukutin is required for maintenance of muscle integrity, cortical histiogenesis and normal eye development. Hum Mol Genet. 2003;12(12):1449-59.

60. Friocourt G, Kanatani S, Tabata H, Yozu M, Takahashi T, Antypa M, et al. Cell-autonomous roles of ARX in cell proliferation and neuronal migration during corticogenesis. J Neurosci. 2008;28(22):5794-805.

61. Friocourt G, Poirier K, Rakić S, Parnavelas JG, Chelly J. The role of ARX in cortical development. Eur J Neurosci. 2006;23(4): 869-76.

62. Sherr EH. The ARX story (epilepsy, mental retardation, autism, and cerebral malformations): one gene leads to many phenotypes. Curr Opin Pediatr. 2003;15(6): 567-71.

63. Colasante G, Simonet JC, Calogero R, Crispi S, Sessa A, Cho G, et al. ARX regulates cortical intermediate progenitor cell expansion and upper layer neuron formation through repression of Cdkn1c. Cereb Cortex. 2015; 25(2):322-35.

64. Folsom TD, Fatemi SH. The involvement of Reelin in neurodevelopmental disorders. Neuropharmacology. 2013;68:122-35.

65. Tissir F, Goffinet AM. Reelin and brain development. Nat Rev Neurosci. 2003;4(6): 496-505.

66. Chen Y, Beffert U, Ertunc M, Tang TS, Kavalali ET, Bezprozvanny I, et al. Reelin modulates NMDA receptor activity in cortical neurons. J Neurosci. 2005;25(36):8209-16.

67. Kato M. Genotype-phenotype correlation in neuronal migration disorders and cortical dysplasias. Front Neurosci. 2015;9:181.

68. Fallet-Bianco C, Laquerrière A, Poirier K, Razavi F, Guimiot F, Dias P, et al. Mutations in tubulin genes are frequent causes of various foetal malformations of cortical development including microlissencephaly. Acta Neuropathol Commun. 2014;2:69.

69. Laquerriere A, Gonzales M, Saillour Y, Cavallin M, Joyē N, Quēlin C, et al. De novo TUBB2B mutation causes fetal akinesia deformation sequence with microlissencephaly: an unusual presentation of tubulinopathy. Eur J Med Genet. 2016;59(4):249-56.

70. Harding BN, Moccia A, Drunat S, Soukarieh O, Tubeuf H, Chitty LS, et al. Mutations in citron kinase cause recessive microlissencephaly with multinucleated neurons. Am J Hum Genet. 2016;99(2):511-20.

71. Barkovich AJ, Ferriero DM, Barr RM, Gressens P, Dobyns WB, Truwit CL, et al. Microlissencephaly: a heterogeneous malformation of cortical development. Neuropediatrics. 1998;29(3):113-9.

72. Poirier K, Martinovic J, Laquerrière A, Cavallin M, Fallet-Bianco C, Desguerre I, et al. Rare ACTG1 variants in fetal microlissencephaly. Eur J Med Genet. 2015;58(8):416-8.

73. Di Donato N, Chiari S, Mirzaa GM, Aldinger K, Parrini E, Olds C, et al. Lissencephaly: expanded imaging and clinical classification. Am J Med Genet Part A. 2017;173(6):1473-88.

74. McGahan JP, Grix A, Gerscovich EO. Prenatal diagnosis of lissencephaly: Miller-Dieker syndrome. J Clin Ultrasound. 1994;22(9): 560-3.

75. Greco P, Resta M, Vimercati A, Dicuonzo F, Loverro G, Vicino M, et al. Antenatal diagnosis of isolated lissencephaly by ultrasound and magnetic resonance imaging. Ultrasound Obstet Gynecol. 1998;12(4):276-9.

76. Kojima K, Suzuki Y, Seki K, Yamamoto T, Sato T, Tanaka T, et al. Prenatal diagnosis of lissencephaly (type II) by ultrasound and fast magnetic resonance imaging. Fetal Diagn Ther. 2002;17(1):34-6.

77. Fong KW, Ghai S, Toi A, Blaser S, Winsor EJT, Chitayat D. Prenatal ultrasound findings of lissencephaly associated with Miller-Dieker syndrome and comparison with pre- and postnatal magnetic resonance imaging. Ultrasound Obstet Gynecol. 2004;24(7): 716-23.

78. Ghai S, Fong KW, Toi A, Chitayat D, Pantazi S, Blaser S. Prenatal US and MR imaging findings of lissencephaly: review of fetal cerebral sulcal development. Radiographics. 2006;26(2):389-405.

79. Leventer RJ, Jansen A, Pilz DT, Stoodley N, Marini C, Dubeau F, et al. Clinical and imaging heterogeneity of polymicrogyria: a study of 328 patients. Brain. 2010;133(Pt 5):1415-27.

80. Stutterd CA, Leventer RJ. Polymicrogyria: a common and heterogeneous malformation of cortical development. Am J Med Genet C Semin Med Genet. 2014;166C(2):227-39.

81. Manzini MC, Walsh CA. The genetics of brain malformations. In: Mitchell KJ (Ed). The Genetics of Neurodevelopmental Disorders. Canada: Wiley-Blackwell; 2015. pp. 129-54.

82. Smigiel R, Cabala M, Jakubiak A, Kodera H, Sasiadek MJ, Matsumoto N, et al. Novel COL4A1 mutation in an infant with severe dysmorphic syndrome with schizencephaly, periventricular calcifications, and cataract resembling congenital infection. Birth Defects Res A Clin Mol Teratol. 2016;106(4): 304-7.

83. Watanabe J, Okamoto K, Ohashi T, Natsumeda M, Hasegawa H, Oishi M, et al. Malignant hyperthermia and cerebral venous sinus thrombosis after ventriculoperitoneal shunt in infant with schizencephaly and COL4A1 mutation. World Neurosurg. 2019; 127:446-50.

84. ERRATA: Intracranial hemorrhage and tortuosity of veins detected on susceptibility-weighted imaging of a child with a type IV collagen α1 mutation and schizencephaly. Magn Reson Med Sci. 2015;14(4):373.

85. Fox NS, Monteagudo A, Kuller JA, Craigo S, Norton ME; Society for Maternal-Fetal Medicine (SMFM). Mild fetal ventriculomegaly: diagnosis, evaluation, and management. Am J Obstet Gynecol. 2018;219(1): B2-B9.

86. Shaheen R, Sebai MA, Patel N, Ewida N, Kurdi W, Altweijri I, et al. The genetic landscape of familial congenital hydrocephalus. Ann Neurol. 2017;81(6):890-7.

87. Ekici AB, Hilfinger D, Jatzwauk M, Thiel CT, Wenzel D, Lorenz I, et al. Disturbed Wnt signalling due to a mutation in CCDC88C causes an autosomal recessive non-syndromic hydrocephalus with medial diverticulum. Mol Syndromol. 2010;1(3): 99-112.

88. Al-Dosari MS, Al-Owain M, Tulbah M, Kurdi W, Adly N, Al-Hemidan A, et al. Mutation in MPDZ causes severe congenital hydrocephalus. J Med Genet. 2013;50(1):54-8.

89. Kousi M, Katsanis N. The genetic basis of hydrocephalus. Annu Rev Neurosci. 2016;39: 409-35.

90. Yamasaki M, Thompson P, Lemmon V. CRASH syndrome: mutations in L1CAM correlate with severity of the disease. Neuropediatrics. 1997;28(3):175-8.

91. Itoh K, Fushiki S. The role of L1cam in murine corticogenesis, and the pathogenesis of hydrocephalus. Pathol Int. 2015;65(2):58-66.

92. Takahashi S, Makita Y, Okamoto N, Miyamoto A, Oki J. L1CAM mutation in a Japanese family with X-linked hydrocephalus: a study for genetic counseling. Brain Dev. 1997;19(8):559-62.

93. Jouet M, Rosenthal A, Armstrong G, MacFarlane J, Stevenson R, Paterson J, et al. X–linked spastic paraplegia (SPG1), MASA syndrome and X–linked hydrocephalus result from mutations in the L1 gene. Nat Genet. 1994;7(3):402-7.

94. Adle-Biassette H, Saugier-Veber P, Fallet-Bianco C, Delezoide AL, Razavi F, Drouot N, et al. Neuropathological review of 138 cases genetically tested for X-linked hydrocephalus: evidence for closely related clinical entities of unknown molecular bases. Acta Neuropathol. 2013;126(3):427-42.

95. Rachel RA, Yamamoto EA, Dewanjee MK, May-Simera HL, Sergeev YV, Hackett AN, et al. CEP290 alleles in mice disrupt tissue-specific cilia biogenesis and recapitulate features of syndromic ciliopathies. Hum Mol Genet. 2015;24(13):3775-91.

96. Iannicelli M, Brancati F, Mougou-Zerelli S, Mazzotta A, Thomas S, Elkhartoufi N, et al. Novel TMEM67 mutations and genotype-phenotype correlates in meckelin-related ciliopathies. Hum Mutat. 2010;31(5): E1319-31.

97. Abdelhamed ZA, Natarajan S, Wheway G, Inglehearn CF, Toomes C, Johnson CA, et al. The Meckel-Gruber syndrome protein TMEM67 controls basal body positioning and epithelial branching morphogenesis in mice via the non-canonical Wnt pathway. Dis Model Mech. 2015;8(6):527-41.

98. Leightner AC, Hommerding CJ, Peng Y, Salisbury JL, Gainullin VG, Czarnecki PG, et al. The Meckel syndrome protein meckelin (TMEM67) is a key regulator of cilia function but is not required for tissue planar polarity. Hum Mol Genet. 2013;22(10):2024-40.

99. Xiao D, Lv C, Zhang Z, Wu M, Zheng X, Yang L, et al. Novel CC2D2A compound heterozygous mutations cause Joubert syndrome. Mol Med Rep. 2017;15(1):305-8.

100. Johnson K, Bertoli M, Phillips L, Töpf A, Van den Bergh P, Vissing J, et al. Detection of variants in dystroglycanopathy-associated genes through the application of targeted whole-exome sequencing analysis to a large cohort of patients with unexplained limb-girdle muscle weakness. Skelet Muscle. 2018;8(1):23.

101. Mirzaa GM, Rivière JB, Dobyns WB. Megalencephaly syndromes and activating mutations in the PI3K-AKT pathway: MPPH and MCAP. Am J Med Genet C Semin Med Genet. 2013;163C(2):122-30.

102. Itoh K, Pooh R, Kanemura Y, Yamasaki M, Fushiki S. Brain malformation with loss of normal FGFR3 expression in thanatophoric dysplasia type I. Neuropathology. 2013;33(6): 663-6.

103. Dicuonzo F, Palma M, Fiume M, Scarpello R, Lefons V, Maghenzani M, et al. Cerebrovascular disorders in the prenatal period. J Child Neurol. 2008;23(11):1260-6.

104. Özduman K, Pober BR, Barnes P, Copel JA, Ogle EA, Duncan CC, et al. Fetal stroke. Pediatr Neurol. 2004;30(3):151-62.

105. Elchalal U, Yagel S, Gomori JM, Porat S, Beni-Adani L, Yanai N, et al. Fetal intracranial hemorrhage (fetal stroke): does grade matter? Ultrasound Obstet Gynecol. 2005;26(3): 233-43.

106. Huang YF, Chen WC, Tseng JJ, Ho ESC, Chou MM. Fetal intracranial hemorrhage (fetal stroke): report of four antenatally diagnosed cases and review of the literature. Taiwan J Obstet Gynecol. 2006;45(2):135-41.

107. Putbrese B, Kennedy A. Findings and differential diagnosis of fetal intracranial haemorrhage and fetal ischaemic brain injury: what is the role of fetal MRI? Br J Radiol. 2017;90(1070):20160253.

108. Kutuk MS, Yikilmaz A, Ozgun MT, Dolanbay M, Canpolat M, Uludag S, et al. Prenatal diagnosis and postnatal outcome of fetal

intracranial hemorrhage. Childs Nerv Syst. 2014;30(3):411-8.

109. Sims ME, Turkel SB, Halterman G, Paul RH. Brain injury and intrauterine death. Am J Obstet Gynecol. 1985;151(6):721-3.

110. Lichtenbelt KD, Pistorius LR, De Tollenaer SM, Mancini GM, De Vries LS. Prenatal genetic confirmation of a COL4A1 mutation presenting with sonographic fetal intracranial hemorrhage. Ultrasound Obstet Gynecol. 2012;39(6):726-7.

111. Garel C, Rosenblatt J, Moutard ML, Heron D, Gelot A, Gonzales M, et al. Fetal intracerebral hemorrhage and COL4A1 mutation: promise and uncertainty. Ultrasound Obstet Gynecol. 2013;41(2):228-30.

112. Vermeulen RJ, Peeters-Scholte C, Van Vugt JJM, Barkhof F, Rizzu P, van der Schoor SRD, et al. Fetal origin of brain damage in 2 infants with a COL4A1 mutation: fetal and neonatal MRI. Neuropediatrics. 2011;42(1):1-3.

113. de Vries LS, Pistorius L, Lichtenbelt KD, Koopman C, Meuwissen MEC, Mancini GMS. COL4A1 Mutation: expansion of the phenotype. Pediatr Res. 2011;70:181.

114. Meuwissen MEC, Halley DJJ, Smit LS, Lequin MH, Cobben JM, de Coo R, et al. The expanding phenotype of COL4A1 and COL4A2 mutations: clinical data on 13 newly identified families and a review of the literature. Genet Med. 2015;17(11):843-53.

115. de Vries LS, Koopman C, Groenendaal F, Van Schooneveld M, Verheijen FW, Verbeek E, et al. COL4A1 mutation in two preterm siblings with antenatal onset of parenchymal hemorrhage. Ann Neurol. 2009;65(1):12-8.

116. Colin E, Sentilhes L, Sarfati A, Mine M, Guichet A, Ploton C, et al. Fetal intracerebral hemorrhage and cataract: think COL4A1. J Perinatol. 2014;34(1):75-7.

117. Papile LA, Burstein J, Burstein R, Koffler H. Incidence and evolution of subependymal and intraventricular hemorrhage: a study of infants with birth weights less than 1,500 gm. J Pediatr. 1978;92(4):529-34.

118. Vergani P, Strobelt N, Locatelli A, Paterlini G, Tagliabue P, Parravicini E, et al. Clinical significance of fetal intracranial hemorrhage. Am J Obstet Gynecol. 1996;175(3 Pt 1):536-43.

119. Pooh RK. The study of early pregnancy with genetic and high-resolution ultrasound. J Perinat Med; 2013.

120. Pooh RK. Sonogenetics in fetal neurology. Semin Fetal Neonatal Med. 2012;17(6):353-9.

Assessment of Fetal Neurobehavior in Special Cases

Panagiotis Antsaklis, Maria Papamichail, Marianna Theodora, George Daskalakis, Asim Kurjak

■ INTRODUCTION

In utero life and particularly fetal brain development and fetal behavior and more specifically assessment and imaging of fetal nervous system is a field of great interest in perinatal medicine with many unanswered questions.[1-4] Human brain development is a very complex, but also extremely structured process commencing the first week after conception and continuing for a very long time, even throughout adult life. Establishing the anatomical integrity of the central nervous system (CNS) is of outmost importance in fetal medicine in order to verify the wellbeing of the fetus, but it is not always enough.[5-9] Motoric disabilities, mental impairment, and behavioral problems can occur even with an anatomical intact CNS, without the presence of any anatomical anomalies.[10-12] So, whenever any of these functional problems occurs, it is always a challenge to identify—if possible—when and how this problem could have happened, especially in cases when suspected to be responsible are antenatal, intrapartum, or postnatal incidents.[13-16] If a specific incident is not identified, environmental factors should also be considered, as it happens for example in cases of prematurity, when the conditions of in-utero life are imitated in order to protect the premature neonate, mainly regarding feeding and nurturing, but still the risk of morbidity and complication

remains high, especially regarding the brain development and nervous function.[17-22] The degree that the fetus may be affected and the degree of neurological compromises in such cases, most of the times it cannot be estimated with the clinical pictures varying significantly, ranging from mild behavioral and learning disabilities to the most severe form of neurological impairment which is cerebral palsy (CP). But even when an anatomical abnormality or variation is detected antenatally, as it happens in the case of fetal ventriculomegaly, for example, we cannot be certain of the degree of fetal compromise, in order to be able to offer a complete counseling to the parents regarding the prognosis. In neonates, children, or adults, certain clinical examinations can show the severity of the neurological damage that may have been caused by an injury, a tumor, or an infection.[23-26] Until recently there were no structured methods of assessing the neurological integrity of the fetus during in-utero life and, therefore, we could not be certain or even distinguish normal from abnormal fetal neurological behavior. As mentioned above, the development and maturation of the fetal nervous system is an extremely structured process and this neuronal development is reflected by certain neurobehavioral patterns of the fetus that correspond to each trimester, or even week of pregnancy.[27-29] The study of this developmental process and mainly being able to recognize the normal fetal neurobehavior that should be expected for each period of pregnancy can help us to understand firstly the normal state for in-utero life. By understanding the normal fetal neurobehavior we could then identify abnormal patterns and if possible link them to different anatomical and chromosomal abnormalities or even various insults that may affect fetal CNS and neurobehavioral integrity.[30-32] Ultrasound technology offered the unique possibility to examine the fetus in utero and detect various anatomical and chromosomal abnormalities. Further evolution of ultrasound technology and particularly three-dimensional (3D) ultrasound allowed us to view the fetus in explicit detail, being able to view fetal parts and characteristics in a similar way that a neonate is looked at, and even further technological advance, four-dimensional (4D) ultrasound, offered the possibility to view all these explicit details in real time. Characteristics such as hand and feet movements, facial alterations, and eye blinking can be assessed prenatally with 4D ultrasound technology, as one would observe and examine a newborn. The first test that succeeded to combine all the parameters and form a scoring system that would assess the fetus in a comprehensive and systematic approach, in the same way that neonatologists perform a neurological assessment in newborns, in order to determine their neurological status during the first days of their life, is the Kurjak's antenatal neurodevelopmental test (KANET) **(Figs. 1 to 4)**. KANET has already been shown to be useful in standardization of neurobehavioral assessment with the potential for antenatal detection of fetuses with severe neurobehavioral impairment. KANET has also succeeded to verify the good neurological outcomes of fetuses that had normal KANET scores, showing a great positive predictive value and offering reassurance for the neurological outcome of these pregnancies.[29-34] The first results prove that the prenatal neurological findings as estimated by KANET test are in concordance with their postnatal outcome **(Fig. 5)**. As already mentioned fetal neurobehavior can be affected by many parameters and can be altered by environmental, racial, and maternal factors, by maternal disease, administration of drugs and neurotropic agents and many other factors.

ETHNICITY AND FETAL BEHAVIOR

Hanaoka et al. studied whether fetuses of different ethnical backgrounds behave differently in utero and alter the assessment of fetal neurobehavior as anthropometric characteristics in the different populations can give different picture, and especially for the Asian population what has been noted is a shorter palpebral fissure, a wider soft nose within wide facial contours, a smaller mouth width, and a lower face smaller than the forehead height, parameters that can differentiate the result.[35-37] The authors applied KANET to Asian (Japanese) and Caucasian (Croatian) population and noted the differences in their scores, and also to the particular parameters that can be different. They calculated the KANET scores for both groups and what they noticed was that although the total KANET scores of both groups were within normal ranges, there was a difference in some parameters that finally altered the score, but not to a statistical significant degree. The parameters of KANET that were noted to have some differences were mainly the following: isolated eye blinking and facial alteration, or mouth opening. As mentioned by the authors, part

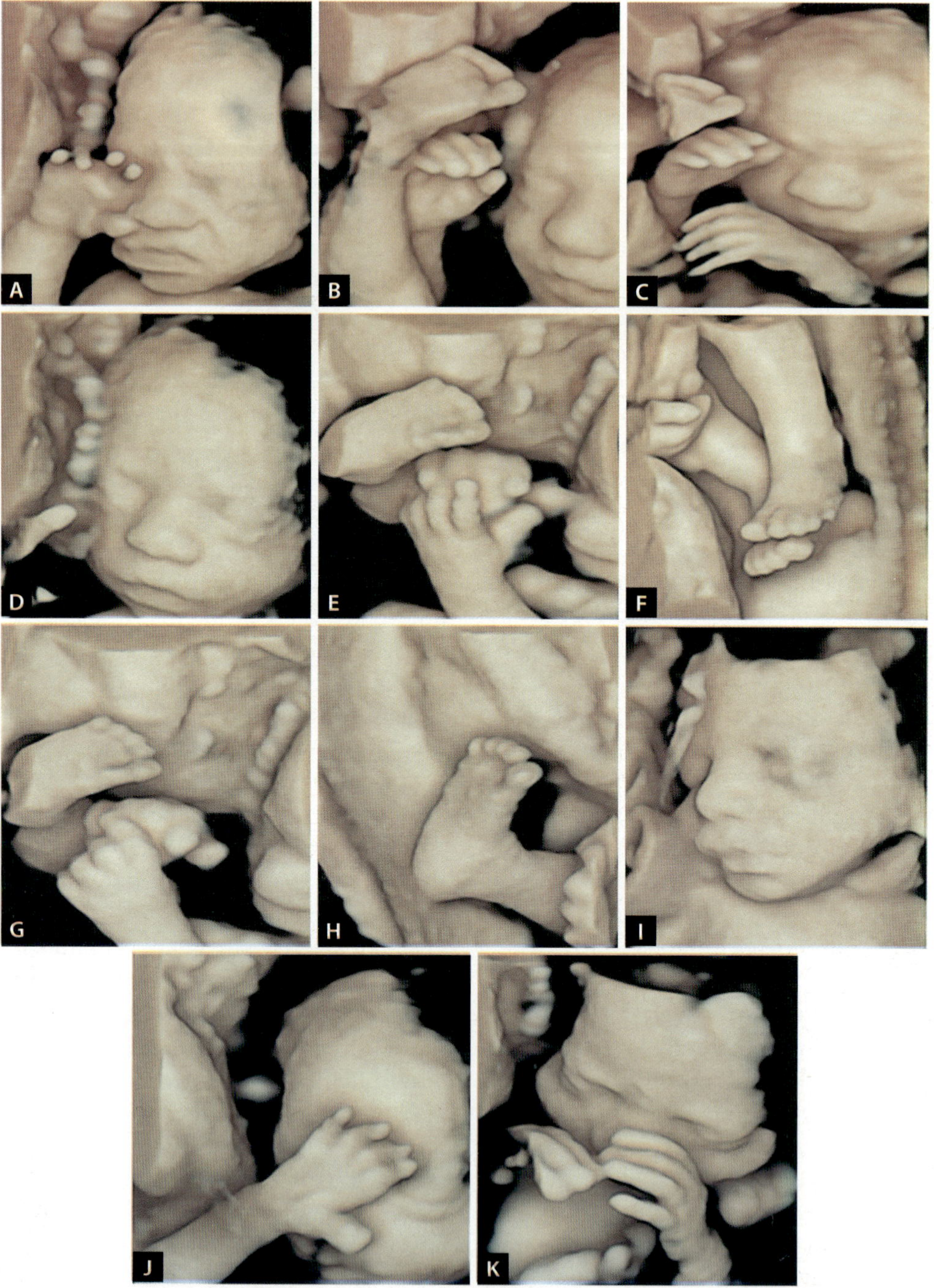

Figs. 1A to K: A complete the Kurjak's antenatal neurodevelopmental test (KANET) with normal score of a fetus at 34 weeks. Most parameters such as leg, hand, and finger movements are seen, and also facial alterations.

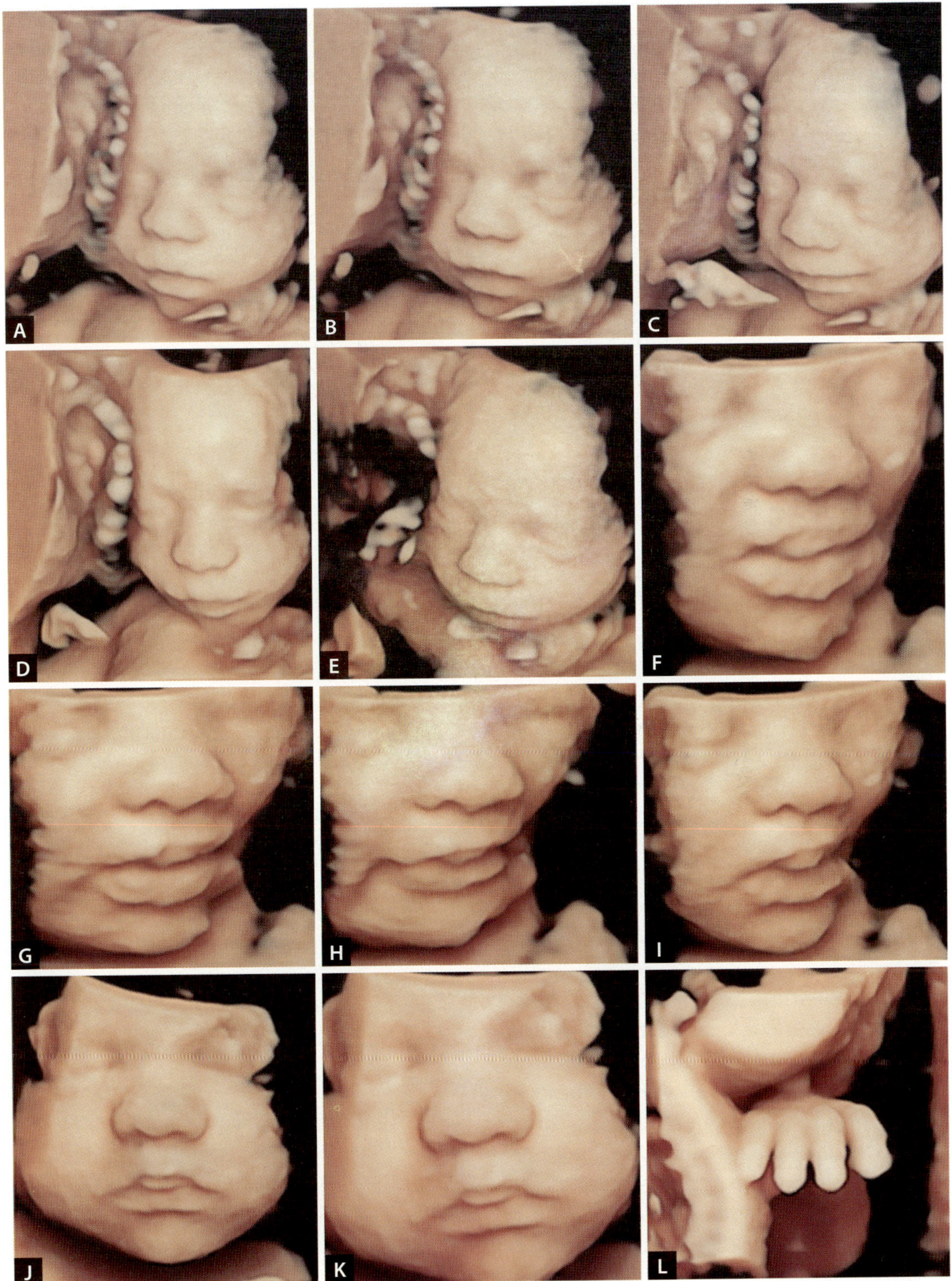

Figs. 2A to L

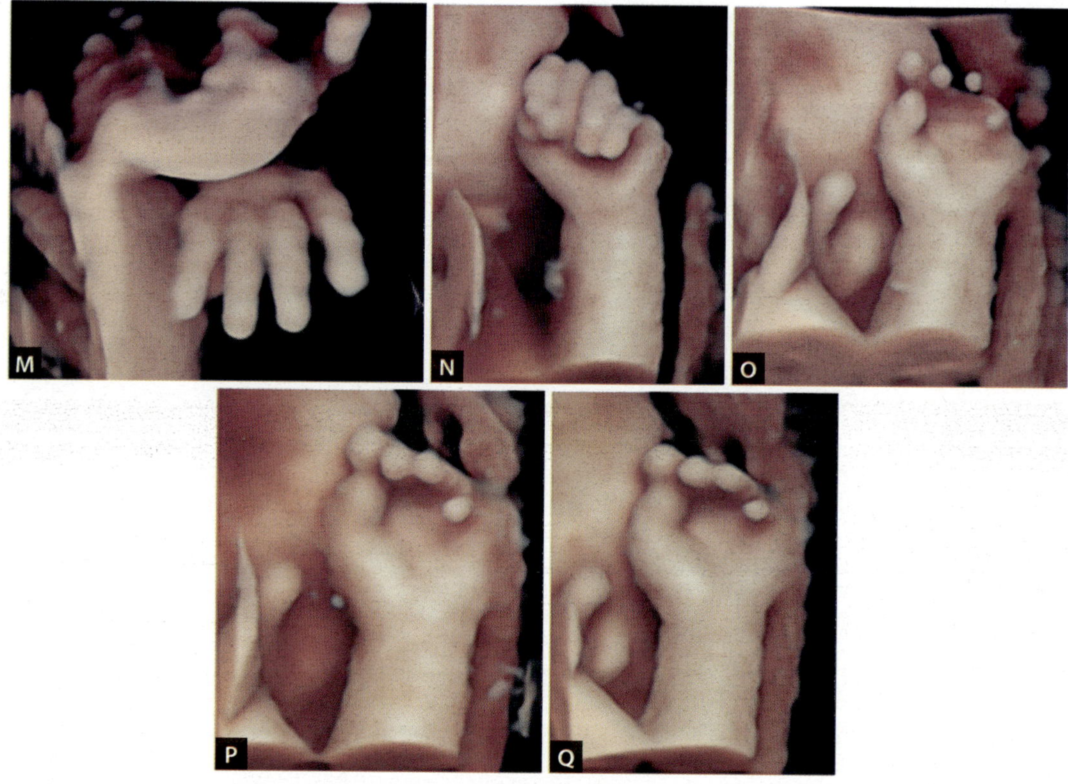

Figs. 2M to Q

Figs. 2A to Q: Facial alterations, finger movements as part of normal the Kurjak's antenatal neurodevelopmental test (KANET) at 36 weeks. Special attention is paid to finger movements as detailed movements are a landmark of adequate neurological integrity of the fetus.

of these differences could be attributed to different anthropometric characteristics which were also mentioned above such as shorter, wider, and shallower noses for the Japanese population and also greater intercanthal width in relation to a shorter palpebral fissure, a smaller mouth width, a lower face, smaller than the forehead height, and a wider, shallower soft nose within wide facial contours. The characteristics of the Caucasian face are high-bridged, long nose, deep-set eyes, and a sharply sculpted face. The authors conclude that even when considering these anthropometric differences ethnicity is a parameter that should be considered when evaluating fetal behavior.

Regarding the remaining parameters of KANET, isolated head anteflexion and isolated leg movement were noted to also differ between the two populations, but not to a statistically significant degree. So, there may be some expected ethnic differences in fetal behavior and they should be kept in mind when assessing fetal neurobehavior, but overall these differences do not affect the final total KANET score (normal, abnormal, and borderline) and the assessment of the fetus, but especially in borderline cases this should be taken into consideration and close follow-up should be continued in these cases.

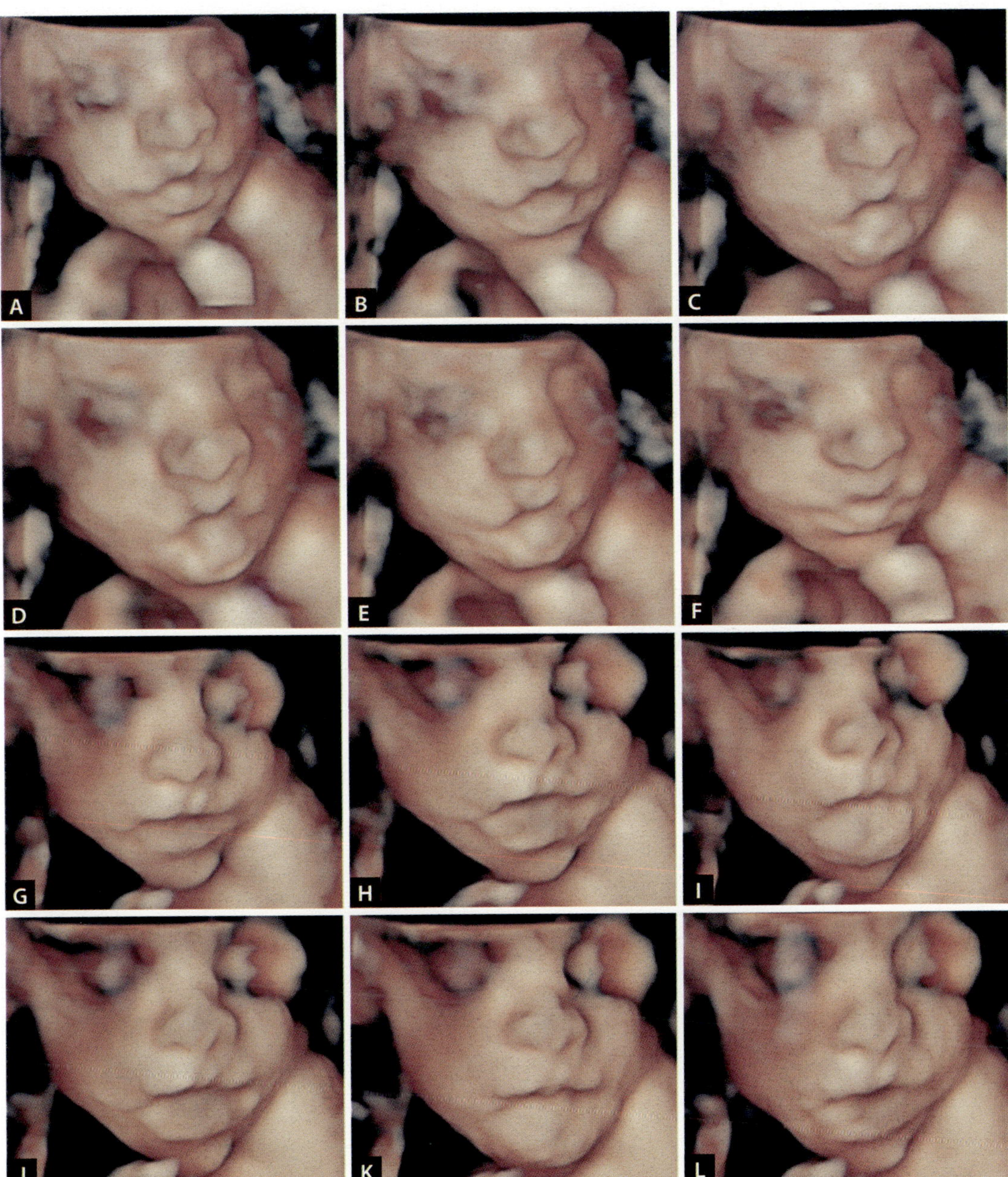

Figs. 3A to L: Fetal facial alterations, grimacing, tongue expulsion, and smiling are important elements that verify neurological integrity of the fetus and important parameters of the Kurjak's antenatal neurodevelopmental test (KANET).

■ FETAL SEX AND FETAL BEHAVIOR

When assessing specific characteristics of newborns, differences have been noted between newborns of different sex and this has been attributed to the different maturational process of the neurobehavior between

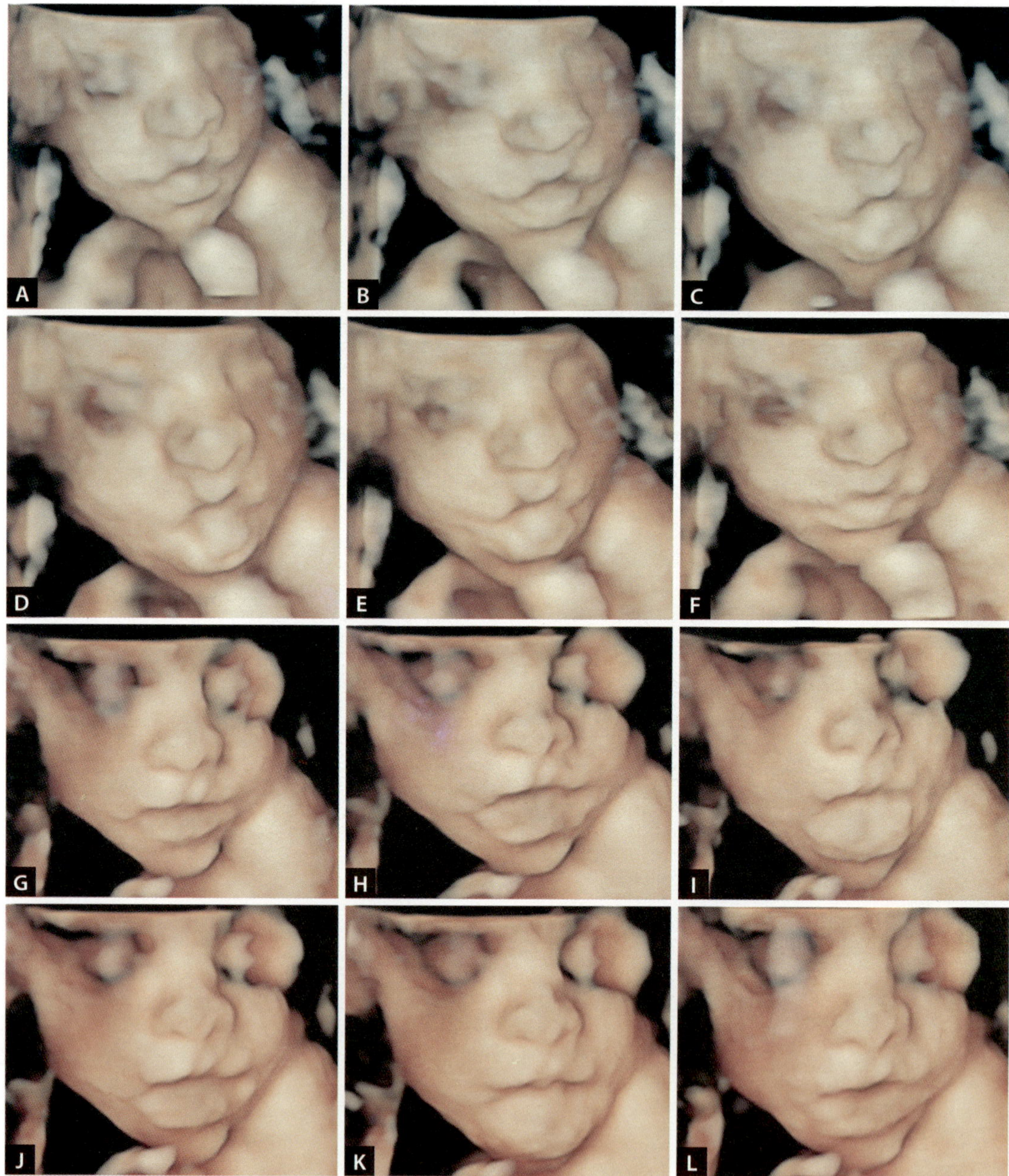

Figs. 4A to L: Fetal mouthing and tongue expulsion as part of the Kurjak's antenatal neurodevelopmental test (KANET) in a fetus at 33 weeks.

the two sexes. Differences in newborns have been noted in startle movements (male newborns are thought to have more frequent movements), in reflex smiles and bursts of rhythmic mouthing (female newborns present them earlier and more frequently), prone head reaction, and grip strength.[38-40] There have been some studies

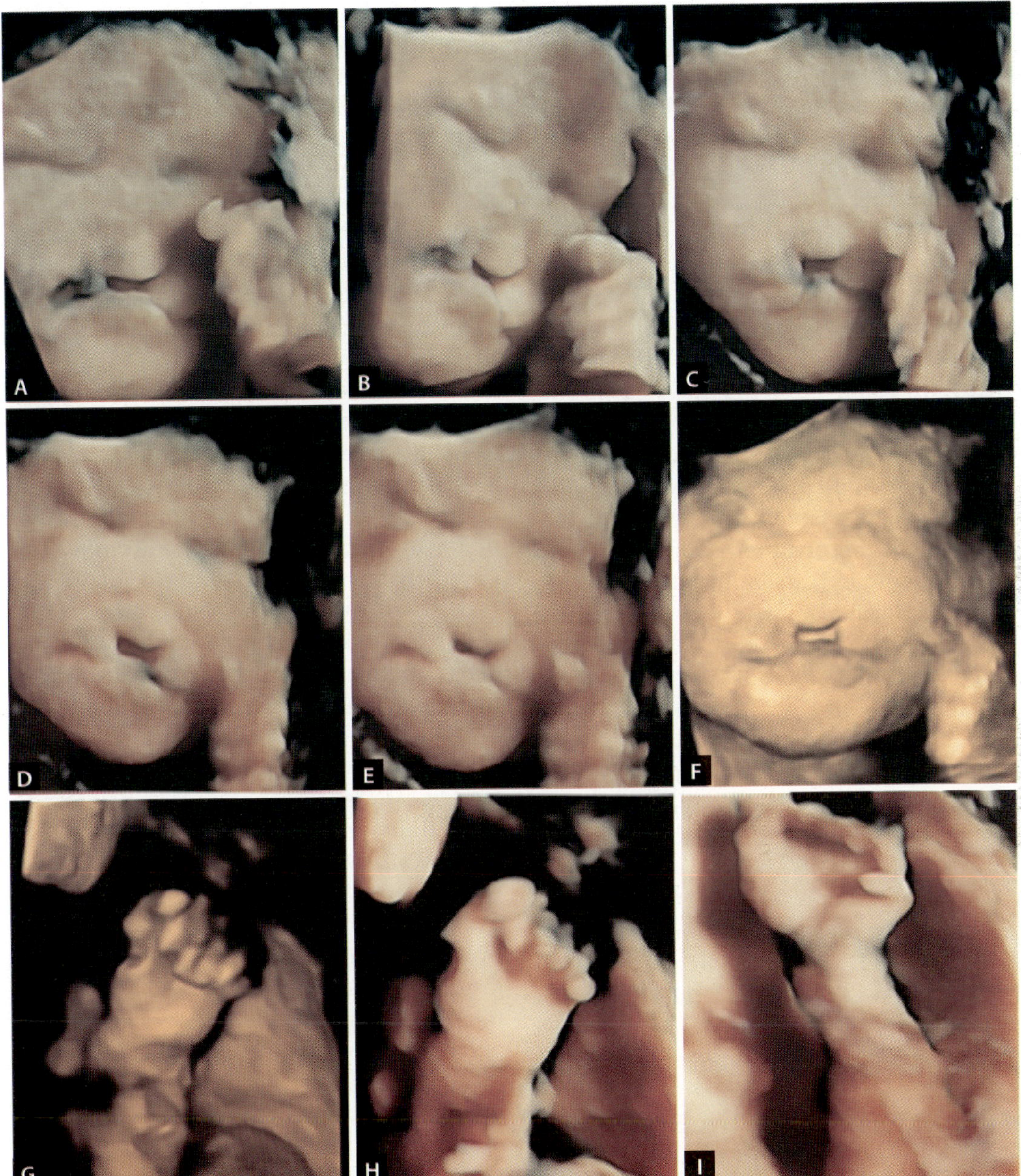

Figs. 5A to I: Fetus with trisomy 13 and abnormal Kurjak's antenatal neurodevelopmental test (KANET). The neonate was delivered and died on day 52 postdelivery.

on sex difference in fetal behavior assessed by two-dimensional (2D) sonography[41-43] or fetal actocardiography using a single wide array Doppler transducer.[44,45] Studies have shown that there may be differences in fetal behavior according to fetal sex and especially mouthing movements (they are increased in female fetuses), while female fetuses appear to require significantly fewer stimuli than males in order to habituate, suggesting that habituation in the human fetus is affected by fetal sex, and these differences have to do with "central type" developmental differences in the nervous system of the fetuses.[46] Taste stimuli of the mother also seem to affect fetuses of different sex in a different way. When pregnant women ingested dark chocolate there was an increase in fetal response and fetal movements, which was more apparent in female fetuses.[47] Hata et al. by using 4D ultrasound and applying KANET for the evaluation of neurobehavior in both male and female fetuses showed that there was no significant difference in the total KANET score between male and female fetuses, and when they further analyzed each parameter of KANET they found no significant difference in none of the eight parameters, concluding that fetal neurobehavioral and developmental process of fetal nervous system have no apparent difference between male and female fetuses.[38] There are studies particularly on neonates[39,40,44] that have shown differences in some parameters of neurobehavior (e.g., general movement, smiling, and mouthing) between males and females, and most of these parameters are parts of the KANET test, but as far as fetuses are concerned these studies used 2D ultrasound to assess fetuses and what is more that could not be confirmed by the only study that assessed fetuses with 4D ultrasound and the complete KANET.

■ DIABETES AND FETAL BEHAVIOR

It has been well established that different maternal or environmental factors can affect the fetal development and fetal neuro-behavior. Especially, for gestational diabetes is a well-known risk factor for both maternal and fetal complications, so that it could affect the fetus either directly or indirectly, by affecting the condition of the mother.[48-50]

Gestational diabetes is a condition that is increasing through the years and is a known risk factor for maternal and fetal complications and affects fetal behavior.[51] In hyperglycemic environment, there is a decrease in the number of fetal movements, and the effect of diabetes on fetal activity could be attributed to immaturity of the development of the sensory-motor response system that characterizes fetuses of diabetic pregnancies, rather than solely a direct effect of glucose levels on the fetus.[52,53] Studies have also shown that fetal breathing and body movements of diabetic pregnancies are decreased and are altered due to poor behavioral organization, even when glycemic control is adequate and often fetuses of diabetic women had higher numbers of fetal breathing movement and fetal heart rate rhythms, but the fetal movements were lower. Studies show that in diabetic pregnancies hypoglycemia rather than hyperglycemia increases fetal activity and that in these pregnancies hyperglycemia is related to a decrease in the frequency of fetal movements.[53-56] However, in most of these studies a structured and homogeneous method of assessing fetal activity was lacking. Antsaklis et al. attempted to assess the fetal behavior of fetuses in conditions of diabetes by applying KANET to fetuses of diabetic mothers.[48] What they showed was that there are identifiable differences in the fetal behavior between diabetic and nondiabetic fetuses with the nondiabetic group having overall higher KANET scores. They also identified which specific parameters—movements differ between the two groups with the biggest difference between the two groups being for isolated eye blinking, facial alterations, and finger movements, while there was also a small difference for isolated hand movements, but this was not statistically significant, concluding that glycemic control affects fetal neurobehavior and possibly early identification of undiagnosed diabetes in pregnancy and good glycemic control may be crucial for fetal neurodevelopment **(Figs. 6A to R)**.

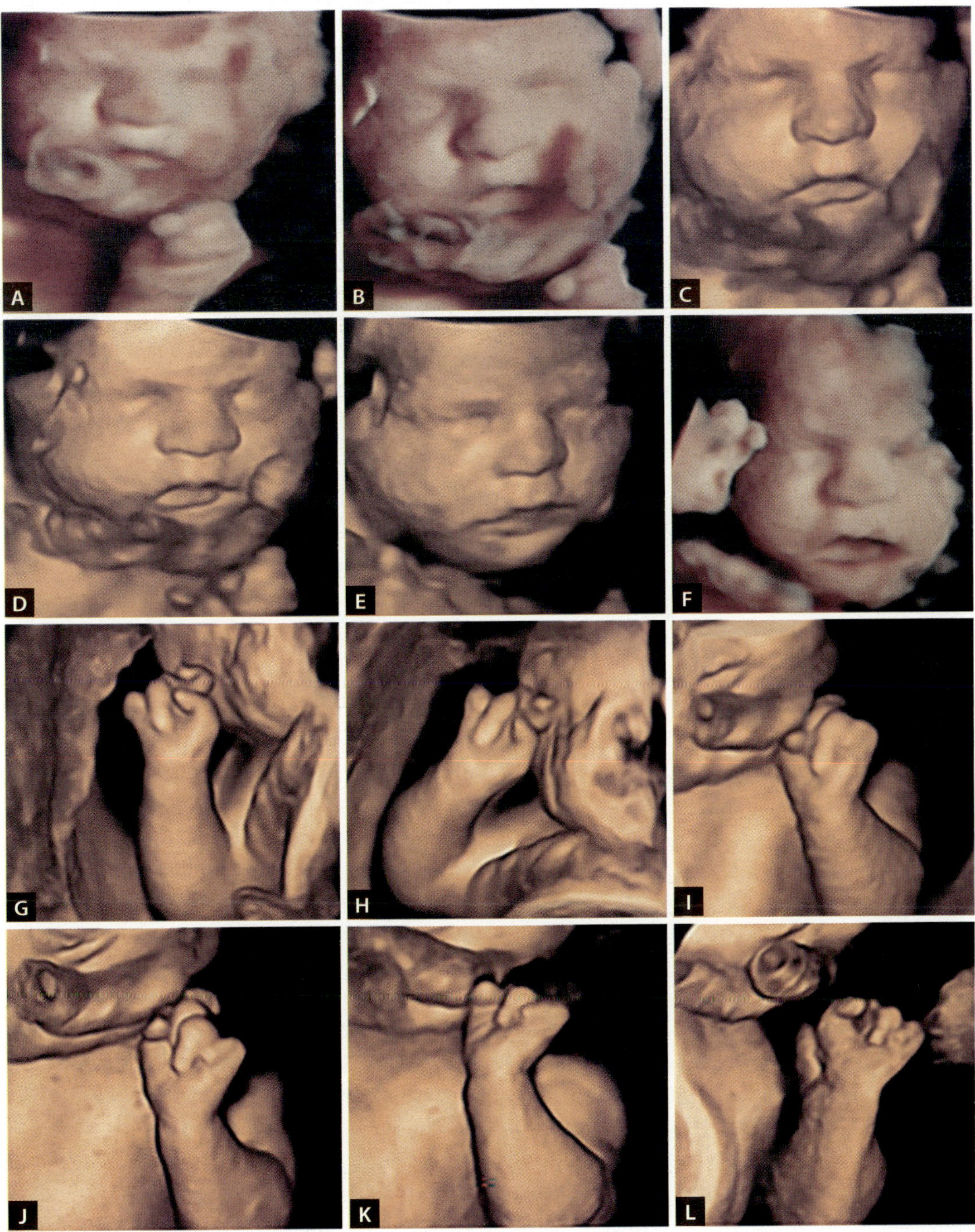

Figs. 6A to L

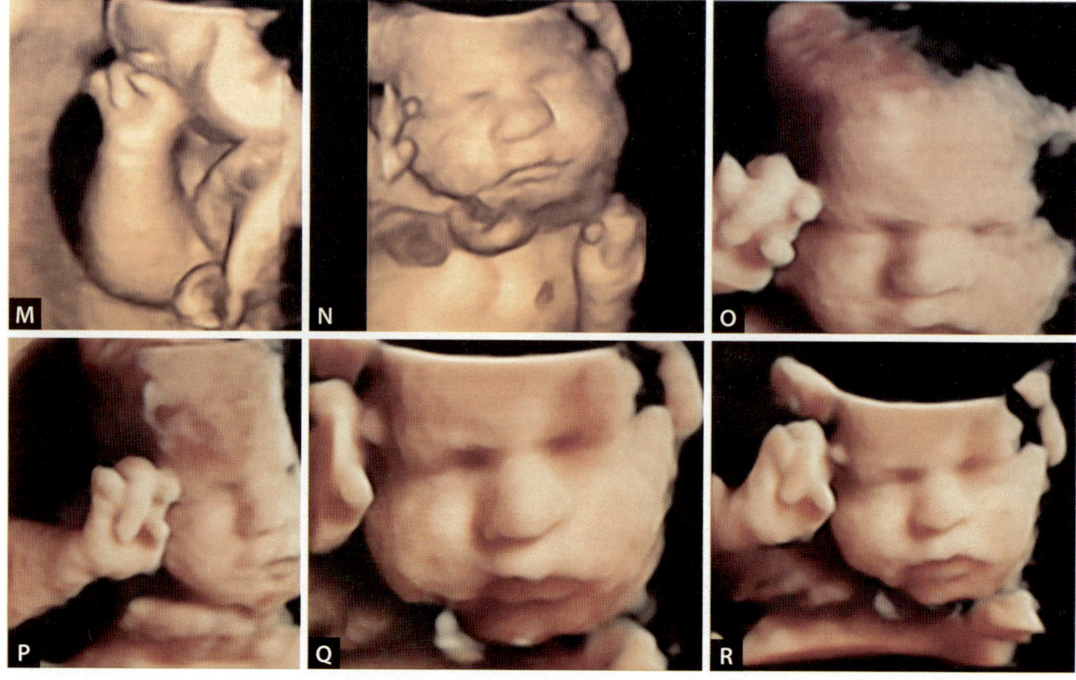

Figs. 6M to R

Figs. 6A to R: Abnormal Kurjak's antenatal neurodevelopmental test (KANET) at 36 weeks in a fetus with metabolic syndrome. The neonate died 1 week after delivery.

HYPOTHYROIDISM AND FETAL BEHAVIOR

Maternal thyroid function is directly related to the development and function of fetal and neonatal neurological system. Thyroid hormones play an important role in the myelination and differentiation of neuronal cells of the fetus and as a result good control of maternal thyroid function, especially during the first week of pregnancy when the fetus is dependent entirely on the maternal thyroid, is important for the formation and development of fetal nervous system and neurobehavior.[57-61] Several studies have shown the significant effect that maternal hypothyroidism, whether overt or subclinical, has on the neurodevelopment and cognitive functions of neonates.[62] Neurophysiological tests on neonates of pregnant women with overt hypothyroidism proved that these neonates are negatively affected and that they have a higher incidence of verbal and nonverbal cognitive delays, but also that motor and intellectual functions are also adversely affected. What is more maternal, hypothyroidism may indirectly affect fetal brain development through pregnancy-related complications as preterm birth, intrauterine growth restriction (IUGR), and CP with their possible detrimental effects on future neurological development of the offspring.[63-65] Amira Dieb et al. showed that fetuses of hypothyroid mothers had lower KANET scores, compared to fetuses of mothers with normal thyroid function.[57] They reported abnormal fetal neurological behavior in cases of overt maternal hypo-thyroidism, proving the importance of well-controlled thyroid function of pregnant women.

PSYCHOTROPIC DRUGS AND FETAL BEHAVIOR

The effect of psychotropic drugs on fetal behavior during pregnancy has been a great challenge in fetal neurology. Prenatal administration of selective serotonin reuptake inhibitors (SSRIs) and antidepressants has been related to neonatal psychiatric, anxiety, and withdrawal symptoms up to 3 years of life and even with cases of autism.[66] It has been reported that fetuses of pregnant women with depression showed differences in their behavior during second and third trimester of pregnancy, as it happened for fetuses of pregnant women who were under treatment with anticonvulsants, with the effects of these drugs being evident even up to school age for these children.[67-72] Even regarding the activity of the fetuses of mothers who had depression there were some differences noted, even for different trimesters. However, all these studies used 2D ultrasonography to evaluate fetal behavior, a technique that limits the assessment of fetal neurobehavior, without structured methods of assessment for the duration of the examination and the parameters that were assessed. Hata et al. used 4D ultrasonography and KANET to assess the fetuses of pregnant women who were under treatment with psychotropic drugs for different conditions [schizophrenia, depression, anxiety, epilepsy, panic disorders, obsessive-compulsive disorder (OCD), personality disorder], and found no significant difference in the total KANET score. There were also no significant differences in any of the eight parameters between the groups, suggesting that psychotropic drugs may not affect fetal behavioral development

in utero. However, their study population was limited (10 cases) and their study group was not homogeneous as it consisted of women with different conditions and under different treatment methods-medications, and these factors were suggested by the authors as a limitation for safe conclusions.

FETAL RESPONSE TO VIBROACOUSTIC STIMULATION

Vibroacoustic stimulation (VAS) has been routinely used in everyday obstetrical clinical practice to stimulate fetuses in order to cause fetal heart rate acceleration during a nonstress test (NST) or biophysical profile, and to detect fetal response and therefore to evaluate fetal wellbeing, fetal hearing impairment, and neurobehavioral development.[73-76] Fetal responses to different stimuli throughout pregnancy and especially during the third trimester have been proposed as a method to assess functional neurodevelopment of the fetus and indirectly to assess the fetal condition and particularly brain maturation and CNS integrity.[76-79] Ogo et al. showed that for fetuses of gestational age <36 weeks VAS did not appear to have a diagnostic value as significant response was not noted in these fetuses, whereas in fetuses after 36 weeks of gestation the response appeared to be notable, and with application of KANET they identified specific changes after VAS, which was significant increase in the frequencies of eye blinking and also in startle movements, and what the authors mentioned was that these changes possibly reflect the functional maturation of the auditory system of the fetus, which does not reach an adequate level before 37 weeks. The decreased maturation of the fetal auditory system appeared to be responsible to the decreased response after VAS to fetuses of gestational age 24–27 weeks, whose auditory system has not yet developed, whereas for later gestational age, that is after 28 weeks, but before 36 weeks (at 28–31 and 32–35 weeks) also had decreased response to VAS as the fetal auditory system has not been completely formed. What is more the authors managed to identify which specific fetal parameters increase in fetuses after 36 weeks after VAS, which was eye blinking and startle movements. This finding was explained by the fact that eye blinking is related to central dopamine system matura-tion, which occurs at about 36 weeks of gestation, while eye blinking and startle movement after 36 weeks of gestation might represent an advanced stage of fetal brain and CNS maturation and response to external stimulation, so that the other parameters of fetal behavior are not altered.

ANTENATAL CORTICOSTEROID ADMINISTRATION AND FETAL BEHAVIOR

Antenatal administration of corticosteroids has been related to a reduction of fetal activity, mainly of body and respiratory movements.[80] It is also well documented that these changes in fetal behavior are not permanent and that they last on average about 1–2 days with a maximum duration reaching up to 4 days.[81] Changes have also been documented regarding the Doppler studies of the fetus, mainly ductus venosus and umbilical Doppler but without affecting the overall uteroplacental circulation.[82] Also, a decrease of the biophysical profile score has been documented after administration of corticosteroids antenatally.[83,84] Beta-methasone has been found to be a stronger risk factor for reduction of fetal movements compared to dexamethasone, although this effect appears to be transient in both cases.[82-85] What is more the effect of corticosteroids on fetal behavior and neurological development

has been proved by studies about direct administration of corticosteroids intrauterine, which caused to the fetus vasoconstriction and hypoxemia, located especially in the area of thalamus, diencephalon and pons. However, the effect of corticosteroid administration as already mentioned is transient and does not appear to alter the overall perinatal outcome, so that decisions regarding management of pregnancy and delivery should be carefully taken when corticosteroids are administered in a pregnancy and their effect may be obvious in the cardiotocograph or the biophysical profile of the fetus to which corticosteroids were administered. Antsaklis et al. studied the effect of corticosteroids on fetal neurobehavior by applying KANET to 65 singleton pregnancies after 28 weeks, who were administered corticosteroids. Compared to the control group, there was an overall decrease of two at the KANET scores when performed 24–48 hours after corticosteroids administration. These reductions of KANET were not reported in the follow-up examination 2 weeks later for the same fetuses. When comparing betamethasone to dexamethasone, dexamethasone appeared to have a smaller effect on KANET score, but this difference was not statistical significant. It is really important, therefore, when applying KANET to have a good knowledge of the maternal history and drug administration that could potentially affect fetal behavior in order to avoid misinterpretations.

CONCLUSION

Verifying the integrity of the fetal nervous system is a very difficult and at the same time very complex procedure. Assessment of fetal anatomy has reached a very high level via 2D, but especially through 3D ultrasound, as has assessment of chromosomal abnormalities of the fetus with molecular genetics, which could affect the nervous motoric, behavioral, and mental status of the fetus. Assessment of fetal neurobehavior has up to a level been standardized with 4D ultrasound and with KANET, a method that by applying 4D ultrasound to the fetus assesses its neurobehavior in real time in a similar way that neonatologists assess the newborn in real life. Many multicentric studies have examined and confirmed the validity of KANET on different populations, both low and high risk. However, on this new field of fetal medicine, fetal neurology and fetal neurobehavior there are still a lot to be discovered and to be learned. Fetal behavior is a very complex situation, susceptible to many genetic, epigenetic, environmental, and anatomical parameters. Common maternal conditions such as maternal diabetes and thyroid disease, administration of medications that are used frequently in pregnancy such as antenatal corticosteroids and psychotropic drugs, or even ethnic and fetal sex differences can alter the way a fetus is behaving. All these parameters should be taken into consideration when fetal neurobehavior is assessed, as we should take into consideration the full maternal medical history. Assessment of fetal neurobehavior opens a new era in fetal medicine, as many of the so-thought routine techniques that we apply in obstetrics could be proved that could be further improved by assessing the fetal neurobehavior at the same time.

■ REFERENCES

1. Yigiter AB, Kavak ZN. Normal standards of fetal behavior assessed by four-dimensional sonography. J Matern Fetal Neonatal Med. 2006;19(11):707-21.

2. Rees S, Harding R. Brain development during fetal life: influences of the intra-uterine environment. Neurosci Lett. 2004; 361(1-3):111-4.

3. Joseph RG. Fetal brain and cognitive development. Dev Rev. 1999;20(1):81-98.

4. Antsaklis P, Antsaklis A, Kurjak A, Chervenak F. The assessment of fetal neurobehavior with four-dimensional ultrasound: The Kurjak Antenatal Neurodevelopmental Test. Donald School J Ultrasound in Obstet Gynecol. 2012;6(4):362-75.

5. Eidelman AI. The living fetus–dilemmas in treatment at the edge of viability. In: Blazer S, Zimmer EZ (Eds). The Embryo: Scientific Discovery and Medical Ethics. Basel: Karger; 2005. pp. 351-70.

6. Stanojevic M, Zaputovic S, Bosnjak AP. Continuity between fetal and neonatal neurobehavior. Semin Fetal Neonatal Med. 2012;17(6):324-9.

7. Kurjak A, Carrera JM, Stanojevic M, Andonotopo W, Azumendi G, Scazzocchio E, et al. The role of 4D sonography in the neurological assessment of early human development. Ultrasound Rev Obstet Gynecol. 2004;4(3):148-59.

8. Strijbis EMM, Oudman I, van Essen P, MacLennan AH. Cerebral palsy and the application of the international criteria for acute intrapartum hypoxia. Obstet Gynecol. 2006;107(6):1357-65.

9. de Vries JIP, Fong BF. Changes in fetal motility as a result of congenital disorders: An overview. Ultrasound Obstet Gynecol. 2007;29(5):590-9.

10. de Vries JIP, Fong BF. Normal fetal motility: An overview. Ultrasound Obstet Gynecol. 2006;27(6):701-11.

11. Kurjak A, Abo-Yaqoub S, Stanojevic M, Yigiter AB, Vasilj O, Lebit D, et al. The potential of 4D sonography in the assessment of fetal neurobehavior—multicentric study in high-risk pregnancies. J Perinat Med. 2010;38(1):77-82.

12. DiPietro JA, Bronstein MH, Costigan KA, Pressmen EK, Hahn CS, Painter K, et al. What does fetal movement predict about behavior during the first two years of life? Dev Psychobiol. 2002;40(4):358-71.

13. Rosier-van Dunné FM, van Wezel-Meijler G, Bakker MP, de Groot L, Odendaal HJ, de Vries

JI. General movements in the perinatal period and its relation to echogenicity changes in the brain. Early Hum Dev. 2010;86(2):83-6.

14. Hata T, Kanenishi K, Akiyama M, Tanaka H, Kimura K. Real-time 3-D sonographic observation of fetal facial expression. J Obstet Gynaecol Res. 2005;31(4):337-40.

15. Kozuma S, Baba K, Okai T, Taketani Y. Dynamic observation of the fetal face by three-dimensional ultrasound. Ultrasound Obstet Gynecol. 1999;13(4):283-4.

16. Kurjak A, Azumendi G, Andonotopo W, Salihagic-Kadic A. Three- and four-dimensional ultrasonography for the structural and functional evaluation of the fetal face. Am J Obstet Gynecol. 2007;196(1):16-28.

17. Kurjak A, Tikvica A, Stanojevic M, Miskovic B, Ahmed B, Azumendi G, et al. The assessment of fetal neurobehavior by three-dimensional and four-dimensional ultrasound. J Matern Fetal Neonatal Med. 2008;21(10):675-84.

18. Kurjak A, Pooh RK, Tikvica A, Stanojevic M, Miskovic B, Ahmed B, et al. Assessment of neurobehavior by 3D/4D ultrasound. In: Pooh RK, Kurjak A (Eds). Fetal Neurology, 1st edition. 2009. pp. 222-85.

19. Kurjak A, Stanojevic M, Andonotopo W, Salihagic-Kadic A, Carrera JM, Azumendi G. Behavioral pattern continuity from prenatal to postnatal life—a study by four-dimensional (4D) ultrasonography. J Perinat Med. 2004;32(4):346-53.

20. Andonotopo W, Kurjak A, Kosuta MI. Behavior of an anencephalic fetus studied by 4D sonography. J Matern Fetal Neonatal Med. 2005;17(2):165-8.

21. Nijhuis JG, Prechtl HF, Martin CB Jr, Bots RS. Are there behavioral states in the human fetus? Early Hum Dev. 1982;6(2):177-95.

22. Lebit FD, Vladareanu R. The Role of 4D ultrasound in the assessment of fetal behavior. Maedica (Bucur). 2011;6(2):120-7.

23. Salihagic-Kadic A, Kurjak A, Medic M, Andonotopo W, Azumendi G. New data about embryonic and fetal neurodevelopment and behavior obtained by 3D and 4D sonography. J Perinat Med. 2005;33(6):478-90.

24. Kurjak A, Azumendi G, Vecek N, Kupesic S, Solak M, Varga D, et al. Fetal hand movements and facial expression in normal pregnancy studied by four-dimensional sonography. J Perinat Med. 2003;31(6):496-508.

25. Andonotopo W, Stanojevic M, Kurjak A, Azumendi G, Carrera JM. Assessment of fetal behavior and general movements by four-dimensional sonography. Ultrasound Rev Obstet Gynecol. 2004;4:103-14.

26. Kurjak A, Stanojevic M, Azumendi G, Carrera JM. The potential of four-dimensional (4D) ultrasonography in the assessment of fetal awareness. J Perinat Med. 2005;33(1):46-53.

27. Kurjak A, Pooh RK, Merce LT, Carrera JM, Salihagic-Kadic A, Andonotopo W. Structural and functional early human development assessed by three-dimensional (3D) and four-dimensional (4D) sonography. Fertil Steril. 2005;84(5):1285-99.

28. Kurjak A, Miskovic B, Andonotopo W, Stanojevic M, Azumendi G, Vrcic H. How useful is 3D and 4D ultrasound in perinatal medicine? J Perinat Med. 2007;35(1):10-27.

29. Andonotopo W, Medic M, Salihagic-Kadic A, Milenkovic D, Maiz N, Scazzocchio E. The assessment of fetal behavior in early pregnancy: comparison between 2D and 4D sonographic scanning. J Perinat Med. 2005;33(5):406-14.

30. Kurjak A, Stanojevic M, Andonotopo W, Scazzocchio-Duenas E, Azumendi G, Carrera JM. Fetal behavior assessed in all three trimesters of normal pregnancy by four-dimensional ultrasonography. Croat Med J. 2005;46(5):772-80.

31. Pooh RK, Ogura T. Normal and abnormal fetal hand positioning and movement in early pregnancy detected by three- and four-dimensional ultrasound. Ultrasound Rev Obset Gynecol. 2004;4(1):46-51.

32. Andonopo W, Kurjak A. The assessment of fetal behavior of growth restricted fetuses by 4D sonography. J Perinat Med. 2006;34(6):471-8.

33. Kurjak A, Andonotopo W, Hafner T, Kadic AS, Stanojevic M, Azumendi G, et al. Normal standards for fetal neurobehavioural developments—longitudinal quantification by four-dimensional sonography. J Perinat Med. 2006;34(1):56-65.

34. Walusinski O, Kurjak A, Andonotopo W, Azumendi G. Fetal yawning assessed by 3D and 4D sonography. Ultrasound Rev Obstet Gynecol. 2005;5(3):210-7.

35. Hanaoka U, Hata T, Kanenishi K, AboEllail MAM, Uematsu R, Konishi Y, et al. Does ethnicity have an effect on fetal behavior? A comparison of Asian and Caucasian populations. J Perinat Med. 2016;44(2): 217-21.

36. Farkas LG, Katic MJ, Forrest CR, Alt KW, Bagic I, Baltadjiev G, et al. International anthropometric study of facial morphology in various ethnic groups/races. J Craniofac Surg. 2005;16(4):615-46.

37. Le TT, Farkas LG, Ngim RCK, Levin LS, Forrest CR. Proportionality in Asian and North American Caucasian faces using neoclassical facial canons as criteria. Aesth Plast Surg. 2002;26(1):64-9.

38. Hata T, Hanaoka U, AboEllail MAM, Uematsu R, Noguchi J, Kusaka T, Kurjak A. Is there a sex difference in fetal behavior? A comparison of the KANET test between male and female fetuses. J Perinat Med. 2016;44(5):585-8.

39. Korner AF. Neonatal startles, smiles, erections, and reflex sucks as related to state, sex, and individuality. Child Dev. 1969;40(4):1039-53.

40. Jacklin CN, Snow M, Maccoby E. Tactile sensitivity and muscle strength in newborn boys and girls. Infant Behav Dev. 1981;4:261-8.

41. de Vries JI, Visser GH, Prechtl HF. The emergence of fetal behavior. III. Individual differences and consistencies. Early Hum Dev. 1988;16(1):85-103.

42. Hepper PG, Shannon EA, Dornan JC. Sex differences in fetal mouth movements. Lancet. 1997;350(9094):1820.

43. de Medina PGR, Visser GHA, Huizink AC, Buitelaar JK, Mulder EJH. Fetal behavior does not differ between boys and girls. Early Hum Dev. 2003;73(1-2):17-26.

44. DiPietro JA, Hodgson DM, Costigan KA, Hilton SC, Johnson TR. Fetal neurobehavioral development. Child Dev. 1996;67(5):2553-67.

45. DiPietro JA, Costigan KA, Shupe AK, Pressman EK, Johnson TR. Fetal neuro-behavioral development: associations with socioeconomic class and fetal sex. Dev Psychobiol. 1998;33(1):79-91.

46. Hepper PG, Dornan JC, Lynch C. Sex differences in fetal habituation. Dev Sci. 2012;15(3):373-83.

47. Tranquilli AL, Lorenzi S, Buscicchio G, Di Tommaso M, Mazzanti L, Emanuelli M. Female fetuses are more reactive when mother eats chocolate. J Matern Fetal Neonatal Med. 2014;27(1):72-4.

48. Antsaklis P, Porovic S, Daskalakis G, Kurjak A. 4D assessment of fetal brain function in diabetic patients. J Perinat Med. 2017;45(6): 711-15.

49. Edelberg SC, Dierker L, Kalhan S, Rosen MG. Decreased fetal movements with sustained maternal hyperglycemia using the glucose clamp technique. Am J Obstet Gynecol. 1987;156(5):1101-5.

50. Cosmi EV, Anceschi MM, Cosmi E, Piazze JJ, La Torre R. Ultrasonographic patterns of fetal breathing movements in normal pregnancy. Int J Gynaecol Obstet. 2003;80(3):285-90.

51. Allen CL, Kisilevsky BS. Fetal behavior in diabetic and nondiabetic pregnant women: an exploratory study. Dev Psychobiol. 1999;35(1):69-80.

52. Mulder EJ, O'Brien MJ, Lems YL, Visser GH, Prechtl HF. Body and breathing movements in near-term fetuses and newborn infants of type-1 diabetic women. Early Hum Dev. 1990;24(2):131-52.

53. Devoe LD, Youssef AA, Castillo RA, Croom CS. Fetal biophysical activities in third-trimester pregnancies complicated by diabetes mellitus. Am J Obstet Gynecol. 1994;171(2):298-303.

54. Kainer F, Prechtl HF, Engele H, Einspieler C. Assessment of the quality of general movements in fetuses and infants of women with type-I diabetes mellitus. Early Hum Dev. 1997;50(1):13-25.

55. Holden KP, Jovanovic L, Druzin ML, Peterson CM. Increased fetal activity with low maternal blood glucose levels in pregnancies complicated by diabetes. Am J Perinatol. 1984;1(2):161-4.

56. Yeoshoua E, Goldstein I, Zlozover M, Wiener Z. Sonographic study of the relationship

between gestational diabetes mellitus and fetal activity. J Matern Fetal Neonatal Med. 2012;25(6):623-6.

57. Dieb A, Salam R, Shaheen D, Shaeer E. Evaluation of foetal neurological behavior in hypothyroid pregnant females - a pilot study. J Matern Fetal Neonatal Med. 2019;32(16):2617-21.

58. Bernal J. Thyroid hormones and brain development. Vitam Horm. 2005;71:95-122.

59. Kooistra L, Crawford S, van Baar AL, Brouwers EP, Pop VJ. Neonatal effects of maternal hypothyroxinemia during early pregnancy. Pediatrics. 2006;117(1):161-7.

60. Henrichs J, Bongers-Schokking JJ, Schenk JJ, Ghassabian A, Schmidt HG, Visser TJ, et al. Maternal thyroid function during early pregnancy and cognitive functioning in early childhood: the generation R study. J Clin Endocrinol Metab. 2010;95(9):4227-34.

61. Li Y, Shan Z, Teng W, Yu X, Li Y, Fan C, et al. Abnormalities of maternal thyroid function during pregnancy affect neuropsychological development of their children at 25-30 months. Clin Endocrinol (Oxf). 2010; 72(6):825-9.

62. Gyamfi C, Wapner RJ, D'Alton ME. Thyroid dysfunction in pregnancy: the basic science and clinical evidence surrounding the controversy in management. Obstet Gynecol. 2009;113(3):702-7.

63. Chevrier J, Harley KG, Kogut K, Holland N, Johnson C, Eskenazi B. Maternal thyroid function during the second half of pregnancy and child neurodevelopment at 6, 12, 24, and 60 months of age. J Thyroid Res. 2011;2011:426427.

64. Pop VJ, Brouwers EP, Vader HL, Vulsma T, van Baar AL, de Vijlder JJ. Maternal hypo-thyroxinemia during early pregnancy and subsequent child development: a 3-year follow-up study. Clin Endocrinol (Oxf). 2003; 59(3):282-8.

65. Nazarpour S, Tehrani FR, Simbar M, Azizi F. Thyroid dysfunction and pregnancy outcomes. Iran J Reprod Med. 2015;13(7):387-96.

66. Hata T, Kanenishi K, AboEllail MAM, Mori N, Koyano K, Kato I, et al. Effect of psychotropic drugs on fetal behavior in the third trimester of pregnancy. J Perinat Med. 2019;47(2):207-11.

67. Sanz EJ, De-las-Cuevas C, Kiuru A, Bate A, Edwards R. Selective serotonin reuptake inhibitors in pregnant women and neonatal withdrawal syndrome: a database analysis. Lancet. 2005;365(9458):482-7.

68. Brandlistuen RE, Ystrom E, Eberhard-Gran M, Nulman I, Koren G, Nordeng H. Behavioral effects of fetal antidepressant exposure in a Norwegian cohort of discordant siblings. Int J Epidemiol. 2015;44(4):1397-407.

69. Boukhris T, Sheehy O, Mottron L, Berard A. Antidepressant use during pregnancy and the risk of autism spectrum disorder in children. JAMA Pediatr. 2016;170(2):117-24.

70. Mezzacappa A, Lasica PA, Gianfagna F, Cazas O, Hardy P, Falissard B, et al. Risk for autism spectrum disorders according to period of prenatal antidepressant exposure: a systematic review and meta-analysis. JAMA Pediatr. 2017;171(6):555-63.

71. Rihtman T, Parush S, Ornoy A. Developmental outcomes at preschool age after fetal exposure to valproic acid and lamotrigine: cognitive, motor, sensory and behavioral function. Reprod Toxicol. 2013;41:115-25.

72. Deshmukh U, Adams J, Macklin EA, Dhillon R, McCarthy KD, Dworetzky B, et al. Behavioral outcomes in children exposed prenatally to lamotrigine, valproate, or carbamazepine. Neurotoxicol Teratol. 2016;54:5-14.

73. Ogo K, Kanenishi K, Mori N, AboEllail MAM, Hata T. Change in fetal behavior in response to vibroacoustic stimulation. J Perinat Med. 2019;47(5):558-63.

74. Spencer JA, Deans A, Nicolaidis P, Arulkumaran S. Fetal heart rate response to vibroacoustic stimulation during low and high heart rate variability episodes in late pregnancy. Am J Obstet Gynecol. 1991;165(1):86-90.

75. D'Elia A, Pighetti M, Vanacore F, Fabbrocini G, Arpaia L. Vibroacoustic stimulation in normal term human pregnancy. Early Hum Dev. 2005;81(5):449-53.

76. Umstad M, Bailey C, Permezel M. Intra-partum fetal stimulation testing. Aust N Z J Obstet Gynaecol. 1992;32(3):222-4.

77. East CE, Smyth RMD, Leader LR, Henshall NE, Colditz PB, Lau R, et al. Vibroacoustic stimulation for fetal assessment in labor in the presence of a nonreassuring fetal heart rate trace. Cochrane Database Syst Rev. 2013;2013(1):CD004664.

78. Arulkumaran S, Talbert D, Hsu TS, Chua S, Anandakumar C, Ratnam SS. In-utero sound levels when vibroacoustic stimulation is applied to the maternal abdomen: an assessment of the possibility of cochlea damage in the fetus. Br J Obstet Gynaecol. 1992;99(1):43-5.

79. Arulkumaran S, Skurr B, Tong H, Kek LP, Yeoh KH, Ratnam SS. No evidence of hearing loss due to fetal acoustic stimulation test. Obstet Gynecol. 1991;78(2):283-5.

80. Mulder EJH, Koenen SV, Blom I, Visser GHA. The effects of antenatal betamethasone administration on fetal heart rate and behavior depend on gestational age. Early Hum Dev. 2004;76(1):65-77.

81. Mushkat Y, Ascher-Landsberg J, Keidar R, Carmon E, Pauzner D, David MP. The effect of betamethasone versus dexamethasone on fetal biophysical parameters. Eur J Obstet Gynecol Reprod Biol. 2001;97(1):50-2.

82. Kelly MK, Schneider EP, Petrikovsky BM, Lesser ML. Effect of antenatal steroid administration on the fetal biophysical profile. J Clin Ultrasound. 2000;28(5): 224-6.

83. Rotmensch S, Liberati M, Vishne TH, Celentano C, Ben-Rafael Z, Bellati U. The effect of betamethasone and dexamethasone on fetal heart rate patterns and biophysical activities. A prospective randomized trial. Acta Obstet Gynecol Scand. 1999;78(6): 493-500.

84. Derks JB, Mulder EJ, Visser GH. The effects of maternal betamethasone administration on the fetus. Br J Obstet Gynaecol. 1995;102(1): 40-6.

85. Mulder EJ, Derks JB, Visser GH. Antenatal corticosteroid therapy and fetal behavior: a randomized study of the effects of betamethasone and dexamethasone. Br J Obstet Gynaecol. 1997;104(11):1239-47.

Cognitive Functions in Pregnant Women

Natalia Lesiewska, Maciej Bieliński

BRAIN CHANGES IN PREGNANT WOMEN

Pregnancy and postpartum is a very specific period in women's life, which is characterized by many physiological changes of an adaptive nature. These changes in women's body are designed to the demands of fetal growth and development, but also they enable pregnant women proper care of the baby after birth. These changes especially affect the reproductive organs and the circulatory system. Nonetheless, functional changes in the brain, mainly understood as neural plasticity, are also very interesting. Data describing brain's changes that occur dynamically during pregnancy come mainly from animal studies. Numerous changes in the structure of the central nervous system (CNS) associated with the activity of female sex hormones were observed for the first time in animal models. The changes found at the cellular level were neurogenesis, synaptic remodeling, and changes (increase and/or decrease) in dendritic morphometry, spine density, and astrocyte density.[1]

Human studies are based primarily on the assessment of brain structure and function before and after pregnancy. Studies comparing women who have given birth with nulliparous ones are also carried out. An interesting neuroimaging study by Hoekzema et al. has shown that pregnancy is associated with reduction of the gray matter volume in regions that support social cognition. These changes were very specific to group of mothers. Moreover, changes in gray matter volume were also associated with the postpartum maternal affection. Based on the observations described, it was concluded that this is an expression of the process of adaptation to motherhood. It is also evidenced that the brain changes induced by pregnancy persist after pregnancy.[2]

Similar observations were made in the study of Chinese researchers who performed the magnetic resonance imaging (MRI) among eight nonpregnant female volunteers and nine women who had vaginal delivery in the first 24 hours after birth. It was found that pregnant women were characterized by cerebral cortex atrophy. Atrophy was ranging from 6 to 13%.[3] The same publication also describes the differences in electroencephalography (EEG) and transcranial Doppler ultrasonography (TCD). Pregnant women showed increased electrical activity of the brain in the middle parietal part and a decrease in the temporoparietal junction. Also, the bilateral pulsation index parameter in the flow through the internal carotid arteries and externally tested with TCD was lower in the pregnant population.[3] The above publications prove the significant influence of pregnancy and motherhood on the structure and functioning of a woman's brain.

Cognitive Functioning in Pregnant Women during Physiological Pregnancy

Physiological changes in a woman's body related to pregnancy result mainly from fluctuations in the level of endogenous hormones and their effects on target cells. These activities are necessary for the maintenance of pregnancy, delivery, and lactation. Careful observations provided information on the functions of individual female hormones during the development of pregnancy and after delivery. Whereas the influence of hormones on the cognitive functioning of the brain is not clear. However, in scientific publications the colloquial term of "pregnancy brain" is utilized.[4]

There are number of reports that indicate changes in the neural structure of the brain regions which are responsible for information storage or processing, and for modulating the emotional response.[5] In contrast, experimental studies do not allow to recognize a global decline in cognitive functions in the pregnant population. Studies by Farrar et al. and Christensen et al. show a decrease in cognitive functioning in individual domains, while maintaining the level of functioning of others.[5,6]

The first study indicated a reduction in spatial recognition memory as a component of executive functions (EFs) in the pregnant group, while no significant correlation of cognitive results with the level of hormones was found.[5] In the second one, (cohort prospective study of nearly 200 pregnant women or mothers) in relation to a large control group, the researchers examined the correlation of pregnancy and motherhood with worse cognitive functioning over many years. The neuropsychological assessment which included the domains of cognitive speed, working memory, immediate and delayed recall, revealed no significant associations between pregnancy and maternity with poorer cognitive outcomes, apart from a worse Digits Backwards score as an element of working memory.[6] It is worth noting that both of these findings concern functions dependent on the activity of the prefrontal cortex of the brain.

An interesting issue is the attempt to determine the relationships between the levels of individual hormones involved in the course of pregnancy. The study on 55 pregnant women analyzed the correlations of the levels of estradiol, progesterone, testosterone, cortisol, and prolactin with the results of a battery of neuropsychological tests. Already in the initial analysis, it was shown that pregnant women in both antenatal and postpartum examinations obtained worse results compared to the control group in the field of verbal recall and processing speed. This study described significant associations of cortisol, prolactin, and estradiol levels, while the nature of the relationship was either linear or inverted-U function (prolactin).[7] The differences in the reports regarding the significance of the influence of pregnancy on the cognitive functioning of pregnant women indicate the validity of further observations, while the reported correlations of hormones with the results of cognitive tests suggest the direction of future research.

COGNITIVE FUNCTIONS IN HYPERTENSIVE DISEASES OF PREGNANCY

Nowadays, the prevalence of hypertensive diseases of pregnancy (HDP) is growing. HDP are responsible for approximately 5–10% of complications during pregnancies throughout the world.[8] With growing gestation, mother's cardiovascular system activates alterations necessary to adapt to changing blood pressure (BP) levels. However, due to many factors (environmental, medical ones) those regulating mechanisms may get depleted and cause greater rise of the BP leading to pathology.[9]

Definition and Classification of Hypertensive Diseases of Pregnancy

Diagnosis of hypertension in pregnancy is made if the value of taken BP exceeds 140 mm Hg systolic or 90 mm Hg diastolic in two measurements separated in time. European guidelines describe the following classification of HDP:

- Preexisting (chronic) hypertension—which appears before pregnancy, during early pregnancy, i.e., before 20 weeks of gestation, or sustains after 6 weeks postpartum.
- Gestational hypertension—which is first diagnosed after 20 weeks of pregnancy and subsides during 6 weeks postpartum.
- Preeclampsia (PE) and eclampsia syndrome—PE is defined as hypertension which develops after 20 weeks of gestation and coexists with at least one of subsequent disorders: proteinuria, thrombocytopenia, renal insufficiency, liver dysfunction, neurologic disorders, hemolysis, or fetal growth restriction. Eclampsia is a severe form of PE characterized as the new onset of tonic-clonic seizures.
- Preeclampsia superimposed of chronic hypertension—defined as development of PE in women with chronic hypertension.[8,10]

Consequences of Hypertensive Diseases of Pregnancy

Hypertensive disorders in pregnancy may cause wide spectrum of complications in many organ systems to both mother and her child, hence they contribute to greater rates of perinatal morbidity and mortality.

Chronic hypertension may predispose to complications such as renal failure, stroke, or respiratory failure, however the greatest consequence associated with this disorder is superimposed PE.[11] Superimposed PE may develop even in 20–40% obstetricians with chronic hypertension.[12] Even higher maternal morbidity and mortality may ensue from superimposed PE in comparison to PE which develops in a woman without the chronic hypertension.[13]

In gestational hypertension the risk of PE estimates around 50% which is linked to many adverse outcomes.[14] Both gestational and chronic hypertension may lead to dangerous perinatal complications like fetal growth restriction, abruption of placenta, which contribute to significantly increased risk of miscarriage, premature birth, or even intrauterine fetal death.[11] Gestational hypertension is the risk factor for the development of chronic hypertension, risk of cardiovascular diseases (CVDs), including myocardial infarction.[15]

Preeclampsia affects organs due to endothelial dysfunction leading to microangiopathy, damaged perfusion, vasoconstriction, and maladaptive response to greater BP in vessels. Therefore, PE may lead to disorders like hepatic failure, acute kidney injury, electrolyte abnormalities, thrombocytopenia, or neurological complications. Eclampsia is the most dangerous complication of PE resulting from encephalopathy owing to hypoperfusion. Apart from seizures, cortical blindness, hemorrhagic stroke (due to coagulopathy), or posterior reversible encephalopathy syndrome (PRES) also pertain to neurological complications.[11]

Similar complications may ensue from superimposed PE, however as we have mentioned, the perinatal risk is greater.

Hypertensive Diseases of Pregnancy and Brain Function

Literature shows that HDP affect many organs in woman's body, including brain, which leads to serious complications. In many guidelines the best medication for gestational hypertension or PE and eclampsia is cessation of the pregnancy—delivery.[16,17]

But let us concentrate a little bit more on brain. HDP, especially PE and eclampsia, inflict great damage to brain, which may lead to stroke, seizures, or temporary blindness. The question is, whether it is possible for HDP to prompt other symptoms which occur even after postpartum period? Those particular symptoms include problems with memory, concentration, or attention, problems with processing information, and hinder daily functioning—namely cognitive functions.

Literature shows evidence that many researchers have tackled the problem of cognitive performance in women whose pregnancies were complicated with HPD.

The study of Postma et al. performed the long-term follow-up study scrutinizing the connection between the history of PE or eclampsia and cognitive functioning in women.[18] They also analyzed the quality of life within their study group. The results indicate that women with the history of PE, perceived cognitive deterioration, worse quality of life, and showed psychological problems in comparison to women with normotensive pregnancies. The study also showed that women who had eclampsia reported even more issues with cognitive functioning. Authors suggest that the possible explanation for these results may stem

from trauma experienced due pregnancy burdened with PE or eclampsia which manifest in significant worrying and feeling acute stress. Such symptoms may contribute to the development of psychiatric pathologies in postpartum period or even in later life, i.e., post-traumatic stress disorder (PTSD) and depression, which are associated with cognitive deterioration.[19-22]

The results of a research conducted by Mielke et al. showed that women with the history of HDP gained worse scores in tests assessing processing speed in comparison to subjects with normotensive pregnancy. However, both groups did not differ regarding EFs, language, or memory. Researchers also evaluated MRI results to search for brain changes. They found that women with history of HDP had both greater brain atrophy and white matter lesions (WMLs).[23]

In a field of cognition, researches show mixed results. In a study of Dayan et al. (who also scrutinized the relation between the history of PE and cognitive deterioration in the long-term follow-up) women with history of PE showed lower scores of cognitive domains such as executive functioning or psychomotor speed, however those results were statistically insignificant.[24] Another data did not show any differences regarding EFs, working memory, or attention between study group and controls.[25] On the contrary, another study found that the history of PE was related to cognitive decline in EFs, as well as in verbal learning and attention.[26]

The association between the history of PE and increased risk of dementia has been proved. The strongest connection was with vascular dementia, however, authors found associations with the heightened risk of Alzheimer's diseases (ADs) as with other subtypes of dementia (although weaker in statistical analysis).[27,28]

How Hypertensive Diseases of Pregnancy Affect Brain?—Putative Mechanisms

Common Risk Factors

Pregnancy itself may be a particular test of women's susceptibility of CVDs development in later life. HDP are risk factors for CVD and also share similar risk factors as CVD.[29,30] The nature of PE is involved with impairment of vessels and in this manner may be connected with greater dementia development in the future. The pathogenesis of PE is associated with endothelial dysfunction and greater inflammatory response.[28] Both factors contribute to the occurrence of plaques in the vessels, leading to atherosclerosis, blockage of small vessels with further angiopathies. In brain, those mechanisms may lead to cerebral lesions and infarctions and hence may explain cognitive declines reported by patients.[31]

White Matter Lesions

Cerebral cortex is perceived as the center of cognitive functions, but another structure with major contribution is white matter. White matter forms neural tracts which are spread throughout the brain. Those tracts form connections between gray matter regions in cortical and subcortical areas, therefore enable conveying information regarding emotion and cognition.[32,33]

Injuries of white matter are associated with cognitive decline and development of dementia.[33] For better classification of white matter involvement in cognitive deterioration, the term of "white matter dementia" was created.[34] Brain injury resulting in demyelination of axons may be responsible for postponed impulse transmission in the brain and hence, contribute to cognitive dysfunction in domains such as EFs, memory, attention, or language processing.[32]

Research showed that WMLs were found more frequently in women with PE and eclampsia than women with a normotensive pregnancy.[35,36] Even though WML are involved in dementia in elderly, yet no evidence shows the clinical consequences of WML in cognitive dysfunction in young women with HDP. Such results may eventuate from neuroplasticity and cognitive reorganization or be the result of inadequate methodology utilized in various studies.

Subjective Cognition

Researches utilizing battery of objective cognitive tests, still show mixed results regarding the connection between cognition and PE. Some authors allude the term of "subjective cognition" to explain the lack of evidence measured in objective tests performed in women who presented worse cognitive functioning in autoquestionnaires.[25] Self-reported cognitive decline may stem from few aspects. Women who were enrolled to studies were too young during the cognitive evaluation. Therefore, lack of evidence regarding cognitive deterioration might be a result of compensatory brain capacity due to young age. Similar explanation might be responsible for the inconsistent results of neuroimaging studies about the connection between WML and cognitive functions after PE.[23,36] However, it is speculated, whether WMLs could be a radiological sign indicating the susceptibility of hypertensive disorder in later life.[37] After reaching elderly stage of life compensatory brain capacity might get depleted and then manifest in cognitive decline.

Cerebral Blood Flow

Pregnancy is challenging for cardiovascular system and requires adaptions like reconfiguration or reconstruction of blood vessels. HDP exert great influence on cerebral blood flow (CBF) even in postpartum period.[38] Women with chronic hypertension and superimposed PE show greater cerebral perfusion pressure and increased resistance of cerebral vessels.[39] Patients with PE have impaired autoregulation mechanisms leading to increased CBF velocity.[40,41] Lack of proper adaptations may result in greater blood-brain barrier (BBB) permeability, heightened hydrostatic pressure, or damage of microvessels. This in turn may lead to microbleeding, cerebral edema, neuroinflammation, and neuronal damage.[42-44] The theory explaining neurologic symptoms in eclampsia involves insufficient autoregulation of CBF which predispose to vasogenic edema and hence to PRES.[45,46] Therefore, impaired autoregulation is linked to poorer cognitive functions and enhanced risk of vascular dementia in the future.[47] It is worth noting that HDP do not cease with delivery, but may exert detrimental consequences in later life.[48]

Blood-Brain Barrier Impairment

Blood-brain barrier is a specialized barrier which maintains brain homeostasis by regulating exchange between blood and cerebral microenvironment. Studies show the connection between increased CBF and greater BBB permeability which may cause damage to the brain.[49,50] Neuroimaging studies proved association between PE/eclampsia and BBB impairment.[51] PE is associated with increased inflammatory response with elevated levels of proinflammatory cytokines like interleukin-6 (IL-6), tumor necrosis factor alpha (TNF-α), and microglia activation.[52] Neuroinflammation may be responsible for deteriorated neurological injury, greater vulnerability to eclampsia-like seizures and contribute to the development of eclampsia.[53,54] Literature shows evidence that neuroinflammation during conditions with raised inflammatory levels influence brain function in domains of learning or memory.[55,56] Moreover, BBB disruption in conjunction with inflammatory mechanisms contribute to cognitive decline.[57] To our knowledge, literature does not provide evidence of the association between neuroinflammation and cognitive decline in women with PE/eclampsia. However, this mechanism may be responsible for symptoms reported by women with history of HDP and for a greater risk of dementia in later life.

GESTATIONAL DIABETES MELLITUS AND BRAIN FUNCTION

Gestational diabetes mellitus (GDM) is a frequent complication during pregnancy. According to International Diabetes Federation (IDF) in 2019 approximately 20 million, or 16% pregnancies worldwide were complicated with hyperglycemia. 1 in 6 births were associated with GDM.[58] Those numbers will be growing, and due to serious consequences associated with GDM, it is crucial to put more effort in order to prevent and to support pregnant women suffering from this disease.

On the molecular basis, GDM develops due to the impairment of β-cells in pancreas as a results of excessive insulin production. The dysfunction is caused by the hyperglycemia and augmented insulin resistance.[59,60]

The state of hyperglycemia may inflict grievous consequences both to mother and her child, for instance: preterm birth, PE, fetal overgrowth resulting in macrosomia, or fetal hyperglycemia which may even lead to stillbirth.[61-65] It is well known that GDM predispose to the development of type 2 diabetes mellitus (T2DM) or CVDs, but also GDM has been linked to greater risk of affective disorders, such as depression.[66]

It has been shown that the relationship between T2DM and depression is bidirectional. T2DM facilitates pathogenesis of depression, and depression is a risk factor for T2DM. Studies show similar connection between GDM and depression.[67] GDM may lead to mood disorders via disturbances in hypothalamic-pituitary-adrenal (HPA) axis, hyperinflammation, or hyperinsulinemia.[68] On the other hand, depression may contribute to further exacerbation of hyperglycemia and glycemic control.[69]

To date, many studies show influence of T2DM on brain function. However, there are none presenting how GDM lead to cognitive impairment. GDM exerts adverse effects on brain in a shorter time period—during pregnancy—in contrast to T2DM. Nonetheless, both diseases show similar consequences, like greater risk of CVD, mood disorders, and obesity. Therefore, GDM and T2DM may affect brain in similar fashion. Moreover, it has been shown that GDM shares similar gene polymorphism as AD. Building on the model of T2DM, I will shortly discuss mechanisms which lead to cognitive deterioration.[70]

Cognitive Dysfunction in Type 2 Diabetes Mellitus

The issue of the development of cognitive deterioration in patients with T2DM has been well studied. Diabetes can lead to functional and structural changes in brain, and thus incur impaired cognitive processing in many domains. Published data show worse performance in speed of information processing, EFs, poorer verbal learning, attention, and psychomotor efficiency.[71,72] Evidence of the Maastricht Aging Study, showed that diabetic patients had greater cognitive decrements in major domains like information processing and word recalling, in comparison to nondiabetic controls in a long-term evaluation.[73]

Along with cognitive decline, it was hypothesized that T2DM might be associated with pathophysiology of dementia. Especially, that factors related to diabetes, i.e., hyperinsulinemia, hyperglycemia, and greater insulin resistance are considered as AD risk factors.[74] It has been shown that patients with T2DM have higher risk of AD development.[75-77] Moreover, T2DM seems to be associated with around 50% greater susceptibility to dementia.[78] Another significant argument pointing to the relationship between T2DM and dementia is that AD has been defined as a "type 3 diabetes". Some researchers utilize this term, because insulin and insulin-like growth factor 1 (IGF-1) take part in neuronal homeostasis and signaling processes within brain. Those processes enable learning and making memories, but in case they are disturbed, they seem to contribute to AD pathogenesis, and neurodegeneration.[77]

Data present associations between cognitive dysfunction and inadequate glycemic control. T2DM patients showed augmented dysfunction in domains such as memory, attention, and psychomotor speed in comparison to subjects with impaired fasting glycemia or normal glucose levels.[79]

Higher levels of glycosylated hemoglobin (HbA1c) are associated with greater cognitive decline. Yaffe et al. showed results indicating that HbA1c correlated with worse scores of Wisconsin Card Sorting Test (WCST) which measures EFs.[80,81] Authors even suggest that HbA1c might be a parameter utilized to predict greater risk of the dementia development in the future.

Literature also show mixed results regarding this topic. Some studies present that dementia develops owing to vascular changes during diabetes, rather than

AD-like alterations within brain.[82-84] Also methodologies of some studies might be responsible for inconsistent results. Complications associated with T2DM and concomitant diseases may affect brain as well and contribute to poorer cognitive functioning, for instance hypertension, visual impairment, stroke, or depression.[85-88] In this manner, different mechanisms (not necessarily associated with T2DM) could influence brain function.

Another issue worth commenting is how soon T2DM exerts adverse alterations in brain and how aging may contribute to cognitive deterioration. Van den Berg et al. performed a study which assessed two groups of patients at two times: at the baseline measurements and after 4 year follow-up. Results demonstrated that, in comparison to healthy controls, patients with T2DM had worse outcomes in processing of information, EFs, and attention. However, over 4 years evaluation, changes in poorer cognitive outcome were rather the results of aging than detrimental influence of diabetes itself.[89] Literature also presents reports indicating rapid cognitive deterioration in T2DM patients within relatively short time of 3–6 years.[90,91] Also in a group of elders T2DM accelerated cognitive dysfunction during 9 years.[92]

Hyperglycemia and Insulin Resistance

Studies suggest that insulin is responsible for adverse brain changes linked to poorer cognitive outcomes. Insulin resistance shows negative correlation with cognitive performance even in individuals without diabetes.[93,94] Another study suggests that insulin resistance may impact brain glucose metabolism and be associated with changes similar to alterations observed in AD.[95]

Insulin resistance is related to hyperinsulinemia and hyperglycemia.[96] Hyperinsulinemia and hyperglycemia are associated with excessive amount of Advanced Glycation End (AGE) products. Those compounds are associated with reduced elasticity of blood vessels and in this mechanism create greater blood flow restriction.[97] Higher glucose levels also contribute to adverse effects within microvascular systems. Within the brain, they may lead to small infarcts in various brain areas, thus may aggravate cognitive processing.[96,98]

Studies present findings between AGEs and pathogenesis of AD. AGEs play role in the formation of fibrillary tangles and amyloid plaques which are responsible for neuronal death and further neurodegeneration processes associated with AD development.[99]

Studies show that reduced neurogenesis, owing to AGEs abundance, complicate forming episodic memory, including verbal and spatial memory.[97] Individuals with prediabetes showed neuropathological changes in comparison to controls with normoglycemia. Increased glucose levels positively correlate with cognitive decline, which may later accelerate age-related cognitive deterioration processes.[100] Study performed by Munshi et al. observed negative correlation with poorer results of tests assessing EFs.[101]

Presented evidence shed light to causes of cognitive deterioration during diabetes. There are factors which influence the degree to which T2DM affects brain. Among them are: the duration of the disease, the level of hyperglycemia and glycemic control, and also presence of concomitant diseases.

Neuroimaging

Many papers present evidence of cognitive impairments in T2DM patients which are expressed in neuropsychological tests and questionnaires. Literature is comprised of neuroimaging studies which scrutinized the relationship between diabetes and structural and functional changes within the brain.

Inappropriate levels of glucose in diabetes were associated with diminished cortical thickness. Studies noted significant reduction of volumetric brain in the area of hippocampus, which is responsible for processes related to memories.[98,102] Similar alterations were observed in frontal lobes which are essential for EFs. Moreover, hyperglycemia may impair cortical and subcortical neuronal pathways. In MRI scans these lesions are presented as white matter hyperintensities. Insulin resistance, HbA1c, and high glucose variability are associated with greater WMLs, which contribute to worse performance in attention, memory, and EFs.[103]

Effects of insulin resistance were evaluated in positron emission tomography (PET) studies. In contrast to healthy controls, individuals with prediabetes showed lower activation in prefrontal regions of cerebral cortex while subjects were performing cognitive tasks. Authors suggest that insulin resistance might be a marker of AD-like cognitive deterioration even before the full onset of mild cognitive impairment (MCI).[95]

To conclude, brain imaging studies show evidence linking T2DM to cortical and subcortical brain shrinkage.[104] Those structural alterations may contribute to cognitive deterioration in diabetic patients.

Importance of Cognitive Functions

Executive functions are responsible for the regulation of human's actions in order to achieve particular goal.[105] Therefore, it is necessary for this cognitive domain to work properly to manage chronic diseases, like T2DM. Regarding EF, patients use them in order to control glycemia levels throughout the day. In order to do that patients have to control themselves and apply proper diet (calculate nutricious values of food), monitor glucose levels, and exercise. During the day many factors may have impact on proper glucose levels, for example, stressful situations. When the daily routine is disturbed, EF is utilized to take proper actions necessary in maintaining intended level of glucose.

In case when EF is deteriorated, T2DM patients may get easily distracted by cues from the environment which can hinder achieving the goal of euglycemia. Such cue can be high-caloric food. When self-control is weakened, there is high chance that patient will stop their diet routine and yield to temptation of eating unhealthy food.

It has been shown that diabetes may also affect work productivity in conjunction with worsened EF (due to hyperglycemia).[106] Also impaired EF may contribute to difficulties with managing emotions. EF may also influence the greater risk of depression development in T2DM.

Similar adjustments in daily routine are required of women with GDM. If insulin resistance or hyperglycemia affect their brain function in similar ways like T2DM, those patients may also struggle in obtaining euglycemia owing to cognitive deterioration. This is particularly important, because complications of GDM are grievous to both mother and her child.

Future Directions

As I have mentioned, glycemic control may affect cognitive performance. Increased glycemia might exert adverse outcomes in brain functioning and result in having difficulties during daily duties or worse quality of life. Pregnancy is a state of greater insulin resistance and higher levels of glucose in blood which are necessary for proper fetal development. During the complication such as GDM, it is essential to commence proper management, not only to prevent consequences related to GDM, but also in order to keep appropriate brain function of the mother.

Unfortunately medical data base lack evidence about how GDM affects cognitive functioning. GDM significantly differs from T2DM and most of all, lasts in the shorter period of time. However, GDM is a risk factor for diabetes development and affects many systems of women body. Therefore, it may influence brain function as well, as contribute to cognitive impairments in later life—for instance those associated with aging. Hence, definitely more, properly planned studies are needed. Those researches should evaluate cognitive factions with follow-up after short and long time. Then, obtained results, would explain to what degree GDM is linked (or not) to cognitive deterioration.

COGNITIVE FUNCTIONS AND OBESITY

As health professionals, currently we are struggling with obesity pandemic. According to World Health Organization (WHO) over 1.9 billion adults were overweight and 650 million of them were obese (2016).[107] Even among children and adolescents overweight is increasing with every year. Around 340 million of them were overweight or obese.

Obesity is considered as a chronic disease with multifactorial pathophysiology. In pregnancy, obesity is very challenging due to adverse outcomes to both mother and fetus. Obesity predispose to complications related to pregnancy like GDM, hypertensive disorders in pregnancy, prolonged labor, disorders in pregnancy, prolonged labor, and greater chance of delivery via cesarean section.[108,109] Moreover, obesity is associated with greater risk of wound infections or postpartum depression.[110]

Concerning fetus, evidence indicate the association between obesity and miscarriage, fetal growth abnormalities (fetal growth restriction and fetal macrosomia), greater risk of preterm birth, stillbirth, or neonatal death after delivery.[109,111-114] Children born from pregnancies complicated with GDM show increased risk of developing obesity, insulin resistance, or diabetes mellitus.[115,116]

Obesity is defined on the basis of body mass index (BMI). In pregnant women the diagnosis of obesity is made if BMI value equals 30 kg/m^2 or more from the calculations using height and weight before pregnancy or from the first trimester of pregnancy (during the first visit).[117]

Cognitive Functions in Obesity

Obesity affects almost every system of human's body and also contributes to worse cognitive processing. Studies showed that patients with excessive BMI had worse results in neuropsychological tests assessing memory, attention, and visuospatial domains.[118-120] In comparison to healthy subjects, overweight individuals demonstrated abnormalities of working memory.[121] Several studies also demonstrated that obesity is a risk factor of developing dementia, even in the independent manner of T2DM.[122-124] Even research of children and adolescents indicates significant differences of cognitive performance between the group of obese and normal-weight participants. Obese children showed deficits in short-term memory and verbal abilities. Furthermore, even neuroimaging studies of obese children show essential abnormalities in brain structure, like WMLs or lower cerebral volume which suggest that excess of adipose tissue may be inflict damage to the developing brain.[125,126]

Data show evidence of putative bidirectional mechanisms between obesity and cognition. Impairments of EFs may contribute to further weight gain. As it has been mentioned before, EF enable control of human's behavior in order to goals. However, disorders of processes which manage self-control may facilitate overconsumption and eating high-caloric food, leading to further weight gain.[127]

Dopaminergic Signaling as a Link between Obesity and Cognitive Factors

Institute of Medicine established gestational weight gain (GWG) guidelines, which are based on the BMI.[128] GWG has been linked to several perinatal and intrapartum complications.[129-131] Therefore, the prevention of GWG is the essential issue which needs more investigation leading to novel prophylactic and therapeutic programs to support women suffering from obesity.

Eating healthy food abundant in vegetables, fruits, and proteins is recommended. However women report troubles with implementing proper diet, due to food cravings, easier access to fast foods, or presence unhealthy food within their environment (i.e., household members have high-caloric diet).[132]

Dopamine (DA) is a key neurotransmitter involved in food intake control. Disturbances in DA signaling within the brain may result in reward-seeking behaviors, have looking for natural rewards as high-caloric food.[133] Several theories which involve dopaminergic signaling, were conceived in order to explain the pathophysiology of obesity.

- Reward surfeit theory suggests that food consumption commence greater reward responsiveness within brain circuits of brain. This mechanism stimulates further overconsumption.[134]

- Incentive sensitization model postulates that repeated intake of highly palatable food containing great amounts of sugar or fat, may increase response within reward regions to cues associated with these type of foods. In this manner, it may explain difficulties with adjusting proper eating habits in overweight women.[135]

- Reward deficit theory indicates that changes within reward circuit in obese persons are associated with lower response to food in comparison with healthy ones. Therefore, obese people consume greater amounts of palatable foods to compromise the deficit.[136]

- Inhibitory control deficit theory demonstrates that individuals with EF dysfunction of inhibitory control are more prone to food cues in the environment and eat more.[137] (This theory explains the bidirectional role of cognitive functions of weight gain in obese people).

- Work of Stice and Yokum showed that gene polymorphisms which modulate neurotransmitter signaling within brain are associated with obesity development.[138,139]

Mechanisms explaining poorer cognitive functioning in obese individuals show mixed results. Among presumed mechanism researches mention obesity-induced low inflammation or microbiota.[140,141] The role of DA transmission is also suggested, because DA plays an essential role in conveying information within cognitive pathways, especially in prefrontal cortex—which is principal brain area of executive functioning.[142] We performed a study scrutinizing the role of *DA* gene polymorphisms, associated with obesity, in cognitive functioning in obese subjects. The results indicated that *DA* gene polymorphisms linked to obesity, contribute to performance of EFs in this group.[143]

Multidimensional Approach of Prevention

Obesity develops due to several mechanisms and is associated with complications affecting brain. Evidence presents that behavioral therapy and psychological interventions may diminish negative role of cognitive factors or mood disturbances supporting further GWG and development obesity-related complications. Novel preventive programs are needed, especially those tackling aspects associated with cognitive dysfunction. Hence, pregnant women will learn new skills enhancing the chance of appropriate weight gain during pregnancy, as well, as possibility of weight loss in her later life.[144,145] Such action could prevent serious complications associated with obesity.

▌DEPRESSIVE DISORDERS AND COGNITIVE FUNCTIONS

Mood disorder is also frequent during pregnancy as during other time of women's life. The definition of perinatal depression points to the occurrence of major or minor depressive episodes during pregnancy or within the first 12 months after the delivery.[146] Symptoms associated with this disease include depressed mood, anhedonia, disruption of sleep, or appetite, having low self-esteem.[147]

Maternal depression is associated with several complications concerning mother and developing fetus.[148,149] Perinatal depression has been associated with greater risk of preeclampsia or preterm birth.[150] Moreover, women experiencing depression during pregnancy tend to care less about themselves and in some cases, may even show risk-taking behaviors.[151,152] To date, many studies show deleterious correlations with fetal brain development and perinatal depression. Children show social and cognitive deficits as well as greater predisposition to neuropsychiatric disorders.[153,154]

Unfortunately, the evidence of depression is growing and often perinatal depression remains missed by healthcare professionals and then, untreated. Therefore, more effort should be put into management and screening of mood disorders in pregnancy.

Cognitive Aspects of Depression

Devastating consequences of maternal depression also include mother's brain function during antenatal and postpartum period. However, literature shows scarce evidence regarding this topic. Research is mostly focused on the function of memory in pregnancy, while one research is related to rodents.[155,156] Some papers do not prove any connections between worse cognitive outcomes and maternal depression.[157-159] Evidence suggest that women report subjective cognitive deterioration due to felt stress and anxiety related to depressive state. Therefore, authors suggest that problems with memory or concentration may arise from symptoms of depression.[158] Maternal depression may exert negative influence on woman's self-assessment rather than inflict cognitive deterioration.[157,159]

Pregnancy is a unique time of woman's life. Along with pregnancy, new challenges occur like different lifestyle or worriness about the newborn. These challenges contribute to greater levels of anxiety and stress and contribute to the development of mood disorders associated with pregnancy. Similarly, enduring stress may predispose to the occurrence of subjective symptoms of cognitive decline.[160]

Studies on nonpregnant individuals show evidence that depressive disorders have negative impact on EFs, namely inhibition control.[161] Neuroimaging studies presented greater amount of WMLs in depressive individuals which may explain cognitive deterioration.[162] Worse processing in inhibition control and working memory (which are the components of EF) may result in difficulties with changing focus from negative stimuli to new information.[163] As a model, imagine the medical consultation between mother with maternal depression and perinatologist about abnormalities found in ultrasound during prenatal diagnosis. During the conversation, mother with depression will mostly focus on potential threat to her unborn child. She will have troubles in changing her attention to proposed methods of treatment after the delivery. Getting to know that something is wrong with a child is grievous for every expecting mother. Nonetheless, women with mood disorders might be more demanding and during making the conversation it is worth knowing, that they might require more time to process received information.

Worse EF performance may result in neglect of self-care and management during pathologies of pregnancies, like taking antipertensive drugs or monitoring glucose levels.[98,105] Hence, obese patients with GDM and depression may have great problems with compliance.

Obesity, Depression, and Diabetes

Due to greater prevalence of obesity, mood disorders, and diabetes, we can describe a standard model of the high-risk pregnant patient: the one who is obese, received inadequate results of oral glucose tolerance test (suggesting gestational diabetes). As I have mentioned earlier, both obesity and diabetes are risk factor for mood disorders. One theory suggests that obesity and depression have same pathophysiology.[164] Results of our study showed the connection between particular dopaminergic genes polymorphisms and greater intensity of depressive symptoms and BMI values, which suggest that one way of common pathogenesis may derives from alternations within dopaminergic signaling.[165]

Term of "metabolic mood disorders" lay emphasis on the interdependence between depression, obesity, and hyperglycemia.[166] Apart from alterations in dopaminergic signaling described above, both diseases are associated with dysregulation of immune system causing inflammation or hormonal dysregulation in HPA axis. Even neuroimaging studies show similar findings like, WMLs, brain shrinkage, or abnormal activity of prefrontal cortex (key element in cognitive processes).[167]

Both depression and metabolic syndrome may have synergistic effect on worse cognitive functions. Study of Sullivan et al. showed that cognitive decline progressed faster in patients with diabetes and depression within 3 years, regardless of glycemic control.[168] Another study shows similar findings—patients with T2DM and depression obtained worse results in memory and EF in comparison to healthy controls and subjects with T2DM.[169]

To conclude, mood disorders may affect cognitive functioning and impair daily living. Growing evidence point to the association with metabolic disorders, i.e., obesity and T2DM, making such patients in need of more health control. Unfortunately, little is known about similar connection in pregnant women due to lack of performed studies. Owing to growing prevalence of metabolic and mood disorders and their deleterious complications, more evidence in this field might significantly improve treatment outcomes and preventing programs in the group of pregnant women.

■ CONCLUSION

In summary, literature show mixed results regarding the influence of pathology of pregnancy on cognitive functions in pregnant women. Such results may ensue from lack of properly performed studies in this group of patients. More research is definitely needed, due to growing prevalence of diseases associated with pregnancy, which could potentially affect brain functions during pregnancy, postpartum, or exert deleterious effects on cognitive functions in later life.

Studies performed in this field may give interesting results, especially that women (during antenatal or postpartum period) report difficulties associated with domains of cognitive functions, like memory. So far, scarce amount of evidence showed by objective neuropsychological tests may result from cognitive brain capacity in young women, or be associated with mood disorders like depression.

Nonetheless, the assessment of cognitive functions in pregnant women, or the evaluation of how pathology of pregnancy affects cognition will bring essential data, which can be later utilized in creating novel preventing and therapeutic programs. Such programs could contribute to better quality of women's life and facilitate complying with recommendations made by healthcare professional.

Cognitive deterioration in pathologies such as, diabetes mellitus, obesity, or hypertensive disorders, shows how the whole body is connected. Even though, there are pathologies related to different organs, they still affect brain function and in this manner may impair processes such as memory, attention, or information processing, which we use every day to fulfill daily tasks and accomplish future goals.

■ REFERENCES

1. Barba-Müller E, Craddock S, Carmona S, Hoekzema E. Brain plasticity in pregnancy and the postpartum period: links to maternal caregiving and mental health. Arch Womens Ment Health. 2019;22(2):289-99.
2. Hoekzema E, Barba-Müller E, Pozzobon C, Picado M, Lucco F, García-García D, et al. Pregnancy leads to long-lasting changes in human brain structure. Nat Neurosci. 2017;20(2):287-96.
3. Luo H, Liang X, Cheng Z, Cai X, Feng F, Zhou H, et al. Effects of normal pregnancy on maternal EEG, TCD, and cerebral cortical volume. Brain Cogn. 2020;140:105526.
4. Henderson VW. Progesterone and human cognition. Climacteric. 2018;21(4):333-40.
5. Farrar D, Tuffnell D, Neill J, Scally A, Marshall K. Assessment of cognitive function across pregnancy using CANTAB: a longitudinal study. Brain Cogn. 2014;84(1):76-84.
6. Christensen H, Leach LS, Mackinnon A. Cognition in pregnancy and motherhood: prospective cohort study. Br J Psychiatry. 2010;196(2):126-32.
7. Henry JF, Sherwin BB. Hormones and cognitive functioning during late pregnancy and postpartum: a longitudinal study. Behav Neurosci. 2012;126(1):73-85.
8. Williams B, Mancia G, Spiering W, Rosei EA, Azizi M, Burnier M, et al.; ESC Scientific Document Group. 2018 ESC/ESH Guidelines for the management of arterial hypertension. Eur Heart J. 2018;39(33):3021-104.
9. Ying W, Catov JM, Ouyang P. Hypertensive disorders of pregnancy and future maternal cardiovascular risk. J Am Heart Assoc. 2018; 7(17):e009382.
10. Brown MA, Magee LA, Kenny LC, Karumanchi SA, McCarthy FP, Saito S, et al.; International Society for the Study of Hypertension in Pregnancy (ISSHP). The hypertensive disorders of pregnancy: ISSHP classification, diagnosis & management recommendations for international practice. Pregnancy Hypertens. 2018;13:291-310.

11. Markham K, Funai EF. Pregnancy-related hypertension. In: Creasy RK, Resnik R, Iams JD, Lockwood CJ, Moore TR, Greene M, et al. (Eds). Creasy and Resnik's Maternal-Fetal Medicine, 7th edition. Philadelphia: Elsevier; 2015. pp. 756-81.

12. Ferrer RL, Sibai BM, Mulrow CD, Chiquette E, Stevens KR, Cornell J. Management of mild chronic hypertension during pregnancy: a review. Obstet Gynecol. 2000;96(5 Pt 2):849-60.

13. Lin CC, Lindheimer MD, River P, Moawad AH. Fetal outcome in hypertensive disorders of pregnancy. Am J Obstet Gynecol. 1982; 142(3):255-60.

14. Report of the National High Blood Pressure Education Program Working Group on High Blood Pressure in Pregnancy. Am J Obstet Gynecol. 2000;183(1):S1-S22.

15. Williams D. Long-term complications of preeclampsia. Semin Nephrol. 2011;31(1): 111-22.

16. Bellamy L, Casas JP, Hingorani AD, Williams DJ. Pre-eclampsia and risk of cardiovascular disease and cancer in later life: systematic review and meta-analysis. BMJ. 2007; 335(7627):974.

17. ACOG Committee on Obstetric Practice. ACOG practice bulletin. Diagnosis and management of preeclampsia and eclampsia. Number 33, January 2002. American College of Obstetricians and Gynecologists. Int J Gynaecol Obstet. 2002;77(1):67-75.

18. Postma IR, Groen H, Easterling TR, Tsigas EZ, Wilson ML, Porcel J, et al. The brain study: cognition, quality of life and social functioning following preeclampsia; An observational study. Pregnancy Hypertens. 2013;3(4):227-34.

19. Gaugler-Senden IPM, Duivenvoorden HJ, Filius A, De Groot CJM, Steegers EAP, Passchier J. Maternal psychosocial outcome after early onset preeclampsia and preterm birth. J Matern Fetal Neonatal Med. 2012;25(3):272-6.

20. Caropreso L, de Azevedo Cardoso T, Eltayebani M, Frey BN. Preeclampsia as a risk factor for postpartum depression and psychosis: a systematic review and meta-analysis. Arch Womens Ment Health. 2020;23(4):493-505.

21. Culpepper L, Lam RW, McIntyre RS. Cognitive impairment in patients with depression: awareness, assessment, and management. J Clin Psychiatry. 2017;78(9):1383-94.

22. Jak AJ, Crocker LD, Aupperle RL, Clausen A, Bomyea J. Neurocognition in PTSD: treatment insights and implications. Curr Top Behav Neurosci. 2018;38:93-116.

23. Mielke MM, Milic NM, Weissgerber TL, White WM, Kantarci K, Mosley TH, et al. Impaired cognition and brain atrophy decades after hypertensive pregnancy disorders. Circ Cardiovasc Qual Outcomes. 2016;9(2 Suppl 1):S70-6.

24. Dayan N, Kaur A, Elharram M, Rossi AM, Pilote L. Impact of preeclampsia on long-term cognitive function. Hypertension. 2018;72(6):1374-80.

25. Postma IR, Bouma A, Ankersmit IF, Zeeman GG. Neurocognitive functioning following preeclampsia and eclampsia: a long-term follow-up study. Am J Obstet Gynecol. 2014;211(1):37.e1-9.

26. Fields JA, Garovic VD, Mielke MM, Kantarci K, Jayachandran M, White WM, et al. Pre-eclampsia and cognitive impairment later in life. Am J Obstet Gynecol. 2017;217(1):74.e1-74.e11.

27. Basit S, Wohlfahrt J, Boyd HA. Pre-eclampsia and risk of dementia later in life: nationwide cohort study. BMJ. 2018;363:k4109.

28. Amaral LM, Cunningham MW Jr, Cornelius DC, LaMarca B. Preeclampsia: long-term consequences for vascular health. Vasc Health Risk Manag. 2015;11:403-15.

29. Bartsch E, Medcalf KE, Park AL, Ray JG; High Risk of Pre-eclampsia Identification Group. Clinical risk factors for pre-eclampsia determined in early pregnancy: systematic review and meta-analysis of large cohort studies. BMJ. 2016;353:i1753.

30. Brouwers L, van der Meiden-van Roest AJ, Savelkoul C, Vogelvang TE, Lely AT, Franx A, et al. Recurrence of pre-eclampsia and the risk of future hypertension and cardiovascular disease: a systematic review and meta-analysis. BJOG. 2018;125(13):1642-54.

31. O'Brien JT, Thomas A. Vascular dementia. Lancet. 2015;386(10004):1698-706.

32. Filley CM, Fields RD. White matter and cognition: making the connection. J Neurophysiol. 2016;116(5):2093-104.

33. Schmahmann JD, Smith EE, Eichler FS, Filley CM. Cerebral white matter: neuroanatomy, clinical neurology, and neurobehavioral correlates. Ann N Y Acad Sci. 2008;1142: 266-309.

34. Filley CM, Franklin GM, Heaton RK, Rosenberg NL. White matter dementia: clinical disorders and implications. Neuro-psychiatry Neuropsychol Behav Neurol. 1988;1(4):239-54.

35. Aukes AM, de Groot JC, Aarnoudse JG, Zeeman GG. Brain lesions several years after eclampsia. Am J Obstet Gynecol. 2009;200(5):504.e1-5.

36. Aukes AM, De Groot JC, Wiegman MJ, Aarnoudse JG, Sanwikarja GS, Zeeman GG. Long-term cerebral imaging after pre-eclampsia. BJOG. 2012;119(9):1117-22.

37. Elharram M, Dayan N, Kaur A, Landry T, Pilote L. Long-term cognitive impairment after preeclampsia: a systematic review and meta-analysis. Obstet Gynecol. 2018; 132(2):355-64.

38. Poston L, McCarthy AL, Ritter JM. Control of vascular resistance in the maternal and feto-placental arterial beds. Pharmacol Ther. 1995;65(2):215-39.

39. Belfort MA, Tooke-Miller C, Allen JC Jr, Varner MA, Grunewald C, Nisell H, et al. Pregnant women with chronic hypertension and superimposed pre-eclampsia have high cerebral perfusion pressure. BJOG. 2001;108(11):1141-7.

40. Oehm E, Reinhard M, Keck C, Els T, Spreer J, Hetzel A. Impaired dynamic cerebral autoregulation in eclampsia. Ultrasound Obstet Gynecol. 2003;22(4):395-8.

41. Williams KP, Wilson S. Maternal cerebral blood flow changes associated with eclampsia. Am J Perinatol. 1995;12(3):189-91.

42. Cipolla MJ. Cerebrovascular function in pregnancy and eclampsia. Hypertension. 2007;50(1):14-24.

43. Hammer ES, Cipolla MJ. Cerebrovascular dysfunction in preeclamptic pregnancies. Curr Hypertens Rep. 2015;17(8):64.

44. Cipolla MJ. The adaptation of the cerebral circulation to pregnancy: mechanisms and consequences. J Cereb Blood Flow Metab. 2013;33(4):465-78.

45. Easton JD. Severe preeclampsia/eclampsia: hypertensive encephalopathy of pregnancy? Cerebrovasc Dis. 1998;8(1):53-8.

46. Donaldson JO. Eclamptic hypertensive encephalopathy. Semin Neurol. 1988;8(3): 230-3.

47. Ogoh S. Relationship between cognitive function and regulation of cerebral blood flow. J Physiol Sci. 2017;67(3):345-51.

48. Jones-Muhammad M, Warrington JP. Cerebral blood flow regulation in pregnancy, hypertension, and hypertensive disorders of pregnancy. Brain Sci. 2019;9(9):224.

49. Johansson BB. Effect of an acute increase of the intravascular pressure on the blood-brain barrier: a comparison between conscious and anesthetized rats. Stroke. 1978;9(6):588-90.

50. Obermeier B, Daneman R, Ransohoff RM. Development, maintenance and disruption of the blood-brain barrier. Nat Med. 2013;19(12):1584-96.

51. Schwartz RB, Feske SK, Polak JF, DeGirolami U, Iaia A, Beckner KM, et al. Preeclampsia-eclampsia: clinical and neuroradiographic correlates and insights into the pathogenesis of hypertensive encephalopathy. Radiology. 2000;217(2):371-6.

52. Szarka A, Rigó J Jr, Lázár L, Beko G, Molvarec A. Circulating cytokines, chemokines and adhesion molecules in normal pregnancy and preeclampsia determined by multiplex suspension array. BMC Immunol. 2010;11:59.

53. Ho YH, Lin YT, Wu CWJ, Chao YM, Chang AYW, Chan JYH. Peripheral inflammation increases seizure susceptibility via the induction of neuroinflammation and oxidative stress in the hippocampus. J Biomed Sci. 2015;22(1):46.

54. Li X, Han X, Bao J, Liu Y, Ye A, Thakur M, et al. Nicotine increases eclampsia-like

seizure threshold and attenuates microglial activity in rat hippocampus through the $\alpha 7$ nicotinic acetylcholine receptor. Brain Res. 2016;1642:487-96.

55. Castanon N, Lasselin J, Capuron L. Neuropsychiatric comorbidity in obesity: role of inflammatory processes. Front Endocrinol (Lausanne). 2014;5:74.

56. Joaquim AF, Appenzeller S. Neuropsychiatric manifestations in rheumatoid arthritis. Autoimmun Rev. 2015;14(12):1116-22.

57. Bowman GL, Dayon L, Kirkland R, Wojcik J, Peyratout G, Severin IC, et al. Blood-brain barrier breakdown, neuroinflammation, and cognitive decline in older adults. Alzheimers Dement. 2018;14(12):1640-50.

58. International Diabetes Federation (Ed). IDF Diabetes Atlas, 9th edition. Brussels: Belgium: International Diabetes Federation; 2019.

59. Weir GC, Laybutt DR, Kaneto H, Bonner-Weir S, Sharma A. Beta-cell adaptation and decompensation during the progression of diabetes. Diabetes. 2001;50(Suppl 1):S154-9.

60. Schwartz R, Gruppuso PA, Petzold K, Brambilla D, Hiilesmaa V, Teramo KA. Hyperinsulinemia and macrosomia in the fetus of the diabetic mother. Diabetes Care. 1994;17(7):640-8.

61. Esakoff TF, Cheng YW, Sparks TN, Caughey AB. The association between birthweight 4000 g or greater and perinatal outcomes in patients with and without gestational diabetes mellitus. Am J Obstet Gynecol. 2009;200(6):672.e1-4.

62. Shostrom DCV, Sun Y, Oleson JJ, Snetselaar LG, BaoW. History of gestational diabetes mellitus in relation to cardiovascular disease and cardiovascular risk fiactors in US women. Front Endocrinol (Lausanne). 2017;8:144.

63. Langer O, Yogev Y, Most O, Xenakis EMJ. Gestational diabetes: the consequences of not treating. Am J Obstet Gynecol. 2005; 192(4):989-97.

64. Peters RK, Kjos SL, Xiang A, Buchanan TA. Long-term diabetogenic effect of single pregnancy in women with previous gestational diabetes mellitus. Lancet. 1996;347(8996):227-30.

65. Tan PC, Ling LP, Omar SZ. The 50-g glucose challenge test and pregnancy outcome in a multiethnic Asian population at high risk for gestational diabetes. Int J Gynaecol Obstet. 2009;105(1):50-5.

66. Byrn M, Penckofer S. The relationship between gestational diabetes and antenatal depression. J Obstet Gynecol Neonatal Nurs. 2015;44(2):246-55.

67. Azami M, Badfar G, Soleymani A, Rahmati S. The association between gestational diabetes and postpartum depression: a systematic review and meta-analysis. Diabetes Res Clin Pract. 2019;149:147-55.

68. Lady K, Williams C, Hansen W, Epstein R. The relationship between gestational diabetes and postpartum depression. Am J Obstet Gynecol. 2013;208(1):S84.

69. von Kanel R, Mills PJ, Fainmam C, Dimsdale JE. Effects of psychological stress and psychiatric disorders on blood coagulation and fibrinolysis: A biobehavioral pathway to coronary artery disease? Psychosom Med. 2001;63(4):531-44.

70. Vacínová G, Vejražková D, Lukášová P, Lischková O, Dvořáková K, Rusina R, et al. Associations of polymorphisms in the candidate genes for Alzheimer's disease BIN1, CLU, CR1 and PICALM with gestational diabetes and impaired glucose tolerance. Mol Biol Rep. 2017;44(2):227-31.

71. Palta P, Schneider AL, Biessels GJ, Touradji P, Hill-Briggs F. Magnitude of cognitive dysfunction in adults with type 2 diabetes: a meta-analysis of six cognitive domains and the most frequently reported neuropsychological tests within domains. J Int Neuropsychol Soc. 2014;20(3):278-91.

72. van den Berg E, Kloppenborg RP, Kessels RPC, Kappelle LJ, Biessels GJ. Type 2 diabetes mellitus, hypertension, dyslipidemia and obesity: a systematic comparison of their impact on cognition. Biochim Biophys Acta. 2009;1792(5):470-81.

73. Spauwen PJJ, Kohler S, Verhey FRJ, Stehouwer CDA, van Boxtel MPJ. Effects of type 2 diabetes on 12-year cognitive change: results

from the Maastricht Aging Study. Diabetes Care. 2013;36(6):1554-61.

74. Matsuzaki T, Sasaki K, Tanizaki Y, Hata J, Fujimi K, Matsui Y, et al. Insulin resistance is associated with the pathology of Alzheimer disease: the Hisayama study. Neurology. 2010;75(9):764-70.

75. Maher PA, Schubert DR. Metabolic links between diabetes and Alzheimer's disease. Expert Rev Neurother. 2009;9(5):617-30.

76. Cheng G, Huang C, Deng H, Wang H. Diabetes as a risk factor for dementia and mild cognitive impairment: a meta-analysis of longitudinal studies. Intern Med J. 2012; 42(5):484-91.

77. Jayaraman A, Pike CJ. Alzheimer's disease and type 2 diabetes: multiple mechanisms contribute to interactions. Curr. Diab Rep. 2014;14(4):476.

78. Biessels GJ, Staekenborg S, Brunner E, Brayne C, Scheltens P. Risk of dementia in diabetes mellitus: a systematic review. Lancet Neurol. 2006;5(1):64-74.

79. Fontbonne A, Berr C, Ducimetire P, Alperovitch A. Changes in cognitive abilities over a 4-year period are unfavorably affected in elderly diabetic subjects: results of the Epidemiology of Vascular Aging Study. Diabetes Care. 2001;24(2):366-70.

80. Yaffe K, Blackwell T, Whitmer RA, Krueger K, Connor EB. Glycosylated hemoglobin level and development of mild cognitive impairment or dementia in older women. J Nutr Health Aging. 2006;10(4):293-5.

81. Cukierman-Yaffe T, Gerstein HC, Williamson JD, Lazar RM, Lovato L, Miller ME, et al.; Action to Control Cardiovascular Risk in Diabetes-Memory in Diabetes (ACCORD-MIND) Investigators. Relationship between baseline glycemic control and cognitive function in individuals with type 2 diabetes and other cardiovascular risk factors: the action to control cardiovascular risk in diabetes-memory in diabetes (ACCORD-MIND) trial. Diabetes Care. 2009;32(2):221-6.

82. Ahtiluoto S, Polvikoski T, Peltonen M, Solomon A, Tuomilehto J, Winblad B, et al. Diabetes, Alzheimer disease, and vascular dementia: a population-based neuropathologic study. Neurology. 2010; 75(13):1195-202.

83. Sonnen JA, Larson EB, Brickell K, Crane PK, Woltjer R, Montine TJ, et al. Different patterns of cerebral injury in dementia with or without diabetes. Arch Neurol. 2009;66(3):315-22.

84. Biessels GJ, Strachan MWJ, Visseren FLJ, Kappelle LJ, Whitmer RA. Dementia and cognitive decline in type 2 diabetes and prediabetic stages: towards targeted interventions. Lancet Diabetes Endocrinol. 2014;2(3):246-55.

85. Moheet A, Mangia S, Seaquist ER. Impact of diabetes on cognitive function and brain structure. Ann N Y Acad Sci. 2015;1353:60-71.

86. Kivipelto M, Helkala EL, Hanninen T, Laakso MP, Hallikainen M, Alhainen K, et al. Midlife vascular risk factors and late-life mild cognitive impairment: a population-based study. Neurology. 2001;56(12):1683-9.

87. DeCarli C, Miller BL, Swan GE, Reed T, Wolf PA, Carmelli D. Cerebrovascular and brain morphologic correlates of mild cognitive impairment in the National Heart, Lung, and Blood Institute Twin Study. Arch Neurol. 2001;58(4):643-7.

88. Hill CD, Stoudemire A, Morris R, Martino-Saltzman D, Markwalter HR. Similarities and differences in memory deficits in patients with primary dementia and depression-related cognitive dysfunction. J Neuropsychiatry Clin Neurosci. 1993;5(3):277-82.

89. van den Berg E, Reijmer YD, de Bresser J, Kessels RPC, Kappelle LJ, Biessels GJ; Utrecht Diabetic Encephalopathy Study Group. A 4 year follow-up study of cognitive functioning in patients with type 2 diabetes mellitus. Diabetologia. 2010;53(1):58-65.

90. Gregg EW, Yaffe K, Cauley JA, Rolka DB, Blackwell TL, Narayan KM, et al. Is diabetes associated with cognitive impairment and cognitive decline among older women? Study of Osteoporotic Fractures Research Group. Arch Intern Med. 2000;160(2):174-80.

91. Hassing LB, Grant MD, Hofer SM, Pedersen NL, Nilsson SE, Berg S, et al. Type 2 diabetes mellitus contributes to cognitive decline

in old age: a longitudinal population-based study. J Int Neuropsychol Soc. 2004; 10(4):599-607.

92. Yaffe K, Falvey C, Hamilton N, Schwartz AV, Simonsic EM, Satterfield S, et al. Diabetes, glucose control, and 9-year cognitive decline among older adults without dementia. Arch Neurol. 2012;69(9):1170-5.

93. Young SE, Mainous 3rd AG, Carnemolla M. Hyperinsulinemia and cognitive decline in a middle-aged cohort. Diabetes Care. 2006;29(12):2688-93.

94. Okereke O, Hankinson SE, Hu FB, Grodstein F. Plasma C peptide level and cognitive function among older women without diabetes mellitus. Arch Intern Med. 2005; 165(14):1651-6.

95. Baker LD, Cross DJ, Minoshima S, Belongia D, Watson GS, Craft S. Insulin resistance and Alzheimer-like reductions in regional cerebral glucose metabolism for cognitively normal adults with prediabetes or early type 2 diabetes. Arch Neurol. 2011;68(1):51-7.

96. Tabák AG, Akbaraly TN, Batty GD, Kivimäki M. Depression and type 2 diabetes: a causal association? Lancet Diabetes Endocrinol. 2014;2(3):236-45.

97. Becker S, Wojtowicz JM. A model of hippocampal neurogenesis in memory and mood disorders. Trends Cogn Sci. 2007;11(2):70-6.

98. Houben K, Dassen FCM, Jansen A. Taking control: working memory training in overweight individuals increases self-regulation of food intake. Appetite. 2016;105: 567-74.

99. Byun K, Bayarsaikhan E, Kim D, Kim CY, Mook-Jung I, Paek SH, et al. Induction of neuronal death by microglial AGE-albumin: implications for Alzheimer's disease. PLoS One. 2012;7(5):e37917.

100. Cukierman-Yaffe T. Diabetes, dysglycemia and cognitive dysfunction. Diabetes Metab Res Rev. 2014;30(5):341-5.

101. Munshi MN, Hayes M, Iwata I, Lee Y, Weinger K. Which aspects of executive dysfunction influence ability to manage diabetes in older adults? Diabet Med. 2012;29(9):1171-7.

102. Ryan CM, van Duinkerken E, Rosano C. Neurocognitive consequences of diabetes. Am Psychol. 2016;71(7):563-76.

103. Wang DQ, Wang L, Wei MM, Xia XS, Tian XL, Cui XH, et al. Relationship between type 2 diabetes and white matter hyperintensity: a systematic review. Front Endocrinol (Lausanne). 2020;11:595962.

104. Biessels GJ, Reijmer YD. Brain changes underlying cognitive dysfunction in diabetes: what can we learn from MRI? Diabetes. 2014;63(7):2244-52.

105. Hofmann W, Schmeichel BJ, Baddeley AD. Executive functions and self-regulation. Trends Cogn Sci. 2012;16(3):174-80.

106. Lavigne JE, Phelps CE, Mushlin A, Lednar WM. Reductions in individual work productivity associated with type 2 diabetes mellitus. Pharmacoeconomics. 2003;21(15): 1123-34.

107. World Health Organization. (2021). Obesity and Overweight. [online] Available from: https://www.who.int/news-room/fact-sheets/detail/obesity-and-overweight [Last accessed on February, 2022].

108. Guelinckx I, Devlieger R, Beckers K, Vansant G. Maternal obesity: pregnancy complications, gestational weight gain and nutrition. Obes Rev. 2008;9(2):140-50.

109. Leddy MA, Power ML, Schulkin J. The impact of maternal obesity on maternal and fetal health. Rev Obstet Gynecol. 2008;1(4):170-8.

110. Sebire NJ, Jolly M, Harris JP, Wadsworth J, Joffe M, Beard RW, et al. Maternal obesity and pregnancy outcome: a study of 287,213 pregnancies in London. Int J Obes Relat Metab Disord. 2001;25(8):1175-82.

111. Catalano PM, Ehrenberg HM. The short- and long-term implications of maternal obesity on the mother and her offspring. BJOG. 2006;113(10):1126-33.

112. Scott-Pillai R, Spence D, Cardwell C, Hunter A, Holmes VA. The impact of body mass index on maternal and neonatal outcomes: a retrospective study in a UK obstetric population, 2004–2011. BJOG. 2013;120(8): 932-9.

113. O'Reilly JR, Reynolds RM. The risk of maternal obesity to the long-term health

of the offspring. Clin Endocrinol (Oxf). 2013;78(1):9-16.

114. Stothard KJ, Tennant PWG, Bell R, Rankin J. Maternal overweight and obesity and the risk of congenital anomalies: a systematic review and meta-analysis. JAMA. 2009;301(6): 636-50.

115. Radzicka-Mularczyk SA, Pietryga M, Brazert J. How mother's obesity may affect the pregnancy and offspring. Ginekol Pol. 2020;91(12):769-72.

116. Lindsay KL, Brennan L, Rath A, Maguire OC, Smith T, McAuliffe FM. Gestational weight gain in obese pregnancy: impact on maternal and foetal metabolic parameters and birthweight. J Obstet Gynaecol. 2018; 38(1):60-5.

117. Vitner D, Harris K, Maxwell C, Farine D. Obesity in pregnancy: a comparison of four national guidelines. J Matern Fetal Neonatal Med. 2019;32(15):2580-90.

118. Bocarsly ME, Fasolino M, Kane GA, LaMarca EA, Kirschen GW, Karatsoreos IN, et al. Obesity diminishes synaptic markers, alters microglial morphology, and impairs cognitive function. Proc Natl Acad Sci U S A. 2015;112(51):15731-6.

119. Smith E, Hay P, Campbell L, Trollor JN. A review of the association between obesity and cognitive function across the lifespan: implications for novel approaches to prevention and treatment. Obes Rev. 2011;12(9):740-55.

120. Gunstad J, Lhotsky A, Wendell CR, Ferrucci L, Zonderman AB. Longitudinal examination of obesity and cognitive function: results from the Baltimore longitudinal study of aging. Neuroepidemiology. 2010;34(4):222-9.

121. Coppin G, Nolan-Poupart S, Jones-Gotman M, Small DM. Working memory and reward association learning impairments in obesity. Neuropsychologia. 2014;65:146-55.

122. Whitmer RA, Gustafson DR, Barrett-Connor E, Haan MN, Gunderson EP, Yaffe K. Central obesity and increased risk of dementia more than three decades later. Neurology. 2008;71(14):1057-64.

123. Hassing LB, Dahl AK, Thorvaldsson V, Berg S, Gatz M, Pedersen NL, et al. Overweight in midlife and risk of dementia: a 40-year follow-up study. Int J Obes (Lond). 2009;33(8):893-8.

124. Anstey KJ, Cherbuin N, Budge M, Young J. Body mass index in midlife and late-life as a risk factor for dementia: a meta-analysis of prospective studies. Obes Rev. 2011; 12(5):e426-37.

125. Miller J, Kransler J, Liu Y, Schmalfuss I, Theriaque DW, Shuster JJ, et al. Neurocognitive findings in Prader-Willi syndrome and early-onset morbid obesity. J Pediatr. 2006;149(2):192-8.

126. Miller JL, Couch J, Schwenk K, Long M, Towler S, Theriaque DW, et al. Early childhood obesity is associated with compromised cerebellar development. Dev Neuropsychol. 2009;34(3):272-83.

127. Stinson EJ, Krakoff J, Gluck ME. Depressive symptoms and poorer performance on the Stroop Task are associated with weight gain. Physiol Behav. 2018;186:25-30.

128. Rasmussen KM, Yaktine AL (Eds). Weight Gain During Pregnancy: Reexamining the Guidelines. Washington, DC: The National Academies Press; 2009.

129. Galtier-Dereure F, Boegner C, Bringer J. Obesity and pregnancy: complications and cost. Am J Clin Nutr. 2000;71(5 Suppl): 1242S-8S.

130. Stotland NE, Hopkins LM, Caughey AB. Gestational weight gain, macrosomia, and risk of cesarean birth in nondiabetic nulliparas. Obstet Gynecol. 2004;104(4):671-7.

131. Hilson JA, Rasmussen KM, Kjolhede CL. Excessive weight gain during pregnancy is associated with earlier termination of breast-feeding among White women. J Nutr. 2006;136(1):140-6.

132. Sui Z, Turnbull DA, Dodd JM. Overweight and obese women's perceptions about making healthy change during pregnancy: a mixed method study. Matern Child Health J. 2013;17(10):1879-87.

133. Baik JH. Dopamine signaling in reward-related behaviors. Front Neural Circuits. 2013;7:152.

134. Stice E, Spoor S, Bohon C, Small DM. Relation between obesity and blunted striatal

response to food is moderated by TaqIA A1 allele. Science. 2008;322(5900):449-52.

135. Robinson TE, Berridge KC. The neural basis of drug craving: an incentive-sensitization theory of addiction. Brain Res Rev. 1993;18(3): 247-91.

136. Volkow ND, Fowler JS, Wang GJ. Role of dopamine in drug reinforcement and addiction in humans: results from imaging studies. Behav Pharmacol. 2002;13(5-6): 355-66.

137. Nederkoorn C, Braet C, Van Eijs Y, Tanghe A, Jansen A. Why obese children cannot resist food: the role of impulsivity. Eat Behav. 2006;7(4):315-22.

138. Yokum S, Marti CN, Smolen A, Stice E. Relation of the multilocus genetic composite reflecting high dopamine signaling capacity to future increases in BMI. Appetite. 2015; 87:38-45.

139. Stice E, Burger K. Neural vulnerability factors for obesity. Clin Psychol Rev. 2019;68:38-53.

140. Bourassa K, Sbarra DA. Body mass and cognitive decline are indirectly associated via inflammation among aging adults. Brain Behav Immun. 2017;60:63-70.

141. Solas M, Milagro FI, Ramírez MJ, Martínez JA. Inflammation and gut-brain axis link obesity to cognitive dysfunction: plausible pharmacological interventions. Curr Opin Pharmacol. 2017;37:87-92.

142. Otero TM, Barker LA. The frontal lobes and executive functioning. In: Goldstein S, Naglieri JA (Eds). Handbook of Executive Functioning. New York: Springer; 2014. pp. 29-44.

143. Bieliński M, Lesiewska N, Junik R, Kamińska A, Tretyn A, Borkowska A. Dopaminergic genes polymorphisms and prefrontal cortex efficiency among obese people - whether gender is a differentiating factor? Curr Mol Med. 2019;19(6):405-18.

144. Blau LE, Hormes JM. Preventing excess gestational weight gain and obesity in pregnancy: the potential of targeting psychological mechanisms. Curr Obes Rep. 2020;9(4):522-9.

145. da Luz FQ, Hay P, Wisniewski L, Cordás T, Sainsbury A. The treatment of binge eating disorder with cognitive behavior therapy and other therapies: an overview and clinical considerations. Obes Rev; 2020.

146. Gavin NI, Gaynes BN, Lohr KN, Meltzer-Brody S, Gartlehner G, Swinson T. Perinatal depression: a systematic review of prevalence and incidence. Obstet Gynecol. 2005;106(5 Pt 1):1071-83.

147. Lee DTS, Chung TKH. Postnatal depression: an update. Best Pract Res Clin Obstet Gynaecol. 2007;21(2):183-91.

148. Van den Bergh BRH, Mulder EJH, Mennes M, Glover V. Antenatal maternal anxiety and stress and the neurobehavioral development of the fetus and child: links and possible mechanisms. A review. Neurosci Biobehav Rev. 2005;29(2):237-58.

149. Goedhart G, Snijders AC, Hesselink AE, van Poppel MN, Bonsel GJ, Vrijkotte TGM. Maternal depressive symptoms in relation to perinatal mortality and morbidity: results from a large multiethnic cohort study. Psychosom Med. 2010;72(8):769-76.

150. Bowen A, Muhajarine N. Prevalence of antenatal depression in women enrolled in an outreach program in Canada. J Obstet Gynecol Neonatal Nurs. 2006;35(4):491-8.

151. Bowen A, Muhajarine N. Antenatal depression. Can Nurse. 2006;102(9):26-30.

152. Bennett HA, Einarson A, Taddio A, Koren G, Einarson TR. Prevalence of depression during pregnancy: systematic review. Obstet Gynecol. 2004;103(4):698-709.

153. Amgalan A, Andescavage N, Limperopoulos C. Prenatal origins of neuropsychiatric diseases. Acta Paediatr. 2021;110(6):1741-9.

154. Maternal depression and child development. Paediatr Child Health. 2004;9(8):575-98.

155. Macbeth AH, Luine VN. Changes in anxiety and cognition due to reproductive experience: a review of data from rodent and human mothers. Neurosci Biobehav Rev. 2010;34(3):452-67.

156. Keenan PA, Yaldoo DT, Stress ME, Fuerst DR, Ginsburg KA. Explicit memory in pregnant women. Am J Obstet Gynecol. 1998;179(3 Pt 1):731-7.

157. Mazor E, Sheiner E, Wainstock T, Attias M, Walfisch A. The association between depressive state and maternal cognitive function in postpartum women. Am J Perinatol. 2019; 36(3):285-90.

158. Zlatar ZZ, Moore RC, Palmer BW, Thompson WK, Jeste DV. Cognitive complaints correlate with depression rather than concurrent objective cognitive impairment in the successful aging evaluation baseline sample. J Geriatr Psychiatry Neurol. 2014;27(3):181-7.

159. Logan DM, Hill KR, Jones R, Holt-Lunstad J, Larson MJ. How do memory and attention change with pregnancy and childbirth? A controlled longitudinal examination of neuropsychological functioning in pregnant and postpartum women. J Clin Exp Neuropsychol. 2014;36(5):528-39.

160. Hohman TJ, Beason-Held LL, Resnick SM. Cognitive complaints, depressive symptoms, and cognitive impairment: are they related? J Am Geriatr Soc. 2011;59(10):1908-12.

161. De Lissnyder E, Koster EHW, Everaert J, Schacht R, Van den Abeele D, De Raedt R. Internal cognitive control in clinical depression: general but no emotion-specific impairments. Psychiatry Res. 2012;199(2):124-30.

162. Dalby RB, Frandsen J, Chakravarty MM, Ahdidan J, Sørensen L, Rosenberg R, et al. Correlations between Stroop task performance and white matter lesion measures in late-onset major depression. Psychiatry Res. 2012;202(2):142-9.

163. Black S, Kraemer K, Shah A, Simpson G, Scogin F, Smith A. Diabetes, depression, and cognition: a recursive cycle of cognitive dysfunction and glycemic dysregulation. Curr Diab Rep. 2018;18(11):118.

164. Lasserre AM, Glaus J, Vandeleur CL, Marques-Vidal P, Vaucher J, Bastardot F, et al. Depression with atypical features and increase in obesity, body mass index, waist circumference, and fat mass: a prospective, population-based study. JAMA Psychiatry. 2014;71(8):880-8.

165. Bieliński M, Jaracz M, Lesiewska N, Tomaszewska M, Sikora M, Junik R, et al. Association between COMTVal158Met and DAT1 polymorphisms and depressive symptoms in the obese population. Neuropsychiatr Dis Treat. 2017;13:2221-9.

166. Mansur RB, Brietzke E, McIntyre RS. Is there a "metabolic-mood syndrome"? A review of the relationship between obesity and mood disorders. Neurosci Biobehav Rev. 2015; 52:89-104.

167. van Duinkerken E, Snoek FJ. Interaction between diabetes and depression: consequences for cognition and the brain. Int J Clin Rev. 2012;23:69-78.

168. Sullivan MD, Katon WJ, Lovato LC, Miller ME, Murray AM, Horowitz KR, et al. Association of depression with accelerated cognitive decline among patients with type 2 diabetes in the ACCORD-MIND trial. JAMA Psychiatry. 2013;70(10):1041-7.

169. Watari K, Elderkin-Thompson V, Ajilore O, Haroon E, Darwin C, Pham D, et al. Neuroanatomical correlates of executive functioning in depressed adults with type 2 diabetes. J Clin Exp Neuropsychol. 2008; 30(4):389-97.

Kurjak's Antenatal Neurodevelopmental Test: Protocol for Evaluating Fetal Neurology In Utero

Panagiotis Antsaklis, Asim Kurjak

◼ INTRODUCTION

Fetal behavior during in utero life is one of the most challenging fields in fetal medicine. The advances of ultrasound technology allow direct observation of the fetus in real time, so that movements, expressions, and fetal reactions can be studied and monitored.[1-3] Since the application of modern technology particularly four-dimensional (4D) ultrasonographic technology allows evaluation of in utero anatomical survey and activity at the same time, with explicit detail. Structured evaluation of the fetus in utero both anatomically and in terms of activity–motility led to the understanding of the pattern and the steps that fetal neurological development goes through every week of gestational age.[4]

Human brain is a very complicated organ both from anatomic and functional point of view, and the developmental process of the human brain starts early during in utero life and carries on for many months or even years after birth, being influenced by many genetic and epigenetic factors.[4] The basic steps of neurodevelopment are demonstrated in **Table 1**. The fact that neurodevelopment is multifactorial and can be affected by many parameters makes it difficult to identify, if disrupted at any time, exactly when did that happen, especially during in utero life. This is even more difficult for preterm infants, particularly for infants of extreme prematurity, which are very sensitive and prone to many incidents that can affect their

TABLE 1: Neurodevelopment: the basic steps.[4]

Neurodevelopment	Age
Initial formation of neurons	3–4 weeks of pregnancy
Formation of prosencephalon	5–6 weeks of pregnancy
Increase of neuron number: • Cerebral • Cerebellar	8–16 weeks of pregnancy 2 months to 1 year after delivery
Migration of neurons: • Cerebral • Cerebellar	14–22 weeks of pregnancy 16–40 weeks of pregnancy
Differentiation of neurons: • Axonal increase • Dendritic increase—synapsis	14 weeks—delivery 6–12 months after birth
Formation of synapsis	From delivery—years after birth
Myelin increase	From delivery—years after birth

neurodevelopment, without being able to identify when exactly the incident occurred, during in utero life, during labor, or sometime after birth, and exactly how severely will it affect it, and when exactly will the problem be diagnosed, as it is mostly diagnosed after birth and sometimes long after birth.[4-6] The main reason why almost all cases of neurological impairment are diagnosed after birth is because there is no standardized method of assessing the fetus neurologically in utero.[6,7] Kurjak's antenatal neurodevelopmental test (KANET) aims to fill in this gap in fetal medicine as the philosophy of this method is to change the way we examine the fetus and with the assistance of 4D ultrasound perform a complete examination as we would do with a neonate.

FROM FETAL MOVEMENTS TO FETAL NEUROBEHAVIOR

Similarly with neonates, fetal cerebral integrity is represented up to a point by its behavior.[8,9] It has been shown that optimal fetal movements are excellent indicators of fetal neurological condition[10-17] and this can be assessed and confirmed with relatively good sensitivity with the classical two-dimensional (2D) ultrasound.[18-21]

De Vries was one of the pioneers who worked on fetal movements and managed to describe and categorize them through gestational age according to each stage of fetal development:

- *Sideways bending*: From seventh to eighth week, subtle movements at one or both fetal poles with very short duration of up to 2 seconds.
- *Startle*: From eighth week. Sharp contraction like movements of the extremities.
- *General movements (GMs)*: From the 8th week. The first complex movements

that involve all body parts. They are not distinctive and have variable pattern and duration.

- *Hiccups*: From 9th week. Irregular spasms of the fetal diaphragm with variable duration, rhythm, or in combination with limb movements.
- *Breathing-like*: From 10th week. Less irregular diaphragmatic mobility that forms characteristic movement of the thorax.
- *Isolated arm or leg movement*: From the 10th week. Variable intensity and duration. Consist of full limb movements including rotating and bending-extending and also movements to and away from the body.
- *Twitches*: Quick single isolated bending and extending movements of limbs and head.
- *Clonic movements*: Quick movements of the limbs 1–3 every second.
- *Head movements—retroflecting*: From 10th week. Irregular movements of the head are of variable speed.
- *Head movements—rotational*: Slow rotational neck movements to either side and back to the midline.
- *Head movements—anteflecting*: Slow, short-lasting small degree anteflexion of the head.
- *Jaw movements*: From 11th week. Irregular movements of the jaw with variable intensity, duration, and degree.
- *Sucking and swallowing*: From 13th week. These movements have a rhythmical pattern that are combined with the swallowing of amniotic fluid.
- *Hand–head contact*: From 10th week. Distinct movement of the upper extremity toward the face with the first movements of the fingers being distinct.

This activity can be further subdivided to:
Movements of hand to:

- Head and mouth
- Close to mouth
- Face
- Close to face
- Eye
- Ear

As development of fetal brain follows a very specific way of development, studies show the type of fetal motility with the overall fetal activity for each trimester could represent an expected or abnormal condition.[21-24] Direct observation of the fetus with 4D ultrasound changed the way fetal behavior is assessed and allowed examination of details that could not be seen before, such facial expressions and detailed finger movements.[24-30]

Many studies have applied 3D and 4D ultrasound in order to study in utero behavior confirming first of all that is possible and which parameters can be indicative of underlying neurological pathology.[31-34] New ultrasonographic technologies and mainly 4D allow examination of fetal condition comparable to how we would examine newborns and develop the behavioral developmental status of the fetus that should be expected for each trimester of pregnancy in order to define which behavioral patterns are normal for each trimester and what could be abnormal.[1-4,18-23,35] KANET was a new method studying fetal neurologic activity real time with direct observation via 4D ultrasonography in accordance to a postnatal assessment.[36-39]

KURJAK'S ANTENATAL NEURODEVELOPMENTAL TEST

Kurjak's antenatal neurodevelopmental test is a new method that studies in utero fetal activity with 4D ultrasound, following almost the same protocol that is used to assess a neonate postnatally so that KANET can define normal fetal behavior for each stage of pregnancy and on the other hand to identify abnormal conditions that could be related to neurologic impairment.[36,48,79] KANET has a general part that includes fetal GMs and the parameters modified by the neonatal assessment, the so-called Amiel-Tison Neurological Assessment at Term (ATNAT) signs.[37,40] KANET test consists of the following characteristics: isolated head anteflexion, overlapping cranial sutures, head circumference, isolated eye blinking, facial alterations, mouth opening (yawning or mouthing), isolated hand and leg movements, and thumb position, gestalt perception of GMs (overall perception of the body and limb movements with their qualitative assessment).[44-49]

Basic principle for KANET is the proven continuity of fetal behavior that exists after birth and the fact that when neonatal activity is compared to fetal activity, they are very similar except for one reflex (Moro's) that depends on gravity,[41,49] and that difference is explained by the lack in gravity between in utero and postnatal life.[6]

Kurjak's antenatal neurodevelopmental test follows standardized protocol, studies show good reproduction between different examiners and a number of minimum cases for training has been established (about 80 cases) which is very acceptable for medical stuff with ultrasound knowledge.[42,43,54] KANET must be applied not earlier than the 28th week of pregnancy and the duration of the test should last about 15–20 minutes, with the test been performed ideally should be performed with the fetus being in active state and not in sleeping mode. In cases that the test cannot be completed, a repeat test should be attempted after half an hour and when still not possible a new test should take part the following day, but not before 14–16 hours.

If the result is characterized pathological or so called borderline, repeat examinations should be scheduled after 15 days. The parameters that have to be more thoroughly examined are movements of the face and of the eyes—"the face is the mirror of the brain" and also fetal movements should be noted **(Figs. 1 to 6)**.[40,42]

The minimum requirements of the ultrasound machine when applying KANET should be, frame rate ≥24 volumes/sec. The latest version of KANET has eight characteristics parameters **(Table 2)**. Accordingly the final score of the test can have three options: (1) abnormal (score number 0–5), (2) borderline (score number 6–13), and (3) normal (score number 14–20) **(Table 3)**. In order for the test to be complete ideally all fetuses undergoing KANET antenatally should also be examined and followed up for 24 months after delivery.

The three groups of the scoring system categorize all cases into low risk, borderline, and high risk, in order to categorize the cases for clinical practice. For pathological cases with severe anatomical or chromosomal abnormalities it has been confirmed that KANET can identify the degree of motoric disability, while in all cases the prognostic value of the test has been verified postnatally, while prognostic value of KANET for neurological impairment has been confirmed in high-risk cases.[50-60]

Success rate of KANET has been calculated to 91–95% and for specific parameters of KANET the completion rate ranged from >85% for eye opening to 100% for mouth opening and isolated leg movement with an almost 100% negative predictive value. Interobserver agreement between two examiners for different components of the KANET test were assessed by calculation of Kappa values which were lowest for the facial expression (K = 0.68) and highest for the finger movements (K = 0.84), proving that KANET test is a reliable method to be used in clinical practice, after appropriate training.

Evolution of Kurjak's Antenatal Neurodevelopmental Test

First form of KANET scoring system as applied by Andonotopo et al.[55] who aimed to assess whether facial expression and body movements could be of any diagnostic value regarding cerebral palsy (CP) in growth restricted fetuses. And noticed decreased behavioral activity in the intrauterine growth restriction (IUGR) fetuses compared to the non-IUGR. This initiated the idea for the development of KANET which started by comparing neonates with neurological impairment and compared them with normal neonates and applied these differences in fetuses by 4D ultrasound, in order to detect these neurological problems prenatally. The first application of KANET was retrospective in low- and high-risk cases. The abnormal KANET scores included four cases with Alobar holoprosencephaly, one with severe hydrocephaly, one with thanatophoric dysplasia, and four cases with multiple severe structural abnormalities. This study **(Table 4)** initiated a cascade of other studies which followed the next years.[25,32]

A recent paper with almost 300 cases showed that most cases with abnormal KANET result ended with stillbirth or opted for termination of pregnancy due to other comorbidities as well. From the remaining pathological KANET results half of them had also a pathological postdelivery neurological assessment, confirming a positive predictive value between KANET. What was also important was the fact that in these cases the facial expressions were characteristically decreased.

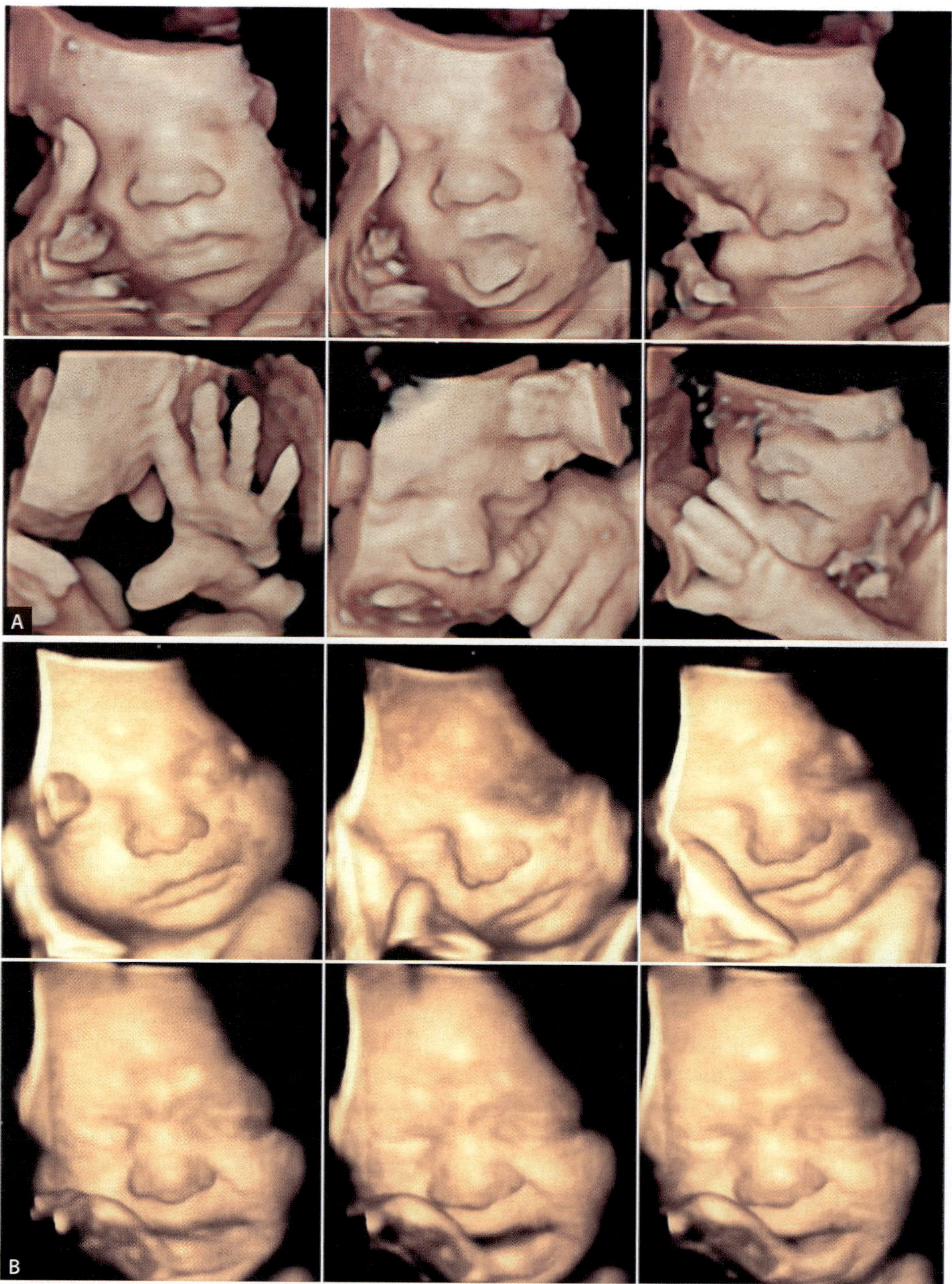

Figs. 1A and B: Pictures that show parameters of Kurjak's antenatal neurodevelopmental test (KANET) especially of the face and hands.

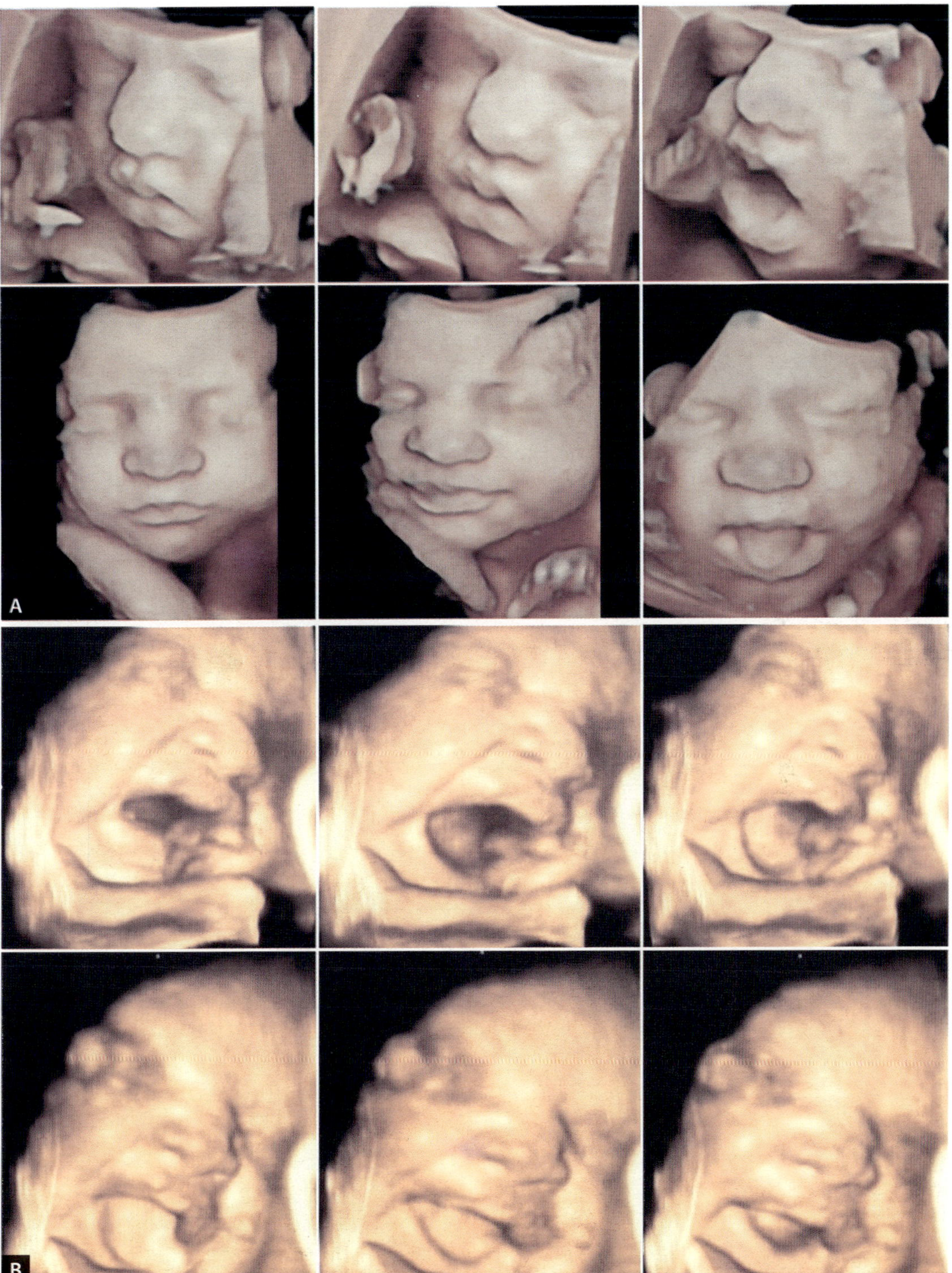

Figs. 2A and B: Parameters of the test that verify the integrity of fetal behavior.

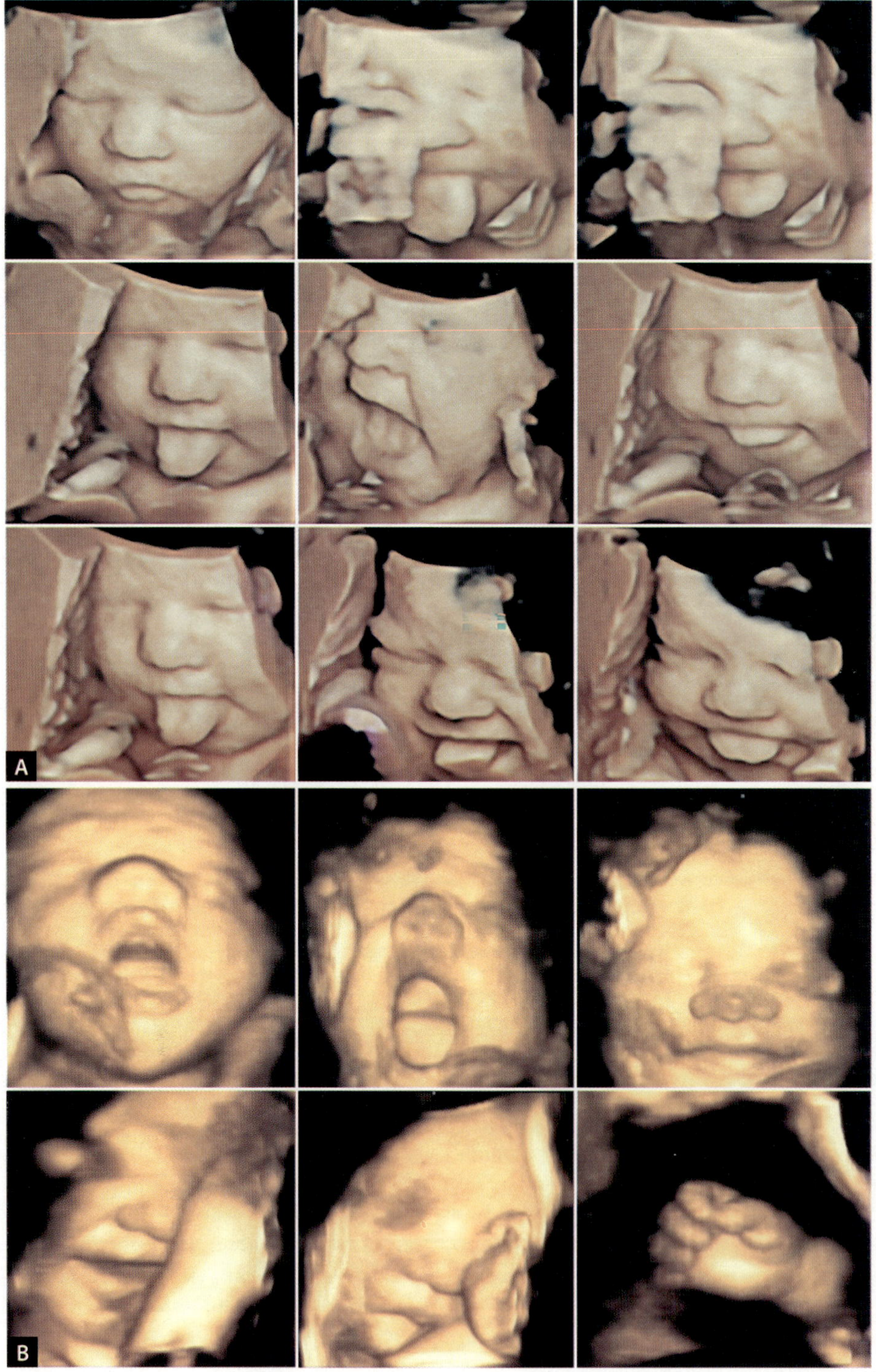

Figs. 3A and B

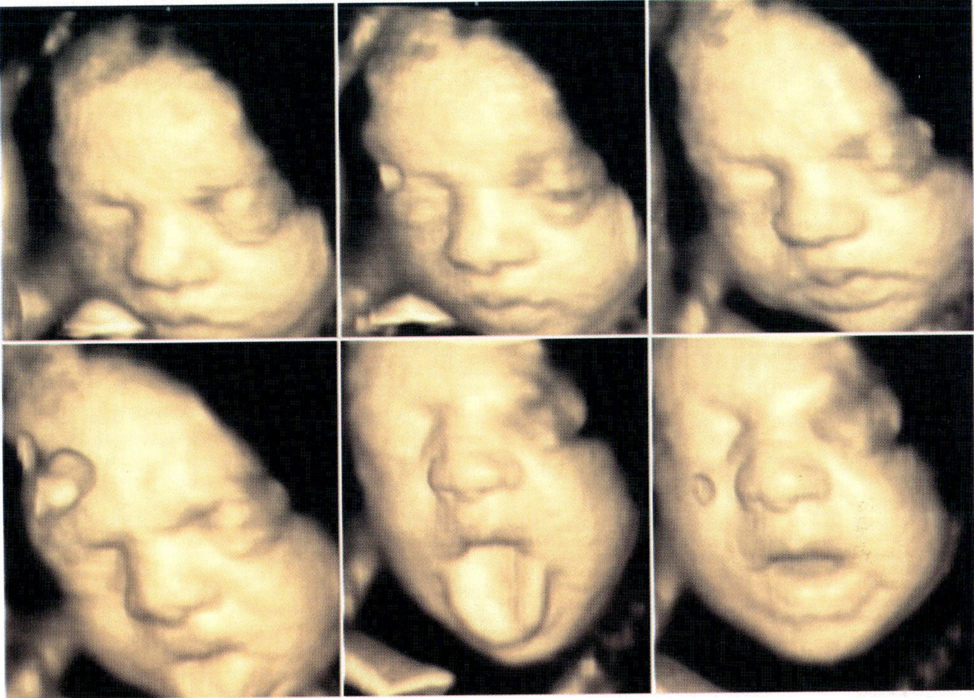

Fig. 3C

Figs. 3A to C: Mouthing and yawning as parts of the fetal assessment that verify the integrity of the fetus.

By studying a fetus with severe central nervous system (CNS) abnormality (acrania) whose mother opted to continue the pregnancy and had follow-ups in the second half of pregnancy, it was observed that as the pregnancy advanced the KANET result was deteriorating and that was attributed to the migration of the CNS centers to the cerebrum, proving the theory that impairment of neurologic status can occur at any stage of pregnancy.[50] In a study where three abnormal cases were identified all of them were confirmed postnatally as they had a chromosomal abnormality.[54]

Through these initial studies it was confirmed that the neonatal examination (ATNAT) showed similar results with the prenatal examination (KANET), confirming the value of KANET. KANET was also applied to high-risk cases of different types of fetal, maternal, or antenatal conditions.[53]

It was shown a difference in these cases compared to normal cases with more characteristic those with past pregnancy that led to neonate with severe neurological impairment while interestingly notable differences were also documented in the group of maternal fever, possibly attributed to chorioamnionitis (56.4%). The conclusion was that the result of KANET is directly related with the neurologic status ante- and postnatally and mainly a pathological score increases the risk of adverse outcome even death. Additionally the good predictive value of the test was confirmed for both for normal and abnormal conditions which can be confirmed postnatally. The good prognostic value of a normal KANET was confirmed in a

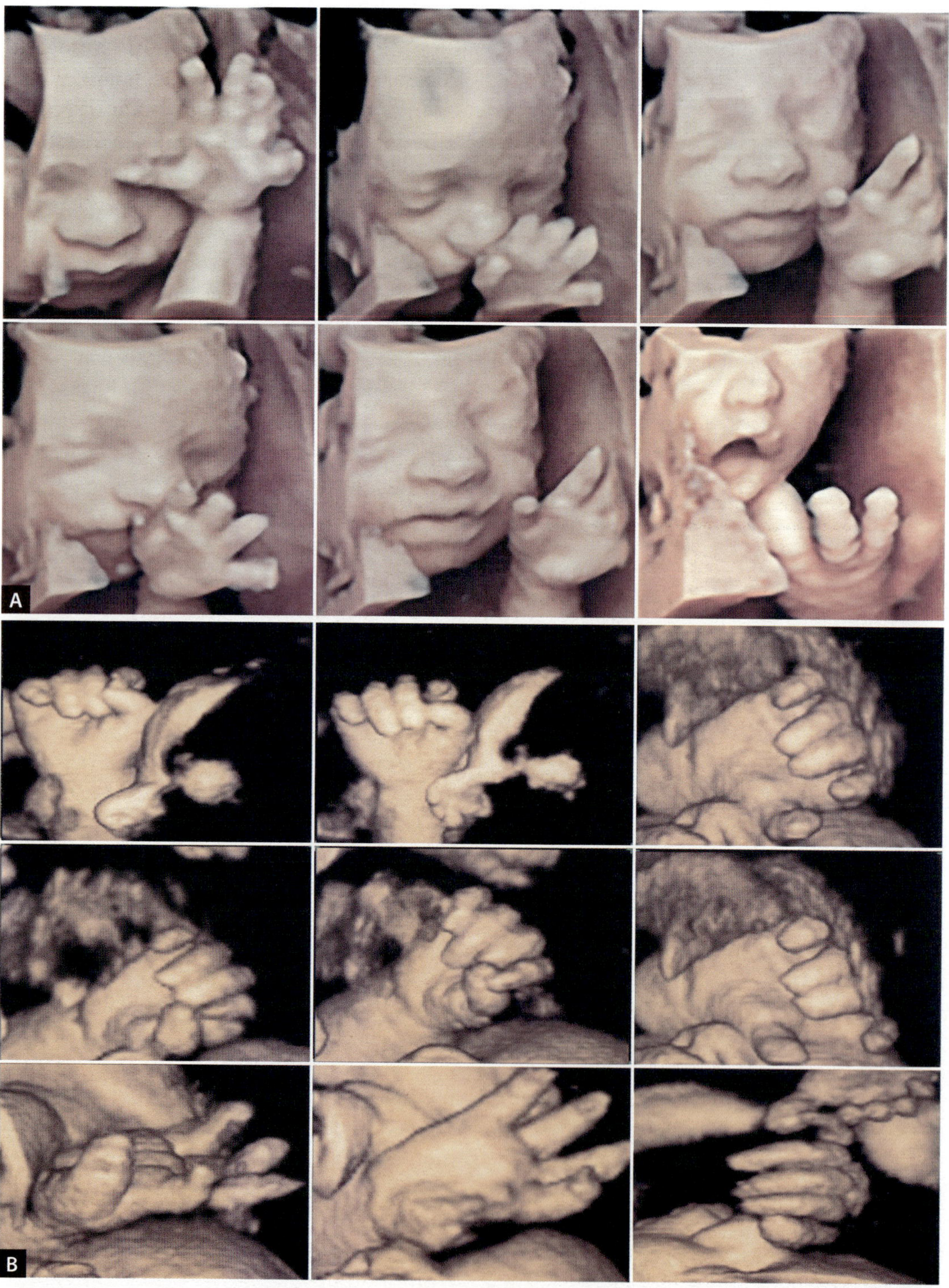

Figs. 4A and B: The fetal activity and especially small movements are important parts of the protocol.

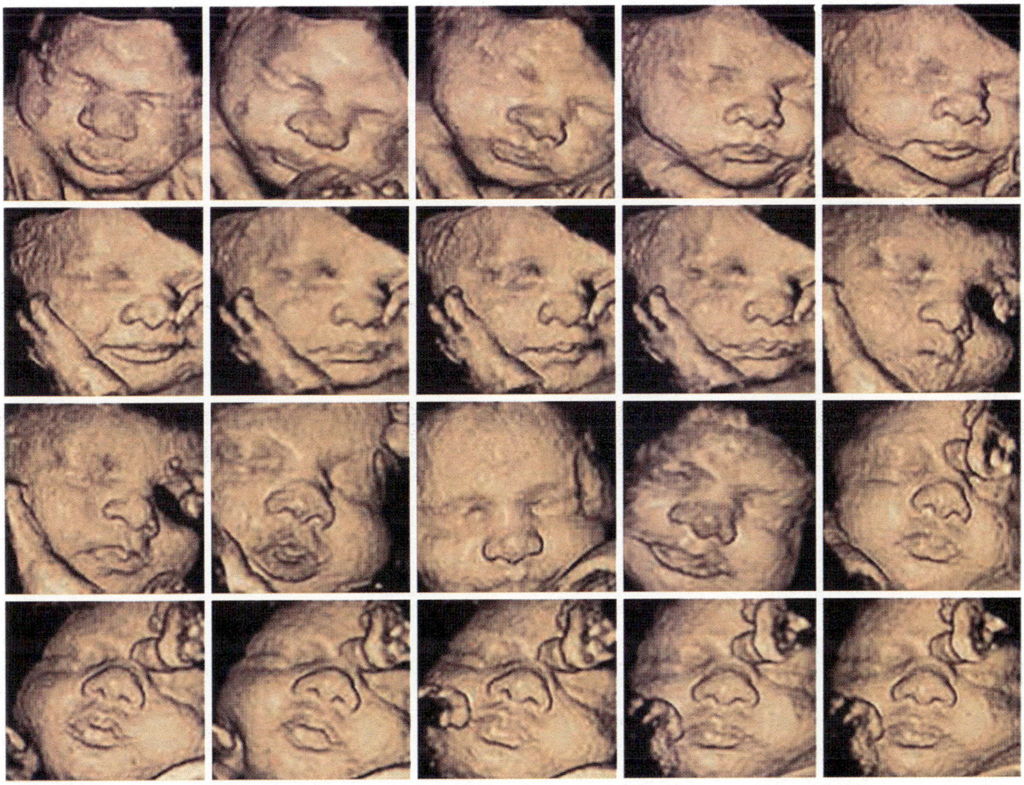

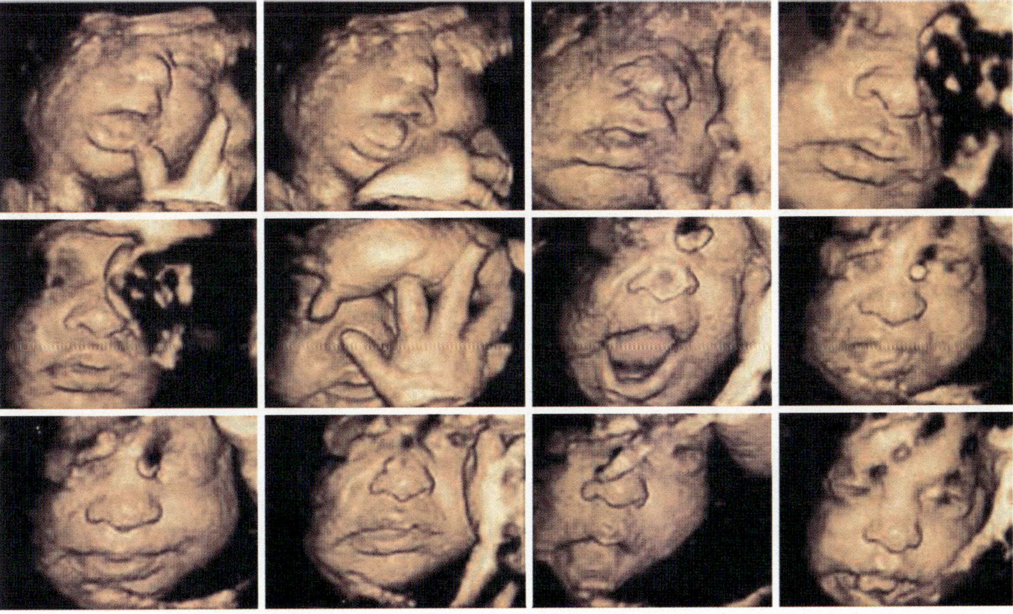

Fig. 5: Third trimester of pregnancy neurobehavior assessment.

Fig. 6: Completion of all parameters for the scoring system of Kurjak's antenatal neurodevelopmental test (KANET).

TABLE 2: The protocol of Kurjak's antenatal neurodevelopmental test (KANET).[43]

Sign	Score 0	Score 1	Score 2	Sign score
Isolated head anteflexion	Abrupt	Small range (0–3 times of movements)	Variable in full range, many alteration (>3 times of movements)	
Cranial sutures and head circumference (HC)	Overlapping of cranial sutures	Normal cranial sutures with measurement of HC below or above the normal limit (–2 SD) according to GA	Normal cranial sutures with normal measurement of HC according to GA	
Isolated eye blinking	Not present	Not fluent (1–5 times of blinking)	Fluency (>5 times of blinking)	
Facial alteration (grimace or tongue expulsion) or Mouth opening (yawning or mouthing)	Not present	Not fluent (1–5 times of alteration)	Fluency (>5 times of alteration)	
Isolated leg movement	Cramped	Poor repertoire or small in range (0–5 times of movement)	Variable in full range, many alteration (>5 times of movements)	

Contd...

Contd...

Sign	Score			Sign score
	0	**1**	**2**	
Isolated hand movement	Cramped or abrupt	Poor repertoire or small in range (0–5 times of movement)	Variable in full range, many alteration (>5 times of movements)	
or Hand to face movements				
Fingers' movements	Unilateral or bilateral clenched fist, (neuro-logical thumb)	Cramped invariable finger movements	Smooth and complex, variable finger movements	
Gestalt perception of GMs	Definitely abnormal	Borderline	Normal	
			Total score	

(GA: gestational age; GM: general movement; SD: standard deviation)

TABLE 3: The scoring system of the test.[43]	
Total score	**Interpretation**
0–5	Abnormal
6–9	Borderline
10–16	Normal

study with 100 cases and a neonatal follow-up up to 3 months.[61]

In attempt to extend this fetal monitoring Lebit et al.[27] started observing fetal behavior from 7 weeks up to 38 weeks and noticed in early pregnancy the fetal activity increases as does the quality of the motility. After 20 weeks the movements in utero become more frequent and variable, as specific motoric skills (facial grimacing and eye blinking) from the second half of the second trimester. As fetal movements decrease during the final weeks of pregnancy, this is due to fetal cerebral maturation, and KANET aims to reflect the different levels of maturation during in utero life.[25-27] Comparing low-risk with high-risk fetuses for neurological problems (ventriculomegaly) by application of KANET, significant differences were shown between the two groups, while the wider the degree of ventriculomegaly, or the presence of other anomalies the lower was the KANET score.[56]

An important finding of this study was that for cases of mild ventriculomegaly with no other findings KANET was normal and that was confirmed postnatally, revealing an additional importance of KANET, for the counseling of pregnancies where an anatomical finding is evident, but the significance of this finding for the neurodevelopment of this neonate is inadequate.

TABLE 4: Summary of studies on fetal neurology.

Author	Year	Study	Study design	Study population	Indication	No.	GA (weeks)	Time (minutes)	Result	Summary
Kurjak et al.[34]	2008	Cohort	Retrospective	High risk	Multiple	220	20–36	30	Positive	Application of a new method for fetal neurology assessment
Kurjak et al.[24]	2010	Multi-center	Prospective	High risk	Multiple	288	20–38	30	Positive	The significance of the test for detection of neurological problems was proven especially in cases where severe abnormalities from CNS or chromosomal abnormalities were also present
Miskovic et al.[54]	2010	Cohort	Prospective	High risk	Multiple	226	20–36	30	Positive	The findings of the test in utero were compared to findings of assessment of neonates postnatally and differences between different risk categories were identified
Talic et al.[53]	2011	Multi-center Cohort	Prospective	High risk	Multiple	620	26–38	15–20	Positive	Pathological antenatal KANET results were found to have strong correlation with adverse fetal or neonatal outcome and distinguish among in utero conditions
Talic et al.[56]	2011	Multi-center Cohort	Prospective	High risk	Ventri-culomegaly	240	32–36	10–15	Positive	The degree of ventriculomegaly was directly related to a poorer outcome and prognosis of the fetus, especially when in combination with ventriculomegaly other comorbidities existed
Honemeyer et al.[61]	2011	Cohort	Prospective	Unselected	Unselected	100	28–38	N/A	Positive	The negative prognostic value of KANET was confirmed

Contd...

Contd...

Author	Year	Study	Study design	Study population	Indication	No.	GA (weeks)	Time (minutes)	Result	Summary
Lebit et al.[27]	2011	Cohort	Prospective	Low risk	Normal 2D examination	144	7–38	15–20	Positive	The in utero development of fetal nervous maturation as expressed by behavioral patterns was clarified for each trimester and period of pregnancy
Abo-Yaqoub et al.[52]	2012	Cohort	Prospective	High risk	Multiple	80	20–38	15–20	Positive	The positive predictive value of KANET was confirmed, as all pathological antenatal results were followed up and confirmed postnatally
Vladareanu et al.[62]	2012	Cohort	Prospective	High risk	Multiple	196	24–38	N/A	Positive	Mixed population of low risk and cases of growth restriction and PTD. The study showed strong correlation of good antenatal result with good postnatal result and vice versa
Honemeyer et al.[63]	2012	Cohort	Prospective	High and low risk	Multiple	56	28–38	30 Max	Positive	The *average KANET score* was proposed by calculating the results of all KANETs that were performed during pregnancy and were related to the time of the day and activity of the fetus
Kurjak et al.[64]	2013	Cohort	Prospective	High and low risk	Multiple	869	28–38	20	Positive	The results were attributed to the different groups of fetus studied with the higher the risk of prognostic factors being directly related to the antenatal KANET and then with the postnatal outcome

Contd...

Contd...

Author	Year	Study	Study design	Study population	Indication	No.	GA (weeks)	Time (minutes)	Result	Summary
Predojević et al.[75]	2014	Case study	Prospective	High risk	IUGR	5	31–39	30	Positive	For growth restricted fetuses the result of the test was predictive when compared to the postnatal outcome and directly related to whether there were Doppler changes in the fetus
Athanasiadis et al.[76]	2013	Cohort	Prospective	Unselected (high and low risk)	Multiple (IUGR, PET, GDM)	152	2nd and 3rd trimester	N/A	Positive	KANET was calculated for each trimester after 28 weeks with differences proven between different groups and findings being confirmed postnatally
Neto et al.[79]	2014	Cohort	Prospective	High and low risk	Multiple	51	3rd trimester	20	Positive	The study confirmed the relationship of high- and low-risk cases and confirmation of postnatal outcome
Hanaoka et al.[80]	2015	Cohort	Prospective	Mixed (Asian and Caucasian)	Multiple	167	3rd trimester	N/A	Positive	Ethnicity impact on KANET was examined without causing difference in the overall result but to certain parameters of the test

(2D: two-dimensional; CNS: central nervous system; GA: gestational age; GDM: gestational diabetes mellitus; IUGR: intrauterine growth restriction; KANET: Kurjak's antenatal neurological test; No.: number of patients; PET: preeclampsia; PTD: preterm delivery)

By comparing two groups (low and high risk for neurological impairment) the parameters that were different were noted and when a pathological KANET result was found that was confirmed at various degrees after delivery, on the other hand a good scoring of KANET or even borderline resulted to a good assessment after delivery. The measurements that were different between the two groups were noted as were the factors that showed no difference.[52]

The Romanian group[62] showed that a low-risk pregnancy is very reassuring for a good neurological outcome confirmed by KANET antenatally when compared with pregnancies that have risk factors (93.4% vs. 75.8%). Fetuses with growth restriction were more prone to have a borderline score especially when Doppler changes were present while the additional factor of threatened preterm labor moved the score from borderline to pathological. Honemeyer et al.[63] failed to detect pathological score but did identify borderlines all in pregnancies with risk factors and aimed to calculate a score that was the sum of all KANETs during pregnancy (average KANET) and also noticed that the time that the assessment takes place may affect the result of the test as the diurnal rhythm of the fetus is also important. Further studies[64] showed the significance that KANET has in order to detect cases at high risk for neurological problems.

Athanasiades and his team also confirmed variations of neurobehavior in high–low risk women with those with diabetes having increased KANET scores in comparison to the other high-risk studied groups.[76]

Neto Raul examined with KANET high-risk cases and showed that for 0 KANET, more common factors to be affected were: isolated head anteflexion, cranial sutures and head circumference, isolated hand movement or hand to face movements, isolated leg movement, and fingers movements. What was also important was the confirmation of positive predictive value of KANET as all abnormal scores belong to groups with risk factors, with none from low and that was confirmed postnatally.[81]

Hanaoka et al. performed a study where they tried to assess the differences of ethnic background on the KANET. What they noticed even in normal scores was a difference between the two populations (Japanese vs. Croatian fetuses) and particularly a difference for four of the parameters. These variations did not affect final score of KANET; however, ethnical differences are something that should be taken under consideration when assessing a fetus.[80]

The Importance of Prompt Detection of Neurological Problems: The Role of KANET

Most neurological problems are detected postnatally or at a time that the problem is very severe-obvious, that is at a time that not much can be done from a therapeutic point of view. The possibility of detecting such a problem earlier or even at the very initial stages, could offer the possibility of an earlier intervention, which could be more effective. KANET is a method that has such a potential and could detect these high-risk fetuses, offer them an appropriate follow-up and when possible an early diagnosis and as a result an early intervention. For physiotherapy it is well known that the earlier it is initiated the better the outcome. A recent Cochrane meta-analysis shows that for preterm infants the earlier the intervention the better the outcome intellectually and motorically and that these improvements are obvious throughout the following years. Whether this could be applied in fetal life or early neonatal life, is still an area of interest, but KANET offers the opportunity to detect these fetuses and initiate further studies. Systematic family home programs for preterm infants for the first year of life showed better results in these individuals compared to cases that did not have that care. The therapies and interventions in cases of neurological impairment are limited, but timely application of these interventions has better results, so prompt diagnosis can offer the chance of prompt intervention with possibly better outcomes.[66-73,77,78]

Application in Clinical Practice

Since the beginning of KANET, the last decade, a great progress has been seen in the area of diagnosis and detection of fetal neurological pathology.[41] Of course more studies are needed and some studies are currently in progress.

The studies that we have until now confirm that KANET is a useful method for assessing in utero behavior, since it offers the opportunity of prompt diagnosis of neurological problems.[26,48,51] Application of this new method and its introduction into clinical practice is feasible, as a method it has been standardized and its positive predictive value has been confirmed, having as a future goal to make KANET part of a more conclusive fetal assessment and therefore more complete counseling of couples with pregnancies that have possible neurological problems.[65] KANET offers opportunity to systematically assess the fetal neurobehavior, collect data of prenatal and postnatal findings, and long-term follow-up, in both high- and low-risk cases, so that hopefully in a few years will have a complete evaluation of fetal neurological status and combine them even with anatomical findings, the significance of which may not be easily understood and explained.

■ CONCLUSION

Fetal neurology, as it is valid for postnatal neurology, is a field of great interest. Especially fetal neurobehavior during in utero life, due to the limited methods that we have to assess the fetus, is an area of great interest. Neurological disorders, even severe ones, such as CP, are almost always diagnosed after delivery, and the question always remains if it could be caused by an intrapartum event, although it has already been clarified by previous studies that >90% of cases of CP have an antenatal origin. All the facts prove that neurological problems are poorly understood and as such difficult to diagnose. In order to diagnose an abnormal condition, we should be able to define normal fetal neurobehavior, something that until recently had not been achieved. KANET by real-time assessment of the fetus allows the assessment of fetal neurobehavior similarly with the examination of a newborn, while also can define the normal fetal neurological profile and detect abnormal conditions. The usefulness of KANET is shown by data of various studies, as a method it has been standardized and it has been introduced into clinical practice with very good results and response. Its importance has been documented for high-risk cases but it also shows benefit for low-risk cases. KANET has come to fill in the gap in fetal neurology and complete fetal assessment especially in cases where there is an anatomical variation or abnormality and cannot be confirmed if clinically can affect the fetus and if yes, at what degree. In these cases the counseling has a gap and a method that examines fetal neurobehavior and not only the anatomy could be of great importance. This new test appeared almost over a decade ago and by now it has been shown by studies that its all statistical markers are very good, it is a method that has been standardized and the teaching process has also been standardized and formalized. KANET could offer the possibility of detecting in utero neurological behavioral problems but also the degree of their severity, and offer them appropriate follow-up, early diagnosis, and the opportunity for a timely intervention, which could lead to a better outcome.

■ REFERENCES

1. Yigiter AB, Kavak ZN. Normal standards of fetal behavior assessed by four-dimensional sonography. J Matern Fetal Neonatal Med. 2006;19(11):707-21.
2. Rees S, Harding R. Brain development during fetal life: influences of the intra-uterine environment. Neurosci Lett. 2004;361(1-3): 111-4.
3. Joseph RG. Fetal brain behavior and cognitive development. Dev Rev. 2000;20(1):81-98.
4. Kurjak A, Carrera JM, Stanojevic M, Andonotopo W, Azumendi G, Scazzocchio E, et al. The role of 4D sonography in the neurological assessment of early human development. Ultrasound Rev Obstet Gynecol. 2004;4(3):148-59.
5. Eidelman AI. The living fetus - dilemmas in treatment at the edge of viability. In: Blazer S, Zimmer EZ (Eds). The Embryo: Scientific Discovery and Medical Ethics. Basel: Karger; 2005. pp. 351-70.
6. Stanojevic M, Zaputovic S, Bosnjak AP. Continuity between fetal and neonatal neurobehavior. Semin Fetal Neonatal Med. 2012;17(6):324-9.
7. Haak P, Lenski M, Hidecker MJC, Li M, Paneth N. Cerebral palsy and aging. Dev Med Child Neurol. 2009;51 [Suppl 4(0 4)]:16-23.
8. Einspieler C, Prechtl HFR. Prechtl's assessment of general movements: a diagnostic tool for the functional assessment of the young nervous system. Ment Retard Dev Disabil Res Rev. 2005;11(1):61-7.
9. Salihagic-Kadic A, Kurjak A, Medić M, Andonotopo W, Azumendi G. New data about embryonic and fetal neurodevelopment and behavior obtained by 3D and 4D sonography. J Perinat Med. 2005;33(6):478-90.
10. Moster D, Wilcox AJ, Vollset SE, Markestad T, Lie RT. Cerebral palsy among term and postterm births. JAMA. 2010;304(9):976-82.
11. Almli CR, Ball RH, Wheeler ME. Human fetal and neonatal movement patterns: gender differences and fetal-to-neonatal continuity. Dev Psychobiol. 2001;38(4):252-73.
12. DiPietro JA, Bronstein MH, Costigan KA, Pressman EK, Hahn CS, Painter K, et al. What does fetal movement predict about behavior during the first two years of life? Dev Psychobiol. 2002;40(4):358-71.
13. DiPetro JA, Hodson DM, Costigan KA, Johnson TR. Fetal antecedents of infant temperament. Child Dev. 1996;67(5):2568-83.
14. DiPietro JA, Costigan KA, Pressman EK. Fetal state concordance predicts infant state regulation. Early Hum Dev. 2002;68(1):1-13.
15. Thoman EB, Denenberg VH, Sievel J, Zeidner LP, Becker P. State organization in neonates: developmental inconsistency indicates risk for developmental dysfunction. Neuropediatrics. 1981;12(1):45-54.
16. St James-Roberts I, Menon-Johansson P. Predicting infant crying from fetal movement data: an exploratory study. Early Hum Dev. 1999;54(1):55-62.
17. Einspieler C, Prechtl HF, Ferrari F. The qualitative assessment of general movements in preterm, term and young infants—review of the methodology. Early Hum Dev. 1997;50(1):47-60.
18. Prechtl HF. Qualitative changes of spontaneous movements in fetus and preterm infant are a marker of neurological dysfunction. Early Hum Dev. 1990;23(3):151-8.
19. de Vries JI, Visser GH, Prechtl HF. The emergence of fetal behaviour. II. Quantitative aspects. Early Hum Dev. 1985;12(2):99-120.
20. de Vries JI, Visser GH, Prechtl HF. The emergence of fetal behaviour. III. Individual differences and consistencies. Early Hum Dev. 1988;16(1):85-103.
21. de Vries JI, Visser GH, Prechtl HF. The emergence of fetal behaviour. I. Qualitative aspects. Early Hum Dev. 1982;7(4):301-22.

22. Nijhuis JG (Ed). Fetal Behaviour: Developmental and Perinatal Aspects. Oxford: Oxford University Press; 1992.

23. Prechtl HF. State of the art of a new functional assessment of the young nervous system. An early predictor of cerebral palsy. Early Hum Dev. 1997;50(1):1-11.

24. Kurjak A, Luetic AT. Fetal neurobehavior assessed by three-dimensional/four-dimensional sonography. Zdrav Vestn. 2010;79(11):790-9.

25. Salihagic-Kadic A, Medic MG, Kurjak A, Andonotopo W, Azumendi G, Hafner T, et al. Four-dimensional sonography in the assessment of fetal functional neuro-development and behavioral patterns. Ultrasound Rev Obstet Gynecol. 2005;5(2): 154-68.

26. Pooh RK, Kurjak A. Assessment of fetal neurobehavior by 3D/4D ultrasound. In: Kurjak A, Pooh RK (Eds). Fetal Neurology. New Delhi: Jaypee Brothers Medical Publishers Pvt. Ltd.; 2009. pp. 222-50.

27. Lebit DF, Vladareanu PD. The role of 4D ultrasound in the assessment of fetal behaviour. Maedica (Bucuar). 2011;6(2): 120-7.

28. Merz E, Abramowicz JS. 3D/4D ultrasound in prenatal diagnosis: is it time for routine use? Clin Obstet Gynecol. 2012;55(1):336-51.

29. Kurjak A, Vecek N, Hafner T, Bozek T, Funduk-Kurjak B, Ujevic B. Prenatal diagnosis: what does four-dimensional ultrasound add? J Perinat Med. 2002;30(1):57-62.

30. Kurjak A, Vecek N, Kupesic S, Azumendi G, Solak M. Four-dimensional ultrasound: how much does it improve perinatal practice? In: Kurjak A, Chervenak FA, Carrera JM (Eds). Controversies in Perinatal Medicine, Studies on the Fetus as a Patient. New York: Parthenon Publishing Group; 2003. p. 222.

31. Andonotopo W, Stanojevic M, Kurjak A, Azumendi G, Carrera JM. Assessment of fetal behavior and general movements by four-dimensional sonography. Ultra Rev Obstet Gynecol. 2004;4(2):103-14.

32. Kurjak A, Carrera JM, Medic M, Azumendi G, Andonotopo W, Stanojevic M. The antenatal development of fetal behavioral patterns assessed by four-dimensional sonography. J Matern Fetal Neonatal Med. 2005;17(6):401-16.

33. Kurjak A, Miskovic B, Andonotopo W, Stanojevic M, Azumendi G, Vrcic H. How useful is 3D and 4D ultrasound in perinatal medicine? J Perinat Med. 2007;35(1):10-27.

34. Kurjak A, Tikvica A, Stanojevic M, Miskovic B, Ahmed B, Azumendi G, et al. The assessment of fetal neurobehavior by three-dimensional and four-dimensional ultrasound. J Matern Fetal Neonatal Med. 2008;21(10):675-84.

35. Morokuma S, Fukushima K, Yumoto Y, Uchimura M, Fujiwara A, Matsumoto M, et al. Simplified ultrasound screening for fetal brain function based on behavioral pattern. Early Hum Dev. 2007;83(3):177-81.

36. Kurjak A, Miskovic B, Stanojevic M, Amiel-Tison C, Ahmed B, Azumendi G, et al. New scoring system for fetal neurobehavior assessed by three- and four-dimensional sonography. J Perinat Med. 2008;36(1):73-81.

37. Gosselin J, Gahagan S, Amiel-Tison C. The Amiel-Tison Neurological Assessment at Term: conceptual and methodological continuity in the course of follow-up. Ment Retard Dev Disabil Res Rev. 2005;11(1):34-51.

38. Amiel-Tison C, Gosselin J, Kurjak A. Neurosonography in the second half of fetal life: a neonatologist's point of view. J Perinat Med. 2006;34(6):437-46.

39. Tomasovic S, Predojevic M. 4D Ultrasound - medical devices for recent advances on the etiology of cerebral palsy. Acta Inform Med. 2011;19(4):228-34.

40. Kurjak A, Stanojevic M, Andonotopo W, Scazzocchio-Duenas E, Azumendi G, Carrera JM. Fetal behavior assessed in all three trimesters of normal pregnancy by four-dimensional ultrasonography. Croat Med J. 2005;46(5):772-80.

41. Stanojevic M, Kurjak A, Salihagic-Kadic A, Vasilj O, Miskovic B, Shaddad AN, et al. Neurobehavioral continuity from fetus to neonate. J Perinat Med. 2011;39(2):171-7.

42. Kurjak A, Andonotopo W, Hafner T, Kadic AS, Stanojevic M, Azumendi G, et al. Normal standards for fetal neurobehavioral

developments—longitudinal quantification by four-dimensional sonography. J Perinat Med. 2006;34(1):56-65.

43. Stanojevic M, Talic A, Miskovic B, V Oliver, Shaddad AN, Ahmed B, et al. An attempt to standardize Kurjak's antenatal neuro-developmental test: Osaka Consensus Statement. Donald School J Ultrasound Obstet Gynecol. 2011;5(4):317-29.

44. Pooh K, Pooh RK. Fetal ventriculomegaly. Donald School J Ultrasound Obstet Gynecol. 2007;1(4):40-6.

45. Kurjak A, Ahmed B, Abo-Yaquab S, Younis M, Saleh H, Shaddad AN, et al. An attempt to introduce neurological test for fetus based on 3D and 4D sonography. Donald School J Ultrasound Obstet Gynecol. 2008;2(4):29-44.

46. Kuno A, Akiyama M, Yamashiro C, Tanaka H, Yanagihara T, Hata T. Three-dimensional sonographic assessment of fetal behavior in the early second trimester of pregnancy. J Ultrasound Med. 2001;20(12):1271-5.

47. Koyanagi T, Horimoto N, Maeda H, Kukita J, Minami T, Ueda K, et al. Abnormal behavioral patterns in the human fetus at term: correlation with lesion sites in the central nervous system after birth. J Child Neurol. 1993;8(1):19-26.

48. Kurjak A, Stanojevic M, Andonotopo W, Salihagic-Kadic A, Carrera JM, Azumendi G. Behavioral pattern continuity from pre-natal to postnatal life—a study by four-dimensional (4D) ultrasonography. J Perinat Med. 2004;32(4):346-53.

49. Stanojevic M, Kurjak A. Continuity between fetal and neonatal neurobehavior. Donald School J Ultrasound Obstet Gynecol. 2008;2(3):64-75.

50. Kurjak A, Abo-Yaqoub S, Stanojevic M, Yigitor AB, Vasilj O, Lebit D, et al. The potential of 4D sonography in the assessment of fetal neurobehavior—multicentric study in high-risk pregnancies. J Perinat Med. 2010;38(1):77-82.

51. Andonotopo W, Kurjak A, Kosuta MI. Behavior of an anencephalic fetus studied by 4D sonography. J Matern Fetal Neonatal Med. 2005;17(2):165-8.

52. Abo-Yaqoub S, Kurjak A, Mohammed AB, Shadad A, Abdel-Maaboud M. The role of 4-D ultrasonography in prenatal assessment of fetal neurobehaviour and prediction of neurological outcome. J Matern Fetal Neonatal Med. 2012;25(3):231-6.

53. Talic A, Kurjak A, Ahmed B, Stanojevic M, Predojevic M, Kadic AS, et al. The potential of 4D sonography in the assessment of fetal behavior in high-risk pregnancies. J Matern Fetal Neonatal Med. 2011;24(7):948-54.

54. Miskovic B, Vasilj O, Stanojevic M, Ivanković D, Kerner M, Tikvica A. The comparison of fetal behavior in high risk and normal pregnancies assessed by four dimensional ultrasound. J Matern Fetal Neonatal Med. 2010;23(12):1461-7.

55. Andonotopo W, Kurjak A. The assessment of fetal behavior of growth restricted fetuses by 4D sonography. J Perinat Med. 2006;34(6):471-8.

56. Talic A, Kurjak A, Stanojevic M, Honemeyer U, Badreldeen A, DiRenzo GC. The assess-ment of fetal brain function in fetuses with ventrikulomegaly: the role of the KANET test. J Matern Fetal Neonatal Med. 2012;25(8):1267-72.

57. Horimoto N, Koyanagi T, Maeda H, Satoh S, Takashima T, Minami T, et al. Can brain impairment be detected by in utero behavioural patterns? Arch Dis Child. 1993;69(1 Spec No):3-8.

58. Morokuma S, Fukushima K, Yumoto Y, Uchimura M, Fujiwara A, Matsumoto M, et al. Simplified ultrasound screening for fetal brain function based on behavioral pattern. Early Hum Dev. 2007;83(3):177-81.

59. Prechtl HF, Einspieler C. Is neurological assessment of the fetus possible? Eur J Obstet Gynecol Reprod Biol. 1997;75(1):81-4.

60. Nijhuis JG, Prechtl HF, Martin CB Jr, Bots RS. Are there behavioural states in the human fetus? Early Hum Dev. 1982;6(2):177-95.

61. Honemeyer U, Kurjak A. The use of KANET test to assess fetal CNS function. First 100 cases. 10th World Congress of Perinatal Medicine 8–11 November 2011. Uruguay. Poster Presentation. p. 209.

62. Vladareanu R, Lebit D, Constantinescu S. Ultrasound assessment of fetal neurobehavior in high-risk pregnancies. Donald School J Ultrasound Obstet Gynecol. 2012; 6(2):132-47.

63. Honemeyer U, Talic A, Therwat A, Paulose L, Patidar R. The clinical value of KANET in studying fetal neurobehavior in normal and at-risk pregnancies. J Perinat Med. 2013;41(2):187-97.

64. Kurjak A, Talic A, Honemeyer U, Stanojevic M, Zalud I. Comparison between antenatal neurodevelopmental test and fetal Doppler in the assessment of fetal well being. J Perinat Med. 2013;41(1):107-14.

65. Kurjak A, Predojevic M, Salihagic-Kadic A. Fetal brain function: lessons learned and future challenges of 4D sonography. Donald School J Ultrasound Obstet Gynecol. 2011;5(2):85-92.

66. Greenwood C, Newman S, Impey L, Johnson A. Cerebral palsy and clinical negligence litigation: a cohort study. BJOG. 2003;110(1):6-11.

67. Strijbis EMM, Oudman I, van Essen P, MacLennan AH. Cerebral palsy and the application of the international criteria for acute intrapartum hypoxia. Obstet Gynecol. 2006;107(6):1357-65.

68. de Vries JIP, Fong BF. Changes in fetal motility as a result of congenital disorders: an overview. Ultrasound Obstet Gynecol. 2007;29(5):590-9.

69. de Vries JIP, Fong BF. Normal fetal motility: an overview. Ultrasound Obstet Gynecol. 2006;27(6):701-11.

70. Rosier-van Dunné FM, van Wezel-Meijler G, Bakker MP, de Groot L, Odendaal HJ, de Vries JI. General movements in the perinatal period and its relation to echogenicity changes in the brain. Early Hum Dev. 2010;86(2):83-6.

71. Hata T, Kanenishi K, Akiyama M, Tanaka H, Kimura K. Real-time 3-D sonographic observation of fetal facial expression. J Obstet Gynaecol Res. 2005;31(4):337-40.

72. Kozuma S, Baba K, Okai T, Taketani Y. Dynamic observation of the fetal face by three-dimensional ultrasound. Ultrasound Obstet Gynecol. 1999;13(4):283-4.

73. Kurjak A, Azumendi G, Andonotopo W, Salihagic-Kadic A. Three- and four-dimensional ultrasonography for the structural and functional evaluation of the fetal face. Am J Obstet Gynecol. 2007;196(1): 16-28.

74. Kurjak A, Talic A, Honemeyer U, Stanojevic M, Zalud I. Comparison between antenatal neurodevelopmental test and fetal Doppler in the assessment of fetal well being. J Perinat Med. 2013;41(1):107-14.

75. Predojević M, Talić A, Stanojević M, Kurjak A, Kadić AS. Assessment of motoric and hemodynamic parameters in growth restricted fetuses - case study. J Matern Fetal Neonatal Med. 2014;27(3):247-51.

76. Athanasiadis AP, Mikos T, Tambakoudis GP, Theodoridis TD, Papastergiou M, Assimakopoulos E, et al. Neurodevelopmental fetal assessment using KANET scoring system in low and high risk pregnancies. J Matern Fetal Neonatal Med. 2013;26(4):363-8.

77. Stanojevic M, Antsaklis P, Salihadic-Kadic A, Predojevic M, Vladareanu R, Vlădăreanu S, et al. Is Kurjak Antenatal Neurodevelopmental Test Ready for Routine Clinical Application? Bucharest Consensus Statement. Donald School J Ultrasound Obstet Gynecol. 2015;9(3):260-5.

78. Spencer-Smith MM, Spittle AJ, Doyle LW, Lee KJ, Lorefice L, Suetin A, et al. Long-term benefits of home-based preventive care for preterm infants: a randomized trial. Pediatrics. 2012;130(6):1094-101.

79. Neto RM, Kurjak A. Recent results of the clinical application of KANET test. Donald School J Ultrasound Obstet Gynecol. 2015; 9(4):420-5.

80. Hanaoka U, Hata T, Kananishi K, AboEllail MAM, Uematsu R, Konishi Y, et al. Does ethnicity have an effect on fetal behavior? A comparison of Asian and Caucasian populations. J Perinat Med. 2016;44(2):217-21.

81. Neto RM. KANET in Brazil: first experience. Donald School J Ultrasound Obstet Gynecol. 2015;9(1):1-5.

Index

Page numbers followed by *f* refer to figure and *t* refer to table